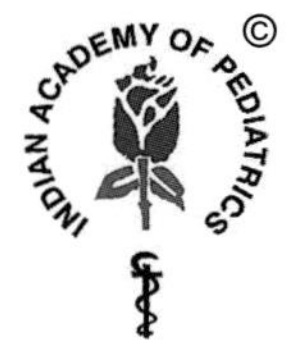

IAP Textbook of Pediatric Allergy

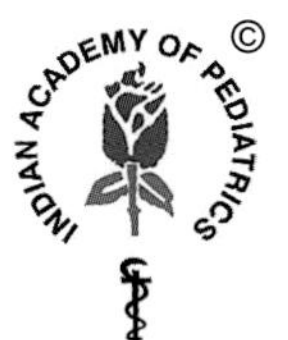

IAP Textbook of Pediatric Allergy

Editors-in-Chief

Neeraj Gupta
DCH DNB FIAP FRCPCH IDPCCM DAA FAAAAI DPSM
Allergist, Pediatric Intensivist, and Sleep Medicine Specialist
Department of Pediatrics
Sir Ganga Ram Hospital
New Delhi, India

Jose Ouseph
MD DCH FIAP DAAI
Professor
Department of Pediatrics
Government TD Medical College
Alappuzha, Kerala, India

Krishna Mohan R
DNB DAA MNAMS ICPP
Consultant Pediatrician and Pediatric Allergist
Department of Health Services
Malappuram, Kerala, India

Executive Editors

Uppin Narayan Reddy
MBBS DCH MD DNB FACI
Professor and Head
Department of Pediatrics
Shadan Institute of Medical Sciences
Hyderabad, Telangana, India

Dhanesh Volvoikar
MBBS MD FACI
Consultant and Pediatric Allergist
Department of Pediatrics
Healthway Hospital
Panaji, Goa, India

Associate Editors

S Narmada Ashok
MD PhD DAA European Certificate of Excellence in Pediatric Allergology
Consultant Pediatrician
Department of Pediatrics
Nalam Medical Centre and Hospital
Vellore, Tamil Nadu, India

Sowmya Nagarajan
DCH DAA FAAAAI European Certificate of Excellence in Pediatric Allergology
Pediatrician, Allergist and Immunologist
Sanjeevini Specialist Clinic and Kangaroo Care Hospitals
Bengaluru, Karnataka, India

Forewords

Neelam Mohan
TU Sukumaran

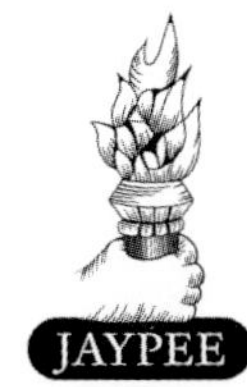

JAYPEE BROTHERS MEDICAL PUBLISHERS
The Health Sciences Publisher
New Delhi | London

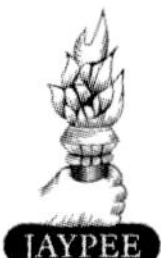

Jaypee Brothers Medical Publishers (P) Ltd

Headquarters
EMCA House, 23/23-B
Ansari Road, Daryaganj
New Delhi 110 002, India
Landline: +91-11-23272143, +91-11-23272703
+91-11-23282021, +91-11-23245672
e-mail: jaypee@jaypeebrothers.com

Corporate Office
4838/24, Ansari Road, Daryaganj
New Delhi 110 002, India
Phone: +91-11-43574357
Fax: +91-11-43574314
e-mail: jaypee@jaypeebrothers.com

Overseas Office
JP Medical Ltd.
83, Victoria Street, London
SW1H 0HW (UK)
Phone: +44-20 3170 8910
e-mail: info@jpmedpub.com

EU GPSR Authorised Representative
Logos Europe, 9 rue Nicolas Poussin
17000, La Rochelle, France
Phone: +33 (0) 6 67 93 73 78
e-mail: contact@logoseurope.eu

Website: www.jaypeebrothers.com
Website: www.jaypeedigital.com

Inquiries for bulk sales may be solicited at: jaypee@jaypeebrothers.com

IAP Textbook of Pediatric Allergy

First Edition: **2026**

ISBN: 978-93-7202-333-6

Printed at: Samrat Offset Pvt. Ltd.

Dedication

To the children—
whose sneezes, wheezes, rashes, and reactions speak volumes beyond clinical symptoms;
who show remarkable resilience through every flare, challenge, and recovery;
and whose courage inspires our unwavering pursuit of safer, healthier, and allergy-free lives.

To the families—
who navigate uncertainty, lifestyle changes, and long-term care with grace, patience, and hope;
your strength fuels our commitment to improving every aspect of allergy management.

To the pediatricians, allergists, nurses, therapists, and healthcare workers across India—
the steadfast guardians in clinics, hospitals, and communities;
your curiosity, compassion, and dedication transform scientific knowledge into healing.

To the pioneers of allergy science in India—past and present—
whose groundwork, vision, and perseverance have illuminated the path for modern pediatric allergy care.

Dedicated to—
All of you for every child comforted,
every family supported,
every life touched,
and every effort that brings us closer to a world where children
breathe, eat, sleep, and live freely—without the burden of allergic disease.

Contributors

Arif Ahmed M MD (Pediatrics) DCH FIAP
EAACI Board Certified in Allergy
Professor and Head
Department of Pediatrics
Shadan Institute of Medical Sciences, Hyderabad
Director and Consultant
Allermy Centre for Allergy and Chest Diseases
Hyderabad, Telangana, India

Barnali Bhattacharya
MD DCH FRSTM&H DPSM
Consultant
Department of Pediatrics
Asthma and Sleep Specialist
Children's Clinic
Pune, Maharashtra, India

Dhanesh Volvoikar MBBS MD FACI
Consultant and Pediatric Allergist
Department of Pediatrics
Healthway Hospital
Panaji, Goa, India

Dipti Pujari MRCPCH MD DNB DCH FACI
European Certificate of Excellence in Pediatric Allergology
Consultant Allergist and Pediatrician
Head
Department of Allergy
Deenanath Mangeshkar Hospital and Research Center
Pujari Pediatric and Allergy Center
Pune, Maharashtra, India

Geetesh Baijal MBBS MD (Pediatrics)
Fellowship in Pediatric Pulmonology
EAACI Certified (Pediatric Allergology and Clinical Immunology)
Pediatric Pulmonologist
Department of Pediatric Pulmonology, Allergy and Sleep Medicine
NH-SRCC Children's Hospital
Mumbai, Maharashtra, India

Hima Mathews P
MBBS DCH DNB DPAA FAAP
Senior Consultant and Allergist
Lisie Hospital
Ernakulam, Kerala, India

Indu Khosla MD DCH RCPCH Fellowship in Pediatric Pulmonology
European Respiratory Diplomate
European Certificate of Excellence in Pediatric Allergology
Consultant Pediatrician and Pulmonologist
Department of Pediatric Pulmonology, Allergy and Sleep Medicine
Nanavati Max Super Speciality Hospital, Mumbai
Narayana Health SRCC Hospital for Children
Director
Dr Indu's Newborn and Childcare Centre
Mumbai, Maharashtra, India

Jefferson Daniel MD DAA
Associate Professor
Department of Pulmonary Medicine
Christian Medical College
Vellore, Tamil Nadu, India

Jijo Joseph John
MD (Pediatrics) FPRD DAA
Professor and Head
Department of Pediatrics
Believers Church Medical College Hospital
Thiruvalla, Kerala, India

Jose Ouseph MD DCH FIAP DAAI
Professor
Department of Pediatrics
Government TD Medical College
Alappuzha, Kerala, India

Karthik Nagaraju
MD DM Critical Care and Pulmonology
Associate Professor
Department of Pediatrics
NIMS Medical College
Jaipur, Rajasthan, India

Krishna Mohan R
DNB DAA MNAMS ICPP
Consultant Pediatrician and Pediatric Allergist
Department of Health Services
Malappuram, Kerala, India

Mangayarkarshi Sinha
DNB (Pediatrics) FACI
Dr Mangai Sinha's Paediatric Clinic
Allergy and Asthma Centre
Navi Mumbai, Maharashtra, India

Mitesh Kakkad
MD (Pediatrics) Diploma (Pediatrics)
Consultant, Pediatric Pulmonologist and Allergist
Neo Children Allergy and Asthma Centre
Ahmedabad, Gujarat, India

Mohammad Ziaul Haque
DTCD DNB Respiratory Medicine DAA
Pulmonologist
Division of Allergy and Immunology
Department of Pulmonology
Apollo Multispecialty Hospital
Kolkata, West Bengal, India

Mohit Poddar MBBS MD FACI
Consultant and Head
Department of Pulmonary and Allergy Services
VN Allergy and Asthma Research Centre
Chennai, Tamil Nadu, India

Mosam Maroo MBBS MD DNB FAAP
Pediatric Allergist
Dr Mosam's Allergy Clinic
Mumbai, Maharashtra, India

Nandana Bala
MBBS MRCPCH (UK) CCT Pediatrics (London Deanery) PG Cert Allergy (Imperial College London)
Consultant Pediatrician and Allergy/ Asthma Specialist
Rainbow Children's Hospital and Prudent Health Specialty Clinic
Bengaluru, Karnataka, India

Narayan Prasad Modi MD (Pediatrics)
Professor and Head
Department of Pediatrics
MKCG Medical College
Berhampur, Odisha, India

Naresh Grover MD FIAP PGPN FACI
Director
Advanced Pediatric and Allergy Management Center, Amritsar
Visiting Consultant
Apollo Cradle Hospital
Amritsar, Punjab, India

Nayan Mani Deka
MD (Pediatrics) DAA (CMC, Vellore)
Consultant Pediatrician and Asthma Allergy Specialist
Department of Pediatrics
Pratiksha Rainbow Children's Hospital
Guwahati, Assam, India

Neeraj Gupta DCH DNB FIAP FRCPCH IDPCCM DAA FAAAAI DPSM
Allergist, Pediatric Intensivist, and Sleep Medicine Specialist
Department of Pediatrics
Sir Ganga Ram Hospital
New Delhi, India

Nihar Ranjan Mishra MD IPSS INSPIRE (USA) FAIMER FACI PGDCR
Additional Professor
Course Director, PDCC Pediatric Allergy
Department of Pediatrics
All India Institutes of Medical Sciences
Kalyani, West Bengal, India

Nimmy Joseph
MBBS DCH DNB (Pediatrics)
Consultant Developmental Pediatrician
Department of Pediatrics
National Institute of Physical Medicine and Rehabilitation
Kallettumkara, Kerala, India

Pawankalyan Pinnamaneni
MD FACI FIAP Fellowship in Pediatric Pulmonology and Sleep (Aus)
Consultant Pediatric Pulmonologist, Allergy and Sleep Specialist
Department of Pediatrics
Dr Pinnamaneni Siddhartha Institute of Medical Sciences and Research Foundation
Pinnamaneni and Anu My Baby Hospital
Vijayawada, Andhra Pradesh, India

R Prasanna
DCH DNB MRCPCH (UK) MRCP (Edin) Diploma in Pediatric Allergy and Asthma
Professor
Department of Pediatrics and Neonatology
SRM Medical College Hospital and Research Centre
Kanchipuram, Tamil Nadu, India

Rama Rajyam Datti MD (Pediatrics)
Diploma in Allergy and Asthma (CMC, Vellore)
Associate Professor
Department of Pediatrics
Paderu Medical College
Visakhapatnam, Andhra Pradesh, India

Reyaz A Malik MBBS MD DPAA
Professor and Head
Department of Pediatrics
SKIMS Medical College
Srinagar, Jammu & Kashmir, India

S Karthikeyan
MBBS DCH DNB FAAP EDPRM Fellowship in Pediatric Pulmonology
Assistant Professor
Department of Pediatrics
KAPV Medical College and Mahatma Gandhi Memorial Government Hospital, Trichy
Consultant Pediatric Pulmonologist and Allergy Specialist
Maa Kauvery Hospital
Trichy, Tamil Nadu, India

S Narmada Ashok
MD PhD DAA European Certificate of Excellence in Pediatric Allergology
Consultant Pediatrician
Department of Pediatrics
Nalam Medical Centre and Hospital
Vellore, Tamil Nadu, India

Saibal Moitra MD PhD FRCP (Edinburgh) FRCP (Glasgow) MAMS DAA FAAAI
Adjunct Professor and Senior Consultant
Division of Allergy and Immunology
Department of Pulmonology
Apollo Multispecialty Hospitals
Kolkata, West Bengal, India

Sanjay Kumar Sahu MD (Pediatrics)
Professor
Department of Pediatrics
Kalinga Institute of Medical Sciences
Bhubaneswar, Odisha, India

Sanjukta De MBBS DCH (Cal) DNB (Pediatrics) DCH (London) MRCPCH (UK) FRCPCH (UK) Diploma in Allergy (UK)
Clinical Director
Department of Pediatrics and Neonatology
Peerless Hospital
Kolkata, West Bengal, India

Shalini Tyagi MD DNB DCH European Certification of Excellence in Pediatric Allergology and Pulmonology
Consultant Allergist and Pediatrician
Asthma and Allergy Centre and MCRD Allergy Centre
Metro Hospital
Noida, Uttar Pradesh, India

Shebna A Khader MD (Pediatrics) DPAA FAAP
Consultant Pediatrician, Pediatric Allergist
Allergo Kidz Pediatric Allergy Clinic
Midtown Medical Centre
Kochi, Kerala, India

Shweta Agarwal FRCOphth FRCS (Ed)
Fellowship in Cornea and Ocular Surface
Senior Consultant
CJ Shah Cornea Services
Dr G Sitalakshmi Memorial Clinic for Ocular Surface Disorders
Medical Research Foundation
Sankara Nethralaya
Chennai, Tamil Nadu, India

Sinchana Bhat MBBS DCH DNB DAA
Consultant Pediatrician and Allergy Specialist
Dr Sinchana's Allergy and Asthma Clinic
Mangaluru, Karnataka, India

Sonia Bhatt MD (Pediatrics) DAA PGCAP (Adolescent Pediatrics)
Professor and Head
Department of Pediatrics
FH Medical College
Agra, Uttar Pradesh, India

Soumyashree Bahalia MD DNB (Pediatrics) DAAI
Senior Resident
Department of Pediatrics
Bhima Bhoi Medical College and Hospital
Gandhrel, Odisha, India

Soundarya M MD ACME DPAA
Pediatric Allergist and Consultant
Department of Pediatrics
KMC Hospital
Mangaluru, Karnataka, India

Sowmya Nagarajan
DCH DAA FAAAAI European Certificate of Excellence in Pediatric Allergology
Pediatrician, Allergist and Immunologist
Sanjeevini Specialist Clinic and Kangaroo Care Hospitals
Bengaluru, Karnataka, India

Spurthi Chitta FAAP (USA) Diplomate of American Board of Pediatrics Fellow Allergy and Asthma (Singapore) Certified EAACI Knowledge Exam
Consultant Allergy and Asthma
Department of Pediatric Allergy and Asthma
Rainbow Children's Hospitals and Avatar Clinics
Hyderabad, Telangana, India

Sugaranjini Galiyugavaradhan
MBBS DO DNB Ophthalmology
Fellowship in Cornea, Refractive Surgery and Ocular Surface Disorders
Associate Consultant
Cornea and Refractive surgery Services
Giridhar Eye Institute
Ernakulam, Kerala, India

Surender Kagithapu MBBS DCH MD (Pediatrics) DPPA ACME
Professor and Head
Department of Pediatrics
GMC Jayashankar Bhupalapally
Kompalle, Telangana, India

Tina N Goel MBBS DNB (Pediatrics)
Consultant Pediatrician and Child Specialist
Kare N Kure Child Clinic
New Delhi, India

Uppin Narayan Reddy MD FACI
Professor and Head
Department of Pediatrics
Shadan Institute of Medical Sciences
Hyderabad, Telangana, India

Vikram Patra DCH MD FACI European Certificate of Excellence in Pediatric Allergology
Consultant
Department of Pediatric Allergy
Allergy Asthma Care Centre, Navi Mumbai
Apollo Hospital and MGM New Bombay Hospital
Navi Mumbai, Maharashtra, India

Vineeth Vijayan PDCC
Pediatric Allergy Fellow
Department of Pediatrics
All India Institutes of Medical Sciences
Kalyani, West Bengal, India

Vipul Sharma MBBS MD DPAA
Principal Consultant
Department of Pediatrics
Max Hospital
Gurugram, Haryana, India

About the Editors

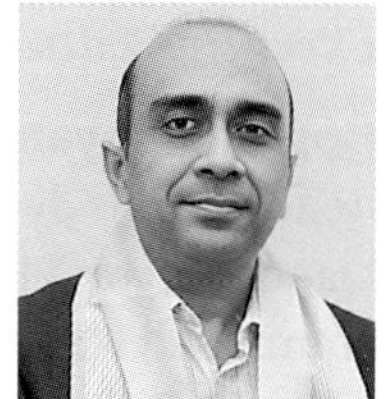

Neeraj Gupta

Neeraj Gupta DCH DNB FIAP FRCPCH IDPCCM, DAA FAAAAI European Certificate of Excellence in Pediatric Allergology *DPSM* is one of India's leading authorities in Pediatric Allergy, with additional expertise in Pediatric Intensive Care, Pediatric Pulmonology, and Sleep Medicine. He is a Senior Consultant and Academic Faculty Member at Sir Ganga Ram Hospital and GRIPMER, New Delhi, India—home to a World Allergy Organization (WAO)-designated Center of Excellence in Allergy. His work has been central to the development and formalization of pediatric allergy as a subspecialty in India.

He is the Founder Director of the Diploma in Pediatric Allergy and Asthma (DPAA), India's first nationally structured training program in this field, and has contributed extensively to academic curricula, national guidelines, and capacity-building initiatives aimed at promoting rational, evidence-based allergy care. He has also served as Chairperson of the IAP Allergy and Applied Immunology Chapter, providing strategic leadership to one of the country's largest pediatric allergy platforms.

An accomplished academician, he has authored over 100 scientific publications and serves as Editor-in-Chief of several landmark texts, including *Comprehensive Textbook of Allergy, Allergy in a Nutshell, and Allergopedia—Clinical Protocols in Pediatric Allergy*. He also leads the *Allergy Bulletin*, a widely read monthly academic publication.

His pioneering contributions include establishing India's first dedicated Pediatric Allergy Laboratory, advancing oscillometry-based research, and expanding access to modern allergy diagnostics and immunotherapy. He is the Founder President of ISAAS (Initiative for Sleep, Asthma and Allergy Sciences), fostering interdisciplinary education and research. A recipient of multiple national and international honors, he is widely respected for his academic leadership, mentorship, and sustained impact on pediatric allergy care.

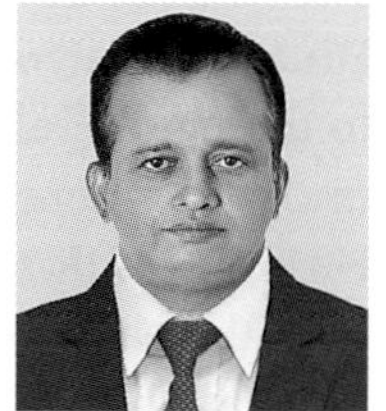

Jose Ouseph

Jose Ouseph MD DCH FIAP DAAI is a Senior Academician and Clinician with over 26 years of dedicated service in pediatric teaching and practice. He is currently serving as Professor, Department of Pediatrics, Government TD Medical College, Alappuzha, Kerala, India, where he has been actively involved in undergraduate and postgraduate teaching and examinations. An alumnus of Government TD Medical College, he completed his MD in Pediatrics from Government Medical College, Kottayam and was awarded the prestigious Fellowship of the Indian Academy of Pediatrics (FIAP) in 2018.

He has held several key leadership positions within the Indian Academy of Pediatrics (IAP) at both state and national levels. His notable roles include State Secretary IAP Kerala, State President of IAP Kerala, and State President of IAP Respiratory Chapter and Environment and Child Health Group. At the national level, he has served as Honorary Secretary and later National Chairperson of the IAP Allergy and Applied Immunology Chapter, and as an Executive Board Member of CIAP on multiple occasions. Currently, he is the South Zone Vice President of CIAP (2026). A respected faculty at numerous national and state conferences, he has made significant contributions to advancing pediatric allergy and respiratory care in India.

Krishna Mohan R

Krishna Mohan R DNB DAA ICPP MNAMS European Certificate of Excellence in Pediatric Allergology is a distinguished Pediatrician and Pediatric Allergist with a strong blend of academic excellence and public health service. He completed his postgraduate training in Pediatrics at the Institute of Maternal and Child Health, Kozhikode, Kerala, India, and subsequently underwent specialized training in Allergy at Christian Medical College, Vellore, Tamil Nadu. He has been serving as a Consultant Pediatrician and Pediatric Allergist in the Kerala Government Health Services since 2009.

He has held several important national academic and leadership roles, including National Chairperson of the Allergy and Applied Immunology Chapter of the Indian Academy of Pediatrics (IAP) in 2024 and Member of ACVIP (2024–25). He is the Honorary Course Director of the DAAI Program (Kerala) under International Asthma Services and Course Director of the Essential Vaccinology Course (IAP Kerala, 2023). He is also a core team member of the IAP-ICP Pediatric Allergy Course and IAP VAC.

An accomplished editor and academician, he is the Chief Editor of *Essentials of Pediatric Allergy* (2021) and *Practicals in Pediatric Allergy* (2025), and has contributed as Associate or Academic Editor to several key IAP publications. A sought-after faculty at national and state forums, he received the Best Doctor Award from the Kerala Government Medical Officers' Association in 2019.

Executive Editors

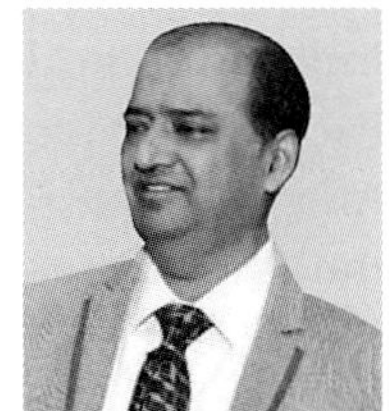
Uppin Narayan Reddy

Uppin Narayan Reddy MBBS DCH MD DNB FACI is a Senior Pediatrician and Allergy Specialist with nearly three decades of academic and clinical experience. He is currently Professor and Head, Department of Pediatrics at Shadan Institute of Medical Sciences, Hyderabad, Telangana, India. He completed his MBBS from Karnataka Medical College, Hubli, DCH from Bangalore Medical College, and MD Pediatrics from Seth GS Medical College and KEM/Wadia Hospital, Mumbai—institutions that shaped his strong academic foundation and clinical rigor.

His interest in respiratory medicine and allergy was nurtured early under the mentorship of stalwarts such as Dr MD Shah, and later strengthened through his association with leaders of pediatric allergy in India. He formally trained in Allergy and Immunology through the Fellowship Program at Saveetha Deemed University, Tamil Nadu, and has since been a committed advocate of ethical, evidence-based allergy care.

He has previously occupied several key leadership positions like Chief organizing Secretary during 5th National PedAllercon at Hyderabad (2017), National Coordinator for CADE Module (2021), CIAP EB Member (2021 and 2024) and Honorary Secretary for National Allergy and Applied Immunology Chapter (2024–25).

A passionate teacher since 1994, he has mentored generations of medical students and pediatricians. His clinical philosophy emphasizes detailed history-taking, rational investigations, preventive counseling, and patient education. Widely respected for his integrity, empathy, and dedication to child health, he continues to inspire young clinicians to practice pediatric allergy with ethics, compassion, and academic excellence.

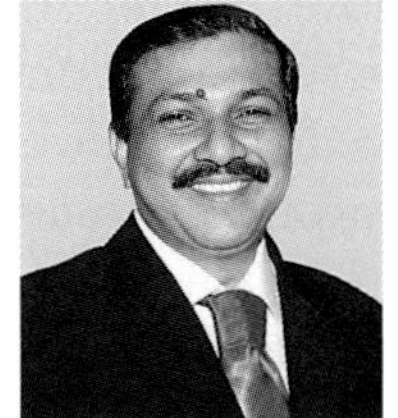
Dhanesh Volvoikar

Dhanesh Volvoikar MD FACI is a committed Clinician and Academician who has devoted himself to the field of allergy since completing his Fellowship in Allergy and Clinical Immunology in 2015 under the mentorship of Dr (Maj.) K Nagaraju at Saveetha University, Chennai, Tamil Nadu, India. He is currently serving as Consultant and Pediatric Allergist, Healthway Hospital, Panaji, Goa, India. Over the past decade, he has been engaged in exclusive allergy practice in Goa, providing specialized and patient-centric allergy care.

He has made significant academic contributions, having authored six chapters in various allergy textbooks. He has also played an important role in the development of allergy guidelines and teaching modules, contributing to the standardization and dissemination of allergy education in India. A regular faculty member at allergy conferences across the country, he is actively involved in teaching and mentoring clinicians with an interest in allergy practice.

In addition to his academic and clinical achievements, he has an illustrious record of medical leadership. He served as Vice President of the Goa State Medical Council for ten years and was the first State Representative to the National Medical Commission in 2020–2021. He is a Past President of the IAP Goa State Chapter and currently serves as the Honorary Treasurer of the Allergy and Applied Immunology Chapter of the Indian Academy of Pediatrics.

Associate Editors

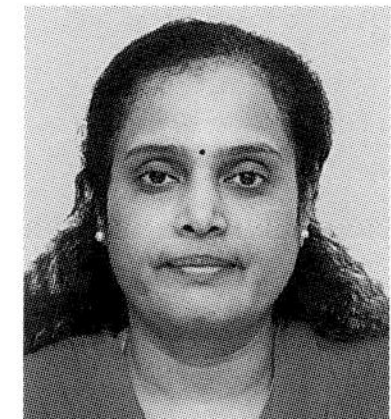
S Narmada Ashok

S Narmada Ashok MD PhD DAA European Certificate of Excellence in Pediatric Allergology is a senior practicing pediatrician from Vellore, Tamil Nadu, India, with special expertise in pediatric asthma and allergy and over two decades of clinical experience. She is currently serving as Consultant Pediatrician, Nalam Medical Centre and Hospital Vellore. She is an alumnus of the prestigious Diploma in Allergy and Asthma (DAA) program jointly conducted by Christian Medical College (CMC), Vellore and the University of Colorado, USA. Demonstrating a strong commitment to academic excellence, she has completed her PhD from VIT University with a focused research interest in asthma.

She is a Fellow of the Indian Academy of Pediatrics (FIAP) and the Royal College of Paediatrics and Child Health (FRCPCH), and has recently earned the EAACI Certification in Allergy, Asthma, and Clinical Immunology. She has been a dedicated faculty member of the DAA course since 2013 and has played a pivotal role in training several pediatric allergy specialists across India. In addition, she serves as faculty for other prestigious programs including DPAA at Sir Ganga Ram Hospital Delhi, DAAI Cochin, and FAAI Rishikesh.

She has numerous publications in national and international journals and has contributed chapters to several academic books. With a keen interest in environmental health, she has also served as Editor of the esteemed *Enrich* newsletter of the IAP Environment Chapter.

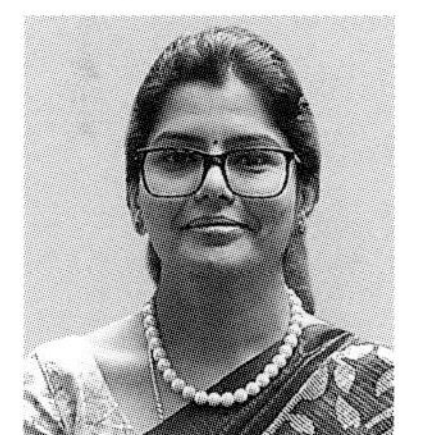
Sowmya Nagarajan

Sowmya Nagarajan DCH DAA FAAAAI European Certificate of Excellence in Pediatric Allergology is a distinguished Consultant Pediatrician, Allergist, and Immunologist based in Bengaluru, Karnataka, India. She holds an MBBS and DCH, along with a Fellowship in Pediatric Allergy and Immunology, Diploma in Allergy and Asthma, and is a Fellow of the American Academy of Allergy, Asthma and Immunology (FAAAI). She has also been awarded the Certificate of Excellence in Allergy by the European Academy of Allergy and Clinical Immunology (EAACI).

She practices at Sanjeevini Specialist Clinic, Motherhood Hospitals, and Narayana Nethralaya, Bengaluru, where she is actively involved in delivering comprehensive and evidence-based allergy care. She has contributed extensively to academic literature with publications in several national and international journals and serves as a reviewer for leading journals in the field of allergy.

A recipient of the EAACI Junior Member Grant, she has undergone advanced clinical exposure at St James's Hospital, Leeds, UK. Her key areas of clinical and research interest include hereditary angioedema, food and drug allergies, and desensitization therapies. She is a sought-after faculty at national and international conferences and is deeply committed to advancing pediatric allergy education and practice.

Founder Chairperson's Address

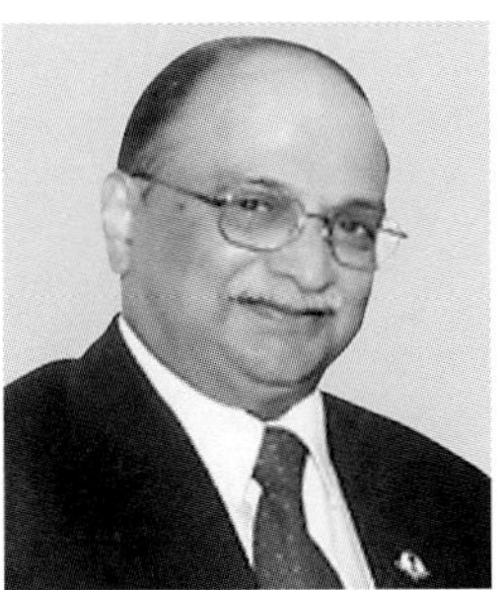

It is with immense joy and deep professional satisfaction that I write this address for the *IAP Textbook of Pediatric Allergy*. As the founder of the IAP Allergy and Applied Immunology Chapter, I have had the privilege of witnessing—firsthand—the remarkable evolution of allergy science in India. What once began as a small, passionate effort to highlight the importance of allergic diseases among children has today grown into a strong national movement. This textbook represents a major milestone in that journey.

Allergic diseases are no longer occasional diagnoses in pediatric practice; they have become common clinical problems affecting millions of children. Rapid urbanization, environmental pollution, changing lifestyles, and climate variability have together created a "perfect storm," contributing to allergies emerging as one of the fastest-growing chronic disorders in our country. While genetic predisposition provides the foundation for allergic diseases, environmental factors play a crucial role in triggering disease expression and may even influence genetic susceptibility over time. There has long been a need for a standardized, India-specific approach to guide both early-career pediatricians and experienced clinicians. This textbook has been developed to address this need.

The editors and contributors have produced a work of exceptional depth and clarity. It blends the fundamental sciences with clinical wisdom, and global evidence with Indian experiences. Importantly, it addresses areas that have long been underrepresented in conventional teaching—indigenous aeroallergens, the impact of pollution and climate change, oscillometry, food allergy trends in Indian infants and children, immunotherapy protocols suited for our settings, and the practical aspects of running an allergy clinic.

This book is not merely a compilation of chapters; it is a reflection of the collective commitment of the Indian pediatric allergy community to elevate our standards of care. It will empower clinicians to make accurate diagnoses, provide timely interventions, support families through chronic disease management, and champion preventive strategies in schools, homes, and communities.

I am deeply proud of the vision, dedication, and teamwork demonstrated by the editorial board under the leadership of Dr Neeraj Gupta, Dr Jose Ouseph, and Dr Krishna Mohan R. Their efforts symbolize what we aspired for when we established this Chapter: To nurture excellence, encourage research, and build a strong foundation for future generations.

I warmly congratulate all authors and editors for this outstanding contribution. May this textbook inspire continued growth, innovation, and compassionate care in pediatric allergy across India.

H Paramesh MD FAAP (USA) FIAP FIAMS FICAAI FPAI
Founder Chairperson
IAP Allergy and Applied Immunology Chapter

From Honorary Secretary General's Desk

It is with great pride and deep satisfaction that I extend my warm wishes to the editorial team and contributors of the *IAP Textbook of Pediatric Allergy*. This book marks an important milestone in our ongoing efforts to strengthen pediatric subspecialty care across India and reflects the growing recognition of allergic diseases as a major public health challenge.

The prevalence of pediatric allergies in our country has risen sharply over the last decade, driven by environmental changes, evolving diets, rapid urbanization, and increasing pollution levels. In this context, the need for a comprehensive, India-centric, and evidence-based resource cannot be overstated. This textbook successfully bridges that gap by providing pediatricians with practical guidance, scientific insights, and structured protocols tailored to the unique allergy patterns seen in Indian children.

I congratulate the Editors-in-Chief—Dr Neeraj Gupta, Dr Jose Ouseph, and Dr Krishna Mohan R—for their visionary leadership in conceptualizing and shaping this volume. I also acknowledge the exceptional efforts of the Executive Editors, Section Editors, and the many distinguished authors whose dedication and expertise have transformed this project into a high-quality academic reference. Their collective commitment embodies the true spirit of academic collaboration and professional excellence.

One of the strongest aspects of this book is its ability to harmonize complex immunological concepts with real-world clinical practice. The content is thoughtfully curated—covering fundamentals, diagnostics, respiratory and food allergies, dermatologic and drug hypersensitivities, immunotherapy, preventive strategies, clinic setup, and future directions. The inclusion of India-specific allergens, pollution factors, component-resolved diagnostics, and practical clinic workflows makes it especially relevant for clinicians working across diverse healthcare settings.

This publication is a testament to the Indian Academy of Pediatrics' dedication to advancing child health through education, standardization, and capacity building. It will undoubtedly empower pediatricians, postgraduate students, allergists, and trainees to deliver more precise, informed, and compassionate care.

My heartfelt appreciation goes to every contributor who helped bring this significant endeavor to fruition. May this textbook serve as a trusted guide and a catalyst for further strengthening pediatric allergy care in our country.

Warm regards,

Yogesh N Parikh MBBS MD FIAP
Associate Professor
Department of Pediatrics
Government Medical College
Surat, Gujarat, India
Honorary Secretary General, IAP (2024–2025)

From President's Desk

It gives me immense pleasure to write this message for the *IAP Textbook of Pediatric Allergy*, a landmark academic contribution that reflects the collective wisdom, scientific rigor, and commitment of our pediatric fraternity. At a time when allergic diseases are rising at an unprecedented pace across India, the need for a comprehensive, evidence-based, and contextually relevant resource has never been more acute. This textbook is therefore both timely and transformative.

Allergic disorders—once considered occasional inconveniences—have now emerged as major contributors to chronic morbidity in children. Their impact spans respiratory, dermatologic, nutritional, and even psychosocial spheres. Against this backdrop, equipping every pediatrician, trainee, and healthcare provider with a structured and practical understanding of allergy care is crucial. This book addresses that need with remarkable clarity and depth.

I congratulate the Editors-in-Chief—Dr Neeraj Gupta, Dr Jose Ouseph, and Dr Krishna Mohan R—along with the Executive Editors and the entire editorial team for steering this ambitious project with exceptional vision and dedication. The meticulous selection of topics, inclusion of India-specific allergens, emphasis on diagnostics, and focus on both foundational sciences and practical management are commendable.

The strength of this book lies in its ability to integrate global evidence with Indian realities. Whether it is the emergence of new aeroallergens, the changing profiles of food allergies, the influence of pollution and climate change, or the evolving landscape of immunotherapy—this textbook provides a reliable compass for clinicians navigating the complex world of pediatric allergy.

I would also like to acknowledge the invaluable contributions of the many authors who have enriched this volume with their expertise. Their commitment to advancing pediatric healthcare is reflected on every page.

This publication perfectly embodies the spirit of IAP—*Serve Children, Colleagues, and Country*. I am confident that this textbook will serve as a trusted guide, an academic companion, and a catalyst for improved allergy care across all corners of India.

My heartfelt compliments go to everyone involved in this extraordinary endeavor. May this book inspire many more initiatives that strengthen pediatric health and nurture the well-being of every child.

Warm regards,

Vasant M Khalatkar MBBS MD FIAP
CIAP President, 2025
Consultant Pediatrician and Neonatologist
Khalatkar Hospital
Nagpur, Maharashtra, India

Message from the IAP National Treasurer's Desk

It gives me immense pleasure to extend my heartfelt congratulations to the editorial team of the *IAP Textbook of Pediatric Allergy*. This comprehensive and timely work reflects the growing commitment of the Indian Academy of Pediatrics to address the rising burden of allergic diseases among children.

Allergy is an area that has long required focused academic attention, structured guidelines, and context-specific clinical insights. This textbook succeeds remarkably in filling that gap by offering a well-organized, evidence-based, and India-relevant resource for pediatricians, postgraduates, and practitioners across diverse healthcare settings.

I applaud the Editors-in-Chief—Dr Neeraj Gupta, Dr Jose Ouseph, and Dr Krishna Mohan R—along with the Executive Editors and all contributors, for their relentless commitment to academic excellence and clinical relevance. Their teamwork has resulted in a publication that combines scientific rigor with practical applicability.

With allergic disorders on the rise due to environmental changes, pollution, and lifestyle transitions, this textbook will serve as a vital tool in guiding correct diagnosis, rational investigations, preventive strategies, and long-term management. It also reinforces the IAP's mission to support pediatricians with high-quality educational materials and standardized approaches to care.

My sincere appreciation goes to the entire team for bringing this invaluable resource to life. I am confident that it will make a lasting impact on pediatric allergy care across the nation.

Warm regards,

Atanu Bhadra MBBS MD
Medical Superintendent
ESI Hospital
Asansol, West Bengal, India
National Treasurer, IAP (2024–2025)

Foreword

It gives me immense pleasure to present the *IAP Textbook of Pediatric Allergy*, a landmark academic contribution that arrives at a pivotal moment for child health in India. Allergic diseases have transitioned from being occasional clinical challenges to becoming one of the most significant public health concerns of our time. Rapid urbanization, changing lifestyles, evolving environmental exposures, and escalating pollution levels have together contributed to an unprecedented rise in allergic disorders among Indian children.

Current estimates suggest that 20–30% of Indian children may be affected by at least one allergic condition, and a 2022 meta-analysis reported the prevalence of childhood asthma in India to be as high as 7.9%. These figures underscore the magnitude of the problem and highlight the urgent need for a comprehensive, evidence-based, and India-centric resource to guide pediatricians in addressing this growing burden.

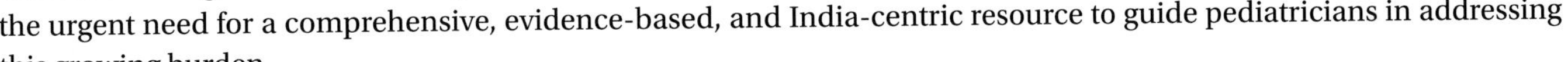

I am particularly pleased that I had the opportunity to engage with the Editors-in-Chief at an early stage and emphasize the necessity of such a textbook, one that integrates scientific foundations, clinical nuances, and real-world challenges of allergy practice in India under a single authoritative umbrella. I sincerely congratulate the editorial leadership—Dr Neeraj Gupta, Dr Jose Ouseph, and Dr Krishna Mohan R, along with the dedicated section editors and chapter authors—for producing a work of exceptional clarity, relevance, and scientific rigor. Their collective effort truly reflects the spirit of academic excellence and collaboration that the Indian Academy of Pediatrics stands for.

Equally commendable is the book's structured and holistic approach, encompassing fundamentals, diagnostics, organ-specific manifestations, preventive strategies, holistic care, and future directions. This thoughtful compilation equips clinicians not only to diagnose and treat allergic disorders but also to prevent disease, counsel families, and empower caregivers—an especially critical aspect in the management of chronic allergic conditions.

For young pediatricians, this textbook will serve as both a learning companion and a practical clinical guide. For experienced practitioners, it will be a valuable reference to enhance day-to-day clinical decision-making. For academicians and researchers, it provides a strong foundation for future research initiatives and policy-level discussions in pediatric allergy.

As we move into 2026 with renewed commitment to child health, this textbook reinforces IAP's leadership in advancing subspecialty care across the country. I am confident that this work will significantly strengthen allergy education in India and contribute meaningfully to better clinical outcomes, reduced disease burden, and improved quality of life for millions of children.

I wholeheartedly endorse the *IAP Textbook of Pediatric Allergy* and congratulate everyone involved in transforming this vision into reality. This book will undoubtedly serve as a cornerstone reference in pediatric allergy for years to come.

Neelam Mohan
DNB (Pediatrics) FRCPCH FIAP Fellwoship in Pediatric Gastroenterology & Hepatology
Sr. Director & HOD, Pediatric Gastroenterology Medanta Hospitals, Gurugram
President, Central Indian Academy of Pediatrics (IAP), 2026

Foreword

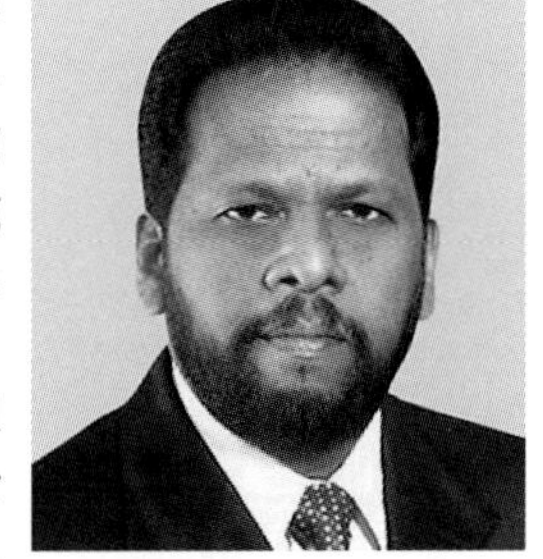

It is a matter of great pride to witness the publication of the *IAP Textbook of Pediatric Allergy*, a timely and transformative contribution to the field of allergy care in India. Over the last decade, our nation has seen a sharp rise in allergic diseases across all age groups—particularly among children. As pediatricians, we stand at the crossroads of growing clinical demand, evolving scientific knowledge, and an urgent need to standardize practice. This textbook arrives as a powerful response to those needs.

What distinguishes this work is its deep commitment to Indian realities. While global literature continues to guide scientific understanding, everyday practice in India requires far more contextualized knowledge—our allergens, our phenotypes, our environmental exposures, our diagnostic limitations, and our sociocultural determinants. This book captures all these elements comprehensively and thoughtfully. From aeroallergen patterns to food allergy trends, from oscillometry and component-resolved diagnostics to pollution-driven disease burden, the content mirrors the cases we encounter in clinics across the country.

The Editors—Dr Neeraj Gupta, Dr Jose Ouseph, and Dr Krishna Mohan R—deserve enormous credit for assembling such a wide and accomplished team of contributors. Their vision is evident in the balanced structure of the book: Foundational immunology, detailed diagnostics, organ-specific disorders, preventive strategies, practical clinic setup, and future directions in biologics and personalized medicine. This makes the textbook not only academically robust but also immensely usable for frontline pediatricians and postgraduate trainees.

As someone who has been closely involved with the growth of the IAP Allergy & Applied Immunology Chapter, I view this textbook as a milestone in our journey. It exemplifies the progress that the allergy community in India has made—moving from fragmented knowledge to structured education, from limited resources to national collaborations, and from individual efforts to unified academic leadership.

I am confident that this book will shape the way pediatric allergy is taught, practiced, and perceived in India. It will strengthen clinical acumen, encourage evidence-based decision-making, and inspire further research in an area of immense public health relevance.

My heartfelt congratulations to the editors and authors for producing a work that will benefit generations of pediatricians and, most importantly, the countless children who suffer from allergic diseases.

TU Sukumaran MBBS DCH MD PhD
Senior Consultant Pediatrics, Caritas Hospital Kottayam, Thellakom, Kerala
Professor of Pediatrics, Pushpagiri Medical College, Tiruvalla, Kerala
Past Chairperson IAP Allergy and Applied Immunology Chapter
National President, IAP 2011

Preface

Allergic diseases in children have emerged as one of the most significant clinical challenges of our time. Rapid urbanization, environmental pollution, changing lifestyles, and evolving dietary patterns have reshaped the epidemiology of allergy in India. Pediatricians now encounter allergies more frequently—and in more complex forms—than ever before. Yet, until now, a comprehensive, India-centric reference dedicated specifically to pediatric allergy was lacking. The *IAP Textbook of Pediatric Allergy* fills this long-felt need.

This textbook represents the collective vision of the Indian Academy of Pediatrics (IAP) to strengthen subspecialty care through structured education, standardized clinical approaches, and context-specific guidance. It brings together leading experts from across the country, each contributing their knowledge, clinical experience, and academic rigor to create a resource that is both authoritative and practical.

The strength of this book lies in its holistic structure. It begins with the fundamentals of immunology and pathophysiology, then progresses through diagnostics, system-wise allergic disorders, food and drug allergies, immunotherapy, preventive strategies, and future directions. The inclusion of India-specific content—such as indigenous aeroallergens, local food allergy trends, pollution-driven disease burden, and diagnostic challenges unique to resource-limited settings—ensures relevance for pediatricians practicing across varied regions of the country.

Particular emphasis has been given to:

- Allergy diagnostics, allergen panels, and advanced testing including oscillometry
- Updated management protocols based on emerging evidence and global best practices
- Preventive care, including primordial, primary, secondary, and tertiary prevention
- Practical aspects of running an allergy clinic, patient education, and community awareness
- Evolving therapeutic options, including biologics and personalized medicine.

This book is the result of months of meticulous planning, writing, reviewing, and refinement. We are deeply indebted to all contributors—chapter authors, section editors, and reviewers—for their expertise and dedication. Their commitment to advancing pediatric allergy care is evident in every chapter.

We extend our heartfelt gratitude to the IAP leadership for their encouragement and support throughout this journey. We also acknowledge the invaluable assistance of M/s Jaypee Brothers Medical Publishers (P) Ltd, New Delhi, India, for their professionalism and commitment to academic excellence.

It is our hope that this textbook will serve as a trusted companion for pediatricians, fellows, postgraduate students, allergists, and family physicians. May it inspire improved diagnosis, timely interventions, rational use of diagnostics, greater awareness, and, most importantly, better outcomes for the countless children living with allergic diseases.

With humility and pride, we present the *IAP Textbook of Pediatric Allergy* to the pediatric fraternity of India.

Editorial Team
IAP Textbook of Pediatric Allergy

Acknowledgments

The creation of the *IAP Textbook of Pediatric Allergy* has been a deeply collaborative effort, and we extend our heartfelt gratitude to all those who made this publication possible.

We are profoundly thankful to the leadership of the Indian Academy of Pediatrics—
Dr Neelam Mohan (President, 2026)
Dr Vasant M Khalatkar (President, 2025)
Dr GV Basavaraja (President, 2024)
Dr Yogesh N Parikh (Honorary Secretary General, 2024–2025)
Dr Atanu Bhadra (National Treasurer, 2024–2025)
for their constant support and encouragement throughout this endeavor.

We express our deep appreciation to all the esteemed *chapter authors, section editors, and peer reviewers* who invested their time, expertise, and clinical insights to craft content that is scientifically robust and clinically meaningful. Their commitment to academic excellence forms the backbone of this textbook.

We are grateful to the *Executive Editors and Associate Editors* for their tireless efforts in ensuring harmony, clarity, and coherence across the chapters.

A special note of appreciation goes to M/s Jaypee Brothers Medical Publishers (P) Ltd, New Delhi, India, particularly the development and production teams, for their professionalism, precision, and support in bringing this book to print with excellence.

Lastly, we extend our gratitude to the families, colleagues, and institutions of all contributors for their continuous encouragement during the creation of this textbook.

This book is dedicated to the thousands of pediatricians across India who work tirelessly to improve the lives of children and to every child whose resilience inspires our pursuit of better care.

Neeraj Gupta
Jose Ouseph
Krishna Mohan R
(Editors-in-Chief)

Contents

1 SECTION

Fundamentals of Allergy

Section Editors: Sanjukta Dey, Soundarya M

1 CHAPTER

Introduction to Allergy

Neeraj Gupta

INTRODUCTION

The term allergy was originally referred for altered reactivity to an external agent. Over the time, the understanding about this entity has improved significantly. Today, it is defined more precisely as a hypersensitivity reaction initiated by specific immunologic mechanisms. Once considered a niche concern, allergy is now recognized as a major global and pediatric health challenge, with its prevalence rising steadily due to environmental change, urbanization, and lifestyle transitions. Advances in immunology, diagnostics, and therapeutics—alongside an evolving understanding of disease mechanisms—have transformed allergy into a multidisciplinary, precision-driven specialty.

DEFINITION AND TERMINOLOGY

The word *allergy* is derived from the Greek terms *allos* ("other") and *ergon* ("work" or "reaction"), coined in 1906 by Clemens von Pirquet to describe an "altered reactivity" of the host to an antigen. Today, the definition is more precise—*Allergy is a hypersensitivity reaction initiated by specific immunologic mechanisms.*

Allergy versus Hypersensitivity

The World Health Organization (WHO) and World Allergy Organization (WAO) classify *hypersensitivity* as *objectively reproducible symptoms or signs initiated by exposure to a defined stimulus at a dose tolerated by normal individuals.* Hypersensitivity may be:

- *Allergic hypersensitivity*—immune-mediated (IgE-mediated, non-IgE-mediated, or mixed)
- *Nonallergic hypersensitivity*—nonimmune mechanisms (e.g., pharmacologic, metabolic)
- Thus, *every allergy is hypersensitivity, but not all hypersensitivity is allergy.*

Atopy

Atopy refers to the genetic tendency to develop allergic diseases such as asthma, allergic rhinitis (AR), and atopic dermatitis (AD), typically associated with heightened IgE responses to common environmental allergens. Not all individuals with atopy manifest clinical allergy, and not all allergies are atopic.

Types of Allergic Reactions

Historically, Gell and Coombs (1963) classified hypersensitivity into four types (I–IV) based on immunological mechanisms. Modern classification recognizes an expanded spectrum of hypersensitivity reactions, including classical types I–IV with further subdivision of type IV, and additional receptor- and chemically-mediated mechanisms.

Type I—Immediate, IgE-mediated

- Classical "allergic" pathway involving allergen-specific IgE bound to high-affinity FcεRI receptors on mast cells and basophils
- *Trigger:* Crosslinking by allergens such as pollens, dust mites, foods, venoms, or drugs
- Rapid onset with release of histamine, leukotrienes, and prostaglandins causing urticaria, rhinitis, asthma, or anaphylaxis
- Primarily driven by type 2 (T2) immune responses but may involve interplay with type IVb mechanisms in chronic disease

Type II—Antibody-mediated cytotoxicity

- IgG or IgM antibodies target antigens on cell surfaces (e.g., drug–cell complexes), activating complement, opsonization, or antibody-dependent cellular cytotoxicity (ADCC).
- *Examples:* Drug-induced cytopenias, hemolytic disease of the newborn, certain transfusion reactions.

Type III—Immune complex-mediated

- IgG/IgM antibodies bind soluble antigens, forming circulating immune complexes that deposit in tissues, activating complement and neutrophils.
- *Examples:* Serum sickness, some drug reactions, hypersensitivity pneumonitis (acute phase)

Type IV—Delayed, T-cell-mediated (now subdivided by dominant immune response)

- *IVa—T1 response:* Th1/Tc1 cells with interferon γ (IFN-γ) and macrophage activation.
  Examples: Allergic contact dermatitis, chronic hypersensitivity pneumonitis, celiac disease
- *IVb—T2 response:* Th2/Tc2 cells, IL-4, IL-5, IL-13, eosinophilia.
  Examples: Chronic asthma, AR, AD, eosinophilic esophagitis
- *IVc—cytotoxic T-cell response:* CD8 T-cell-mediated killing via perforin/granzymes.
  Examples: Stevens-Johnson syndrome, toxic epidermal necrolysis
- *IVd—neutrophil-dominated:* T-cell-driven neutrophilic inflammation.
  Example: Acute generalized exanthematous pustulosis (AGEP)
- *Other possible mechanisms—p-i concept (pharmacological interaction with immune receptors):* Some drugs can bind directly and reversibly (noncovalently) to immune receptors without the need for prior hapten formation. This direct interaction—either with a specific T-cell receptor (TCR) or a human leukocyte antigen (HLA) molecule—can, in conjunction with TCR-HLA interaction, activate T cells, induce cytokine secretion, and trigger cytotoxic responses. This mechanism helps explain the strong HLA associations seen in certain drug hypersensitivity reactions.

Type V—stimulatory receptor-mediated

- Antibodies act as agonists to cell-surface receptors, altering function.
- *Example:* Graves' disease [thyroid-stimulating hormone (TSH) receptor stimulation]

Type VI—inhibitory/blocking receptor-mediated or metabolic dysregulation

- Antibodies inhibit receptors or interfere with metabolic pathways.
- *Example:* Myasthenia gravis (acetylcholine receptor blockade)

Type VII—direct chemical/toxin-induced cell activation

- Tissue or immune cell activation without a classical antigen-specific immune response, often by small reactive chemicals or drugs acting directly on receptors or ion channels.
- *Example:* Non-IgE-mediated mast cell activation by radiocontrast media

Clinical relevance:

- Multiple types can coexist in the same disease (mixed-pattern hypersensitivity), and endotypes can shift over time.
- For pediatric allergy, type I reactions dominate in conditions like asthma, food allergy, and anaphylaxis, but type IVb mechanisms drive chronic allergic inflammation, and other types (II, III, IVc, IVd) are important in specific drug or contact allergies.
- Understanding this expanded classification aids in precise diagnosis, targeted therapy (including biologics and immunotherapy), and anticipatory guidance.

Clinical Scope of the Term

In pediatrics, the term "allergy" is often used colloquially by caregivers to mean any adverse reaction to food or the environment. Clinicians must clarify whether the reaction is immune-mediated to avoid misdiagnosis and inappropriate restrictions.

HISTORICAL EVOLUTION OF ALLERGY

The understanding of allergic diseases has undergone a remarkable transformation over the last century, evolving from vague notions of "idiosyncrasy" to the modern science of immunologically mediated hypersensitivity **(Fig. 1)**.

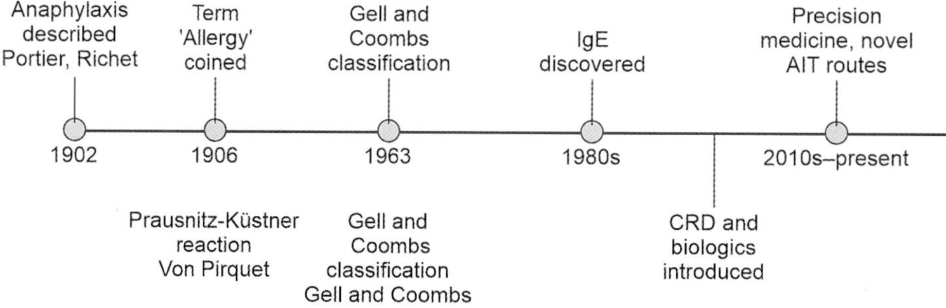

Fig. 1: Timeline of allergy milestones. (AIT: allergen-specific immunotherapy; CRD: component-resolved diagnostics)

BIRTH OF THE TERM

In *1906*, the Austrian pediatrician *Clemens von Pirquet* introduced the term *allergy*, combining the Greek *allos* (other) and *ergon* (work) to describe altered reactivity to environmental agents. Initially, it encompassed both protective immunity and harmful hypersensitivity.

Early Discoveries in Allergic Mechanisms

The early 20th century saw recognition of *hay fever*, *asthma*, and *anaphylaxis* as clinical entities. Landmark events include the following:

- *1902:* Portier and Richet describe anaphylaxis during jellyfish toxin studies (Richet was later awarded the Nobel Prize in 1913).
- *1921:* Prausnitz and Küstner demonstrate the transferability of allergic sensitivity via serum, indicating a circulating factor (later identified as IgE).
- *1930s–40s:* Skin prick testing becomes a clinical diagnostic tool.

Immunoglobulin E Era

A major breakthrough occurred in *1966–1967*, when *Kimishige and Teruko Ishizaka* and *Johansson & Bennich* independently identified *IgE* as the key mediator of immediate allergic reactions. This discovery cemented the immunologic basis of allergy and guided the development of specific IgE diagnostics.

Classification Framework

In *1963*, *Gell and Coombs* proposed their now-classic classification of hypersensitivity reactions into four types, linking pathophysiology with clinical syndromes.

Advances in Therapy

The second half of the 20th century brought standardized allergen extracts, safer *subcutaneous allergen immunotherapy (SCIT)*, and later *sublingual immunotherapy (SLIT)*. Antihistamines evolved from sedating first-generation agents to second-generation drugs with improved safety profiles.

Modern Era: Precision Allergy Medicine

The 21st century introduced *component-resolved diagnostics (CRD)*, *biologics* (e.g., anti-IgE, anti-IL-5), and *novel immunotherapy routes* such as *epicutaneous (EPIT)* and *intralymphatic (ILIT)* administration. Understanding of *endotypes* has refined disease classification and treatment. Globally, allergy care is now an interdisciplinary specialty integrating immunology, pulmonology, dermatology, and gastroenterology.

Pediatric Allergy in India

India's allergy landscape evolved later than in the West. Early work focused on asthma epidemiology and aeroallergen surveys. The last two decades have seen the establishment of dedicated pediatric allergy clinics, Indian allergen panels, and indigenous research on aeroallergen and food allergy patterns, albeit with challenges in training and infrastructure. Recently, some tertiary care state-of-art centers have been designated as "Centre of Excellence" by the WAO due to their pioneer work in the field.

SCOPE OF ALLERGY AS A DISCIPLINE

Allergy is not a confined subspecialty—it is an interdisciplinary domain that bridges *immunology, pediatrics, pulmonology, dermatology, otolaryngology, ophthalmology, gastroenterology*, and even *psychiatry*. The complexity of allergic disorders stems from the immune system's interaction with genetic predisposition, environmental triggers, and developmental changes, making the pediatric population a uniquely dynamic focus of care.

Breadth of Clinical Conditions

The scope encompasses multiple organ systems:

- *Respiratory allergy*—AR, asthma, hypersensitivity pneumonitis
- *Food allergy*—IgE-mediated, non-IgE-mediated (e.g., food protein-induced enterocolitis), and mixed disorders (eosinophilic esophagitis)
- *Skin allergy*—AD, urticaria, contact dermatitis
- *Drug allergy*—immediate and delayed hypersensitivity to antibiotics, nonsteroidal anti-inflammatory drugs (NSAIDs), vaccines
- *Insect venom allergy*—rare but potentially life-threatening in children
- *Ocular allergy*—seasonal and perennial allergic conjunctivitis, vernal keratoconjunctivitis

This diversity requires an integrated diagnostic and therapeutic approach.

PEDIATRIC CONSIDERATIONS

Children differ from adults in several respects:

- Immune system immaturity alters disease expression and progression.

- Growth, nutrition, and psychosocial development are directly impacted by chronic allergic disease.
- Allergic conditions often evolve over time—the "atopic march" (progression from eczema to food allergy to respiratory allergy) illustrates this natural history.

Pediatric allergy management must therefore focus on early diagnosis, prevention, and long-term monitoring.

Multidisciplinary Collaboration

Optimal allergy care demands collaboration among:

- *Pediatricians and allergists*—primary diagnosis and long-term management
- *Pulmonologists*—advanced airway management in asthma
- *ENT surgeons*—surgical interventions in chronic rhinosinusitis with polyposis
- *Dermatologists*—severe eczema and chronic urticaria
- *Gastroenterologists*—eosinophilic gastrointestinal diseases
- *Ophthalmologists*—sight-threatening ocular allergy

In India, this collaborative model is emerging, with growing recognition of allergy as a distinct academic discipline.

Expanding Frontiers

Emerging areas include:

- *Precision medicine*—identifying phenotypes/endotypes for targeted therapy
- *Biologics*—monoclonal antibodies against IgE, IL-4/13, IL-5, TSLP
- *Allergen immunotherapy innovations*—epicutaneous, intralymphatic, recombinant allergens
- *Climate change and pollution research*—understanding their impact on pediatric allergy trends

As the following chapters will detail, the scope of allergy extends well beyond symptom control to encompass prevention, education, and research—particularly vital in a country like India with a rising allergy burden.

GLOBAL BURDEN OF ALLERGIC DISEASES

Allergic diseases have emerged as a global public health challenge, affecting individuals across all ages, ethnicities, and socioeconomic strata. The *WAO* estimates that up to *30–40% of the global population* suffers from one or more allergic disorders, with a consistent upward trajectory over the past five decades.

Epidemiological Trends

- *Asthma:* Affects ~262 million people globally (WHO, 2019), with prevalence varying from <5% in some rural areas to >20% in urban centers of high-income countries
- *AR:* Estimated to affect *10–30% of adults* and up to *40% of children* worldwide, with a significant overlap with asthma
- *AD:* Global prevalence in children ranges from 5 to 20%, with higher rates in industrialized nations
- *Food allergy:* Affects 6–8% of children in high-income countries, with peanut, milk, egg, and tree nut allergy being most common
- *Anaphylaxis:* Lifetime prevalence estimated at 0.05–2%, with increasing hospital admissions in many countries

The *ISAAC (International Study of Asthma and Allergies in Childhood)* program, conducted in over 100 countries, documented dramatic variations—often with higher prevalence in developed nations, but with rapidly rising rates in developing countries undergoing urbanization.

Drivers of the Global Increase

Multiple hypotheses attempt to explain this rise:

- *Urbanization and westernized lifestyles*—reduced microbial exposure (hygiene hypothesis) and increased pollution
- *Dietary changes*—lower intake of fresh fruits/vegetables, higher processed food consumption, altered gut microbiome
- *Climate change*—extended pollen seasons, altered allergenicity
- *Indoor environments*—dust mites, mold, pet allergens, poor ventilation.

Genetic predisposition remains important, but environmental and lifestyle shifts play a dominant role in recent epidemiologic changes.

Economic and Psychosocial Impact

Allergic diseases cause a substantial *economic burden*—both direct (medical care, medications) and indirect (school/work absenteeism, productivity loss). For example:

- Asthma accounts for billions in annual healthcare costs in high-income countries.
- AR, though often underappreciated, is linked to reduced academic performance and impaired quality of life.

The psychosocial impact—chronic symptoms, dietary restrictions, activity limitations, and anxiety—can be particularly profound in children and their families.

Inequities in Global Care

While high-income countries face high prevalence but have advanced diagnostic and therapeutic resources, many low- and middle-income countries (LMICs) have rising prevalence with limited infrastructure, workforce, and access to medicines. This disparity underscores the need for global collaboration in allergy prevention and management.

ALLERGY BURDEN IN INDIA

India, with its diverse geography, climate, and cultural practices, presents a unique landscape for allergic diseases. While historically considered uncommon, allergies are now recognized as a significant and growing pediatric health issue. The *ISAAC Phase III* and *INSEARCH* studies have provided key epidemiological insights, revealing both regional variation and an overall rising trend.

Prevalence and Patterns

- *Asthma:* Prevalence in Indian children aged 6–7 years is ~5–8%, with higher rates (10–15%) in adolescents (13–14 years) in urban centers such as Delhi, Bangalore, and Kolkata
- *AR:* Affects 10–20% of children, often underdiagnosed or misattributed to recurrent viral infections
- *AD:* Prevalence estimates range from 2 to 6% but may be underestimated due to limited dermatology access in rural areas
- *Food allergy:* Traditionally considered rare, but emerging data show clinically significant IgE-mediated food allergies, particularly to milk, egg, wheat, legumes, and certain fruits
- *Ocular allergy:* Vernal keratoconjunctivitis is relatively more common in India, particularly in hot, dry regions.

Regional and Environmental Influences

The spectrum and severity of allergic diseases vary by:

- *Geographic zone:* Coastal areas with high humidity favor dust mite proliferation; arid zones see more pollen-induced allergy.
- *Urban versus rural:* Urbanization correlates with higher prevalence, likely due to pollution, reduced microbial exposure, and indoor allergen load.

TABLE 1: Estimated prevalence of common allergic disorders in India.

Disease	*India (children)*	*Global average (children)*
Asthma	5–15%	7–20%
Allergic rhinitis	10–20%	10–30%
Atopic dermatitis	2–6%	5–20%
Food allergy	<2% (confirmed)	6–8%
Ocular allergy (VKC)	1–3%	<1% (VKC specifically)

- *Pollution:* Outdoor air pollutants ($PM_{2.5}$, NO_2) and indoor pollutants (biomass fuel smoke) are significant contributors, with seasonal peaks post Diwali and during crop residue burning.

Challenges in Diagnosis and Management

- *Under-recognition:* Symptoms are often attributed to infections or "seasonal change."
- *Limited access to specialists:* Few certified allergists; pediatric allergy is an emerging field.
- *Diagnostic gaps:* Allergen panels may not reflect regional sensitization patterns.
- *Therapeutic limitations:* Allergen immunotherapy and biologics remain underutilized due to cost, awareness, and infrastructure constraints.

Comparative Overview

Table 1 contrasts the estimated prevalence of key allergic diseases in India with global averages.

THE WAY FORWARD FOR INDIA

Addressing the allergy burden in India requires:

- *Awareness campaigns* for early recognition
- *Region-specific epidemiological studies* and allergen mapping
- *Training programs* for pediatricians and primary care physicians
- *Policy support* for air quality improvement and access to diagnostics and therapeutics

CONCLUSION

Allergy, once considered a niche concern, has become a major pediatric health priority worldwide, including in India. From von Pirquet's early concept of "altered reactivity" to the era of precision medicine, the field has evolved into a multidisciplinary, evidence-driven specialty. The global burden of allergic diseases continues to rise, driven by environmental change, urbanization, and lifestyle transitions, with India showing similar trends but unique epidemiological patterns.

For pediatricians, early recognition, accurate diagnosis, and evidence-based management are critical—not only to alleviate symptoms but also to alter the disease course and improve quality of life. In India, the challenge is twofold: Increasing prevalence and limited specialist resources. The way forward lies in awareness, capacity building, research tailored to local needs, and policy advocacy. This textbook aims to equip clinicians with the knowledge and tools to advance pediatric allergy care, ultimately shaping healthier futures for children.

KEY POINTS

- *Expanded classification of allergic reactions:* Modern immunology recognizes several types of hypersensitivity reactions beyond the classic Gell and Coombs I–IV, incorporating antibody-, cell-, receptor-mediated, and direct chemical activation mechanisms.
- *Global burden and trends:* Up to 30–40% of the global population is affected by allergic disorders, with rising prevalence driven by urbanization, pollution, dietary shifts, and climate change.
- *Pediatric allergy in India:* Indian children show increasing rates of asthma (5–15%), AR (10–20%), and emerging food allergies; regional patterns are influenced by geography, humidity, and pollution.
- *Multidisciplinary nature of allergy care:* Effective management requires collaboration among pediatricians, allergists, pulmonologists, dermato logists, ENT specialists, gastroenterologists, and ophthalmologists.
- *Future directions:* Precision medicine, biologics, novel allergen immunotherapy routes (EPIT, ILIT), and region-specific epidemiological research are key to improving outcomes, especially in resource-limited settings like India.

SUGGESTED READING

1. Asher MI, Montefort S, Björkstén B, Lai CKW, Strachan DP, Weiland SK, et al. Worldwide time trends in the prevalence of symptoms of asthma, allergic rhinoconjunctivitis, and eczema in childhood: ISAAC phases one and three repeat multicountry cross-sectional surveys. Lancet. 2006;368(9537):733-43.
2. Jutel M, Agache I, Zemelka-Wiacek M, Akdis M, Chivato T, Del Giacco S, et al. Nomenclature of allergic diseases and hypersensitivity reactions: Adapted to modern needs: An EAACI position paper. Allergy. 2023;78(11):2851-74.
3. Mahesh PA, Moitra S, Mabalirajan U, Garg M, Malamardi S, Vedanthan PL, et al. Allergic diseases in India - Prevalence, risk factors and current challenges. Clin Exp Allergy. 2023;53(3):276-94.
4. Papadopoulos NG, Custovic A, Cabana MD, et al. Pediatric allergy: Where have we been and where are we going? Pediatr Allergy Immunol. 2019;30(1):19-27.
5. Pawankar R, Canonica GW, Holgate ST, Lockey RF, Blaiss MS. WAO White Book on Allergy: Update 2023. Milwaukee, WI: World Allergy Organization; 2023.
6. Pawankar R. Allergic diseases and asthma: A global public health concern and a call to action. World Allergy Organ J. 2014;7:12.
7. Sehgal S, Gupta N, Dadha P, Nagarajan S, Gupta R, Jain Verma M, et al. Understanding the burden of food allergy among urban and rural school children from north India. World Allergy Organ J. 2024;17(6):100916.
8. Singh AB, Shahi S. Aeroallergens in clinical practice of allergy in India— ARIA Asia-Pacific Workshop report. Asia Pac Allergy. 2011;1(2):91-102.
9. Vedanthan PK, Christopher DJ, Gupta N. Allergy training in India. Clin Exp Allergy. 2022;52(7):833-5.
10. von Pirquet C. Allergie. Münch Med Wochenschr. 1906;53:1457–8.

2 CHAPTER

Immunology of Allergy

Saibal Moitra, Mohammad Ziaul Haque

INTRODUCTION

Allergy is a hypersensitive immune response to ordinarily harmless environmental substances known as allergens. These allergens can include pollen, dust mites, animal dander, certain foods, insect venoms, and drugs. Allergic reactions occur when the immune system mistakenly identifies these innocuous substances as threats, triggering a cascade of immunological events that result in symptoms ranging from mild irritation to life-threatening anaphylaxis. Understanding the immunology of allergy involves unravelling the complex interactions between the innate and adaptive immune systems, particularly focusing on the roles of immunoglobulin E (IgE), mast cells, basophils, eosinophils, and T helper 2 (Th2) cells. This chapter delves into the cellular and molecular mechanisms underlying allergic responses, the genetic and environmental factors that predispose individuals to allergy, and the immunopathology that characterizes various allergic diseases.

ETIOPATHOGENESIS

Allergy is a complex interplay of genetic predisposition, environmental exposures, and immune system dysregulation, leading to an abnormal hypersensitive response to otherwise harmless antigens known as allergens.

Genetic Factors

Genetic susceptibility plays a crucial role in the development of allergic diseases. A family history of atopy (the genetic tendency to develop allergic diseases) increases the risk significantly. Multiple genes are implicated in allergy susceptibility, including those regulating immune responses such as cytokine production [interleukin-4 (IL-4), IL-5, IL-13], IgE synthesis, and barrier functions of the skin and mucosa (e.g., filaggrin gene mutations in atopic dermatitis). These genetic factors influence the balance between T helper cell subsets and the propensity to mount a Th2-skewed immune response, which is characteristic of allergy.

Environmental Factors

Environmental exposures interact with genetic predispositions to trigger allergic sensitization. Common environmental factors include the following:

- *Allergens:* Pollens, dust mites, molds, animal dander, foods, insect venoms, and certain drugs.
- *Pollution:* Air pollutants like diesel exhaust particles can enhance allergic sensitization and exacerbate symptoms.
- *Infections:* Early-life infections and microbial exposures can influence immune system development and either protect against or promote allergy (the "hygiene hypothesis").
- *Lifestyle:* Changes in diet, increased urbanization, and indoor living conditions may affect allergen exposure and immune responses.

Immune Mechanisms

The hallmark of allergy is a type I hypersensitivity reaction mediated by IgE. The pathogenesis proceeds through two key phases: (1) Sensitization phase and (2) effector phase.

Sensitization Phase

Upon first exposure, allergens are taken up by antigen-presenting cells (APCs), especially dendritic cells, which process and present allergenic peptides to naïve $CD4^+$ T cells in lymphoid tissues. In genetically predisposed individuals, these T cells differentiate into Th2 cells under the influence of cytokines like IL-4. Th2 cells secrete IL-4, IL-5, and IL-13, promoting B cells to switch antibody production toward IgE specific to the allergen. These IgE antibodies bind to FcεRI receptors on mast cells and basophils, "arming" them for subsequent allergen encounters.

Effector Phase

Upon re-exposure to the allergen, cross-linking of IgE on mast cells and basophils triggers their activation and

Flowchart 1: Immunological cascade of allergy.

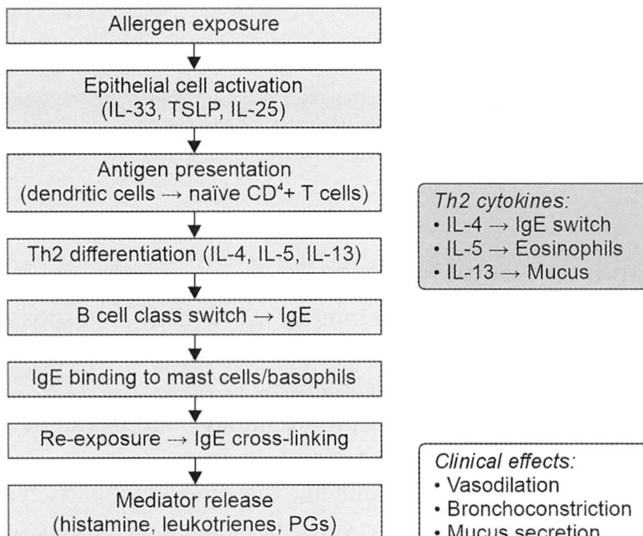

degranulation. This releases histamine, prostaglandins, leukotrienes, and other inflammatory mediators that cause the clinical symptoms of allergy such as vasodilation, bronchoconstriction, mucus secretion, and recruitment of eosinophils and other inflammatory cells **(Flowchart 1)**. The chronicity and severity of allergic inflammation are maintained by persistent Th2 responses and the involvement of eosinophils and other immune cells, leading to tissue remodeling and damage in diseases like asthma and atopic dermatitis.

TH1/TH2 BALANCE

The balance between T helper 1 (Th1) and Th2 immune responses plays a crucial role in the development of allergic diseases. Th1 cells are primarily involved in cell-mediated immunity and protect against intracellular pathogens by producing cytokines like interferon-gamma (IFN-γ). In contrast, Th2 cells promote humoral immunity and are responsible for allergic inflammation by secreting cytokines such as IL-4, IL-5, and IL-13. These cytokines drive IgE production, eosinophil activation, and mucus secretion—all hallmarks of allergic responses. In allergic individuals, there is a shift toward a Th2-dominant immune profile, which leads to hypersensitivity to harmless environmental antigens. This Th2 skewing may be influenced by genetic predisposition and environmental factors such as reduced microbial exposure in early life, as proposed by the hygiene hypothesis. A well-regulated immune system maintains a proper Th1/Th2 balance, preventing overreaction to nonpathogenic antigens. Therapeutic strategies in allergy often aim to restore this balance by suppressing Th2 activity or enhancing regulatory and Th1 responses.

Role of Cytokines

Cytokines play a central role in the development and regulation of allergic responses by mediating communication between immune cells and directing the type of immune reaction. In allergic individuals, the immune response is skewed toward a Th2 profile, which is driven by key cytokines. IL-4 is crucial for initiating and maintaining the Th2 response and promoting class switching in B cells to produce allergen-specific IgE antibodies. IL-5 plays a major role in the recruitment, activation, and survival of eosinophils, which contribute to tissue inflammation and damage in conditions such as asthma and atopic dermatitis. IL-13, along with IL-4, enhances mucus secretion and airway hyperreactivity, especially in allergic asthma. IL-9 supports mast cell proliferation and IgE-mediated responses. In addition, cytokines like IL-33, TSLP (thymic stromal lymphopoietin), and IL-25, released by epithelial cells upon allergen exposure, act as "alarmins" that further amplify the Th2 response. These cytokines not only contribute to the initiation of the allergic reaction but also sustain chronic inflammation. Therefore, targeting specific cytokines has become a key strategy in treating allergic diseases, as seen with biologics like anti-IL-4Rα (dupilumab) and anti-IL-5 (mepolizumab).

IgE Synthesis

Immunoglobulin E synthesis is a hallmark event in allergic sensitization and is driven by a Th2-skewed immune response. Upon first exposure to an allergen, APCs (such as dendritic cells) process the allergen and present it to naïve $CD4^{+}$ T cells in the lymphoid tissues. In atopic individuals, these T cells differentiate into Th2 cells under the influence of IL-4. Th2 cells then secrete cytokines, primarily IL-4 and IL-13, which stimulate B cells to undergo class-switch recombination from producing IgM or IgG to producing IgE. This process occurs through activation-induced cytidine deaminase (AID) and CD40–CD40L interaction between B and T cells. The newly synthesized allergen-specific IgE antibodies bind to high-affinity FcεRI receptors on the surface of mast cells and basophils, sensitizing these cells. Upon subsequent exposure to the same allergen, cross-linking of IgE on these cells leads to their activation and degranulation, releasing histamine and other mediators that produce allergic symptoms. Thus, IgE synthesis is central to the pathogenesis of type I hypersensitivity reactions.

IMMUNE TOLERANCE IN ALLERGY

Immune tolerance refers to the immune system's ability to recognize and ignore harmless substances, such as food proteins or environmental allergens, without mounting an immune response. In healthy individuals, tolerance is maintained through mechanisms involving regulatory T cells (Tregs), which suppress allergen-specific Th2 responses and promote the production of anti-inflammatory cytokines like IL-10 and transforming growth factor-beta (TGF-β). These cytokines help prevent IgE class switching and inhibit mast cell and eosinophil activation. Additionally, the induction of IgG4 antibodies, which can block allergen binding to IgE (known as "blocking antibodies"), contributes to immune tolerance. In allergic individuals, this tolerance is broken or insufficient, leading to hypersensitivity responses. Restoring tolerance is the main goal of allergen-specific immunotherapy (AIT), which gradually exposes patients to increasing doses of allergens to shift the immune response from Th2 dominance toward Treg activity and immune regulation. Promoting tolerance is a promising strategy for long-term management and potential prevention of allergic diseases.

CONCLUSION

The immunology of allergy represents a finely tuned yet dysregulated interaction between genetic susceptibility, environmental exposures, and immune mechanisms. Central to this process is the skewing of the immune response toward a Th2-dominated profile, driving IgE synthesis and activation of effector cells such as mast cells, basophils, and eosinophils. The resulting release of inflammatory mediators accounts for the clinical manifestations of allergic disease, while persistent immune activation leads to chronic inflammation and tissue remodeling. Understanding these mechanisms not only provides insights into the pathogenesis of allergic disorders but also opens avenues for targeted therapies—ranging from biologics to immunomodulatory interventions—aimed at restoring immune tolerance and achieving long-term disease control.

KEY POINTS

- *Genetic and environmental interplay:* Atopy arises from a complex interaction between genetic predisposition (e.g., cytokine and barrier function gene variants) and environmental exposures such as allergens, pollutants, and early-life microbial encounters.
- *Th2-skewed immune response:* Allergic disease is driven by a shift toward Th2 dominance, with key cytokines (IL-4, IL-5, IL-13) orchestrating IgE production, eosinophil recruitment, mucus hypersecretion, and airway hyperreactivity.
- *IgE-mediated sensitization and effector phases:* Sensitization involves allergen presentation to Th2 cells and IgE class switching in B cells; re-exposure triggers mast cell/basophil activation, releasing histamine and other mediators.
- *Role of epithelial "alarmins":* Cytokines such as IL-33, TSLP, and IL-25 released from damaged epithelial cells amplify Th2 inflammation and sustain allergic pathology.
- *Immune tolerance as a therapeutic goal:* Tregs, IL-10, TGF-β, and IgG4 antibodies maintain tolerance to harmless antigens; AIT seeks to restore this balance and reduce long-term disease burden.

SUGGESTED READING

1. Abbas AK, Lichtman AH, Pillai S. Cellular and Molecular Immunology, 8th edition. Philadelphia: Elsevier; 2014.
2. Akdis CA, et al. Allergic disease mechanisms: From molecules to therapeutic strategies. J Allergy Clin Immunol. 2020;145(5):1189-204.
3. Franklin Adkinson Jr. N, Bochner BS, Wesley Burks A, Busse WW, Holgate ST, Jr. Lemanske RF, et al. Middleton's Allergy: Principle and Practice, 8th edition. New York: Mosby; 2013.
4. Muraro A, Lemanske Jr RF, Castells M, Torres MJ, Khan D, Simon HU, et al. Precision medicine in allergic disease—food allergy, asthma, and more. J Allergy Clin Immunol Pract. 2022;10(1):57-69.
5. Murphy K, Weaver C. Janeway's Immunobiology, 9th edition. London: Garland Science; 2017.

3 CHAPTER

Pathophysiology of Allergic Diseases

Sanjukta De

INTRODUCTION

Allergic diseases such as atopic dermatitis (AD), allergic rhinitis (AR), asthma, seasonal allergies, and food allergy (FA) are manifestations of dysregulated immune system resulting from either intolerance or poor tolerance to harmless exogenous stimuli or allergens. Allergic reactions involve various types of hypersensitivity reactions involving antibodies, immune cell-mediated, tissue-driven, or metabolic mechanisms resulting in the development of the observed symptoms in various parts of the body such as skin, lungs, and gastric system and other symptoms. An understanding of the underlying mechanisms allows for the development of more effective and targeted treatment plans, better patient outcomes, including faster recovery, reduced relapse rates, and improved overall well-being.

The genetic predisposition to develop allergy is defined as atopy; however, it does not represent the current understanding of allergy pathophysiology, and hence its use has become redundant in recent times. This is partly owing to the various endotypes or underlying mechanisms that further complicate the observed allergic traits. In addition, various environmental factors such as pollution, infection, or even lifestyle changes can interact with various genetic elements (genes, regulatory proteins) to exacerbate allergic diseases. These modulations further add to the complexity of allergic pathophysiology and have led to the understanding of phenotypes versus endotypes.

HYPERSENSITIVITY TYPES

The classical hypersensitivity reactions are a secondary immune response occurring in an individual presensitized to the allergen. As per the EACCI 2001 guidelines, hypersensitivities have been divided into the following categories: IgE-mediated and non-IgE-mediated reactions. IgE-mediated disorders include atopic and nonatopic conditions (e.g., insect sting, food allergies, drugs, helminths). The non-IgE-mediated disorders are cell-mediated reactions such as those mediated by T-lymphocytes (contact dermatitis), IgG-mediated (allergic alveolitis), and other immune cells, such as eosinophils (gastroenteropathy). Nonallergic reactions do not involve immune mechanisms.

The updated 2025 EACCI guidelines covers the classical Gel and Coombs classification of hypersensitivity and incorporates newer findings on T-cell responses (types IVa–d), tissue-driven mechanisms (types V and VI), and direct chemical response (type VII) **(Table 1)**. This updated nomenclature aims to highlight the complexity of allergic diseases along with the various endotypes that can overlap simultaneously or evolve over time.

Classification of Hypersensitive Reactions

Type I Hypersensitivity

Type I hypersensitivity is characterized by two main phases: Sensitization phase and effector phase. During sensitization, there is an asymptomatic contact with the allergen (e.g., pollen, dust mites, peanuts) which results in activation of circulating B lymphocytes to form IgE-secreting plasma cells and memory cells. The naïve $CD4^+$ T helper $(Th)^0$ cells differentiate into Th2 cells; the latter in turn secrete cytokines, particularly interleukin (IL)-4 and IL-6, which along with other co-stimulatory surface signals promote stimulation of IgE-producing B cells. IgE binds via the Fc fragment to its high-affinity FcεRI receptor on mast cells and basophils which are the main effector cells of type I hypersensitive reaction. Upon re-exposure, the same allergen crosslinks the membrane-bound IgE molecules on sensitized mast cells and basophils, resulting in degranulation wherein the various inflammatory mediators released result in increased vascular permeability and smooth muscle contraction which results in vasodilation, mucus secretion, itching, and pronounced bronchoconstriction.

Extensive activation of mast cells causes release of histamine which acts mainly via the H1 receptors leading to smooth muscle contraction in the lungs and intestine as well as results in vascular permeability as observed in

TABLE 1: Updated nomenclature of hypersensitivity reactions (EACCI 2025).

	Antibody-mediated hypersensitization (Immediate)			***Cell-mediated hypersensitization (Delayed)***			
Hypersensitivity types	***Type I***	***Type II***	***Type III***	***Type IVa***	***Type IVb***	***Type IVc***	***Type IVd***
Cell types	B cells: IgE (Th)^0: Th2	B cells, IgG, IgM	B cells, IgM, IgG Immune complexes	Th1	Th2	Primarily CD8$^+$	CD4$^+$, CD8$^+$
Cytokines involved	IL-4, IL-5, IL-6, IL-13	–	IL-1, IL-6, TNF-α	IFN-γ and TNF-α	IL-4, IL-5, IL-9, IL-13, IL-31	IL-17A, IL-17F, IL-21, IL-22, GM-CSF	IL-8, GM-CSF
Effector cells	Mast cells, basophils: histamine, serotonin, etc.	NK cell, eosinophil, Mϕ, neutrophil	Basophils, mast cells, platelets, Mϕ, neutrophil, monocytes	Mϕ	Mast cells, basophils, eosinophils	Mϕ	Neutrophils
Examples	AD, asthma, AR, food allergy, drug allergy	Chronic urticaria, penicillin-induced hemolytic anemia and autoimmune hemolytic anemia, myasthenia gravis, thyroiditis	Serum sickness, SLE, glomerulonephritis, RA, farmers' lung	Contact dermatitis, AD, AR, asthma, drug allergy	AD, asthma, contact dermatitis, food allergy, drug allergy	Contact dermatitis, GVHD, asthma, drug allergy	Drug allergy, pustular eruptions, Behcet's disease
Tissue-Driven Hypersensitization							

Contd...

Contd...

Hypersensitivity types	***Type V***	***Type VI***	***Type VII***
Dysregulation type	Epithelial barrier, leaky junctions	Metabolic-induced immune dysregulation	Chemical substance-induced cellular and inflammatory response
Mediators and mechanisms	• ILC2s • Mutation of filaggrin and disruption of epithelial barrier, microbial dysbiosis • Immune modulation by alarmins, TSLP, IL-25, and IL-33 • Epigenetic modulation	• Increased release of proinflammatory mediators and airway inflammation in obese patients; modification of gut, oral, and lung microbiome • Leaky barrier sites in the gut enable immune cells to migrate to distant organs causing inflammation in those areas • Metabolites such as tryptophan metabolites, short-chain fatty acids contribute to allergy development	• Inhibition of COX-1 and release of eicosanoid mediators in susceptible individuals (PGs, and LTs) • LTC4, LTD4, and LTE4 • Anaphylactoid reactions, increased MRGPRX2 expression • Release of histamine, TNF, • PGD2, and β-hexosaminidase
Examples	Asthma, AR, celiac disease, CRS, AD, FPIES	Obesity and asthma, histamine-mediated allergic responses	AERD, idiosyncratic reactions (drug-induced)

(AD: atopic dermatitis; AERD: aspirin-exacerbated respiratory diseases; AR: allergic rhinitis; CRS: chronic rhinosinusitis; COX-1: cyclooxygenase-1; FPIES: food protein-induced enterocolitis syndrome; GM-CSF: granulocyte-macrophage colony-stimulating factor; GVHD: graft-versus-host disease; IFN-γ: interferon-gamma; Ig (E, G, M): immunoglobulin (type E, G, M); IL: interleukin; ILC: innate lymphoid cells; LTs: leukotrienes; Mϕ: macrophage; NK: natural killer; PGs: prostaglandins; RA: rheumatoid arthritis; SLE: systemic lupus erythematosus; Th: T helper lymphocytes; TNF-α: tumor necrosis factor-alpha) anaphylaxis. Histamine released in the blood plasma has a short half-life of typically 20 minutes and can be as low as 6 minutes, post which they are rapidly degraded and eliminated by diffusion, explaining the transient effect of hypersensitivity reactions.

Type II Hypersensitivity

Type II hypersensitivity or humoral cytotoxic immune response are cytotoxic reactions medicated by humoral antibodies such as IgM or IgG. In this type of classic hypersensitivity drug-dependent-type reaction, the drug or its metabolite binds to proteins on the cell membrane which results in the formation of the antibodies. The antibody and drug-membrane protein complex bind and activate complement or are being bound by the Fc fragment gamma receptor (FcγR) on the effector cell such as an NK cell, eosinophil, macrophage (Mϕ), or neutrophil, finally inducing cytolysis.

The mechanisms of sensitization leading to the development of IgG antibodies are unclear. However, once the complex is formed, they are destroyed by the following methods such as complement-mediated cytolysis, antibody-dependent cell-mediated cytotoxicity (ADCC), phagocytosis, antibody-mediated cellular dysfunction, or antibody-mediated cellular dysfunction (a noncytotoxic mechanism). A few examples of type II hypersensitivity include chronic urticaria, penicillin-induced hemolytic anemia, autoimmune hemolytic anemia, myasthenia gravis, and thyroiditis.

Type III Hypersensitivity

Type III hypersensitivity or immune complex-mediated hypersensitivity is initiated owing to inefficient elimination of immune complexes which are deposited in various tissues to trigger an immune response followed by complement activation and inflammatory reactions. The immune complexes formed in vessels and tissues can be bound by the FcγR of mast cells and other leukocytes leading to their activation. Complement activation results in neutrophil recruitment and other inflammatory cells which release inflammatory mediators and enzymes contributing to the clinical symptoms of type III hypersensitivity. Examples include serum sickness, glomerulonephritis, rheumatoid arthritis, farmers' lung, and systemic lupus erythematosus (SLE).

Type IV Hypersensitivity

Type IV hypersensitivity or delayed-type hypersensitivity (DTH) is an umbrella term that encompasses various T cell-mediated immune responses such as Th1 or Th17 cells. During sensitization, APCs process and present the allergen to Th cells resulting in clonal expansion of Th1 cells. The sensitized T cells ($CD4^+$ helper and $CD8^+$ cytotoxic) release cytokines that attract and activate other immune cells leading to inflammation. These reactions are delayed, typically appear over 48–72 hours after exposure to antigen. Type IV hypersensitivity is further classified into four types, types IVa to IVd (detailed in **Table 1**), depending on the type of T cell involved and the cytokines or chemokines produced. Examples include contact dermatitis (e.g., nickel allergy) and some cases of chronic allergic eczema.

Type V Hypersensitivity

Recent findings on the phenotypes and endotypes of mucosal/cutaneous inflammatory diseases such as AR, allergic rhinoconjunctivitis (ACR), AD, asthma, or food protein-induced enterocolitis syndrome revealed that they result from altered barrier function of the skin or mucosa that leads to the activation of the underlying immune system leading to chronic inflammation. Mutations in filaggrin (FLG), a keratin-binding protein, play a key role in epidermal homeostasis and can predispose individuals to AD and asthma. In AR and asthma, the tight junctions in the airway mucosa were also found to be disrupted. Microbial dysbiosis reportedly found in the leaky epithelial barrier along with bacterial translocation has been associated with the exacerbation of allergic symptoms.

Type VI Hypersensitivity

Obesity and diabetes which result from metabolic dysregulation have shown to exert create epithelial barriers wherein the immune cells activated at the epithelial barriers can travel to distant sites and cause a cascade of inflammatory reaction in that area. In the circulation, the acute-phase reactants such as chemokines and cytokines increase metabolic burden and these mechanisms are observed in obese asthmatics which are relatively distinct from those observed in nonobese patients. Lately multiple immune-modifying metabolites have also been identified in various allergic diseases.

Type VII Hypersensitivity

This type of hypersensitivity describes direct cellular and inflammatory responses to chemical substances wherein direct interaction of chemicals with immune cells trigger an inflammatory response without the need for antibody involvement or prior sensitization. The chemicals reportedly can directly activate mast cells or Mψ and therefore cause inflammation. Type VII hypersensitivity represents a shift in understanding how chemicals can trigger immune responses, emphasizing the direct role of the innate immune system and the potential for direct chemical-immune cell interactions. Examples include insulin autoimmune syndrome (also known as Hirata's disease), aspirin-exacerbated respiratory diseases (AERD), and idiosyncratic reactions.

ALLERGEN PRESENTATION

Allergen Capture and Processing

Antigen presenting cells (APCs), such as dendritic cells (DCs), macrophages, and B cells, play a crucial role in bridging between the innate and adaptive immune responses. Upon exposure to allergens, APCs engulf or internalize the allergens by phagocytosis or other endocytic pathways. Antigen processing is a process wherein foreign protein antigens are broken down into its peptides and thereafter presented on the surface of APCs bound to major histocompatibility cells (MHC). Interaction between the MHC and the corresponding T cell receptor (TCR) drives the differentiation of naïve $CD4^+$ T cells into Th2 phenotype and subsequently mount the specific cellular immune response. In AD, for example, barrier dysfunction owing to FLG mutations permits transcutaneous sensitization. The keratinocytes release cytokines such as cytokines called alarmins such as thymic stromal lymphopoietin (TSLP) and IL-33 which act on DCs and Langerhans cells influencing their maturation and migration from the epidermis to the lymph nodes where they present the antigens to T cells. Cytokines such as IL-4 and IL-13 are also produced in AD which further amplify the Th2 immune response and contribute to disease progression.

Two classical pathways have been described for the processing of antigens, namely the *cytosolic pathway* for endogenous antigens and the *endocytic pathway* for exogenous antigens employing the MHC I and MHC II, respectively.

T Cell–B Cell Interaction

T cell–B cell interaction is crucial to class switching and in particular the production of IgE molecules. The interaction between T cells and B cells together with the cytokine signals triggers class switch recombination (CSR). CSR is a process wherein the B cell changes the type of antibody it produces, for example, from IgM to IgE. The signals from Th2 cells, particularly IL-4 and CD40L, are crucial for inducing CSR to the IgE isotype T cells and also exhibit switching wherein its phenotype changes in response to environmental signals which involves a shift from its naïve state to an effector state (e.g., Th1, Th2, or cytotoxic T cell), to a memory state, or even to a T regulatory (Treg) state. It can also involve changes in the TCR specificity or changes in metabolic pathways.

EPIGENETICS

Alterations in gene expression without altering the DNA sequence are called epigenetics. These modifications are mostly post-translational and can be mediated by DNA methylation and histone modifications and also influenced by environmental factors. The modifications and classical epigenetic modifications include DNA methylation and histone modifications induced by methylation, acetylation, phosphorylation, and ubiquitination. Histone methylation and acetylation are probably more extensively studied.

DNA Methylation

DNA methylation involves covalent addition of a methyl group to a cytosine base within the CpG dinucleotides. This process of methylation varies across cell types and developmental stages, thereby influencing which genes are active or silenced in a cell.

Histones

Histones can be *acetylated* at lysine residues and are mediated by histone deacetylases (HDACs).

microRNAs and Noncoding RNAs

Post-transcriptional control elements such as microRNAs (miRNAs) have been identified recently as nonclassical epigenetic regulators of gene expression.

Impact of Epigenetics on Allergy Pathophysiology

Epigenetics can influence various aspects of allergy development such as differentiation of Th2 cells which are crucial in allergic inflammation as well as the function of Treg cells which help maintain tolerance.

Epigenetics explains why patients with the same genetic predisposition experience varied disease severity or develop different allergic conditions. For example, studies have shown that differential methylation of DNA at the promoter region of IL-4 or interferon (IFN)-γ locus was responsible for why some patients had asthma versus those who did not have asthma. Similar epigenetic modifications were observed in other allergic conditions such as AR and food allergies (cow's milk, peanuts, etc.).

Impact of Epigenetics on Early-life Environment

Environmental, dietary, and microbial exposures in early life help shape immune tolerance and influence genetic predisposition. Epigenetic modulations mediate how early-life exposures can influence immune development. For example, maternal smoking and diet can alter methylation patterns in key immune genes like *IL-4*, *FOXP3*, and *IFN-γ*, potentially affecting allergy risk in offspring. These changes can potentially alter the body's ability to mount specific immune responses impacting risk of atopy in early childhood. For example, hypermethylation of the *IFN-γ* gene can suppress Th1 responses and potentially result in an imbalanced Th2 response.

DNA methylation patterns in cord blood have shown to be associated with the development of AD later in childhood. Some of the methylation patterns have shown to persist from cord blood into mid-childhood suggesting a potential link to the progression of atopic march (AM).

Altered DNA methylation patterns in the epidermal layer of the skin in AD reportedly influence the overall methylation signature and can contribute to other atopic diseases. Therefore, understanding the role of DNA methylation in AM could lead to early identification of individuals at risk of developing allergic diseases, thereby allowing timely interventions to potentially prevent or mitigate its progression.

Microbiome and Epigenetics

The *hygiene hypothesis*, proposed by David Strachan in 1989, suggests that early exposure to infections and a less clean environment can lead to a diverse gut microbiome and may confer protection against atopy. Microbiome and its metabolites such as short-chain fatty acids (SCFAs) can influence epigenetic modifications (DNA methylation and histone modifications). Microbial dysbiosis in early life alters SCFA production which in turn impacts histone acetylation in Treg cells, compromising immune tolerance. It has been observed that lack of microbial exposure can lead to epigenetic changes that promote an inflammatory immune response, increasing the likelihood of developing allergies and other immune-related conditions. Epigenetic epidemiology suggests that early-life exposure to diverse microbiomes can lead to epigenetic modifications that promote immune tolerance and reduce the risk of allergic diseases.

Epigenetic mechanisms therefore will shed light on understanding how environmental factors interact with the genes to shape the development and progression of allergic diseases. These modifications can serve as biomarkers to predict if an individual is susceptible to develop allergic disease and predict the response to therapy as well as disease progression. This will shape precision medicine in the future to tailor treatments specific to individual based on their unique characteristics, genetic makeup, environment, and lifestyle.

ATOPIC MARCH OR ATOPIC MULTIMORBIDITY

Atopic march refers to sequential development of allergic diseases in children and usually starts with AD and thereafter progressing to FA, AR, and asthma in a certain route occurring within the same individual progressively as the child becomes older.

Timelines and Clinical Patterns of Atopic March

The AM can be categorized chronologically as follows:

- *0–2 years:* AD/eczema and FA (milk, egg, peanut)
- *2–5 years:* AR and wheezing
- *5–15 years:* Asthma and multiple aeroallergen sensitivities.

It has been observed that this temporal pattern is not always sequential. Furthermore, the severity of AD/eczema can correlate with the likelihood and severity of subsequent allergic conditions. Not everyone with AD/eczema will lead to exert the full AM.

Various mechanisms and endotypes have been identified that drive the AM:

- It has been observed that the primary diver is a *leaky skin barrier* owing to FLG mutations observed in eczema/AD that allows transcutaneous sensitization.
- *Early food sensitization* is a crucial step in the development of FA. The process involves systemic priming of naïve CD4$^+$ T helper cells into Th2 phenotype driven by IL-4 eventually leading to the production of IgE antibodies, which is a key player in allergic reactions.
- *IL-33 and TSLP* play crucial roles in initiating and driving the AM and contribute to allergic memory by influencing epigenetic modifications.
- Further, *altered microbiome* and *immune dysregulations* complicate the clinical picture of AM.

The traditional concept of AM has been questioned by newer studies which indicate that the evolutionary pathway of allergic diseases is far more multifaceted and does not entirely align with the classical AM theory.

Atopic Multimorbidity

Only a bare 3.1% of atopic children exhibit AM and newer studies emphasize the concept of atopic multimorbidity **(Flowchart 1)** concept instead of AM. In 2014, Belgrave and colleagues employed a Bayesian approach to model the trajectory of allergic diseases amongst 10,000 children in the United Kingdom. After assessing three models to study the allergic diseases such as eczema, wheeze, and AR and their symptoms, they postulated a multimorbidity framework. They argued that allergic disease progression cannot be defined by a cause-and-effect linear model and that there is diversity inherent in allergic phenotypes.

Flowchart 1: Multimorbidity associated with atopic march—interplay of systemic and tissue-specific factors along with various endotypes complicate the allergy trajectory.

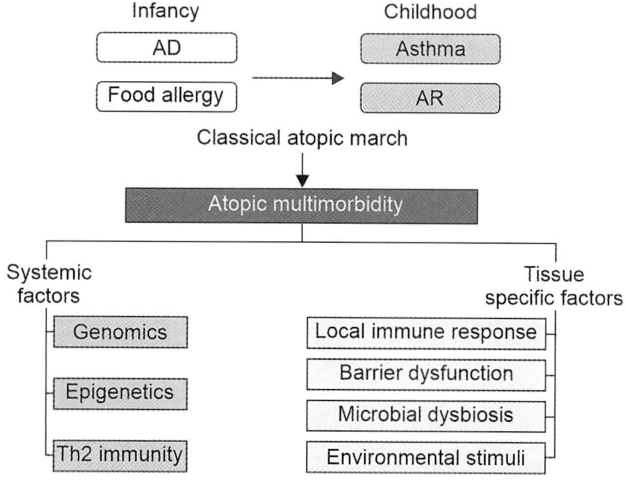

(AD: atopic dermatitis; AR: allergic rhinitis)

Various factors that complicate this trajectory are rooted to the loss of epidermal barrier homeostasis, primarily linked to FLG mutations resulting in leaky barrier and microbial dysbiosis and thereby result in AD. Mutations in FLG are also linked to peanut FA.

Thymic stromal lymphopoietin is a cytokine that stimulates the production of IL-4, IL-5, and IL-13 from naïve CD$^+$ T cells. Increased expression of TSLP has been observed not only in patients with AD but also in the airways of patients with asthma and nasal passages in individuals with AR. Further, children with altered skin barrier show compromised antiviral IFN production and their skin reflects increased colonization by *Staphylococcus aureus*.

Exposome Hypothesis

Exposome hypothesis has been postulated which states that environmental pollution resulting from various toxic substances including microplastics can impact not only epidermal barrier, but also intestinal epithelial barrier and lung barrier function by breakdown of the intercellular junction proteins in the lung.

In a genome-wide association study (GWAS) comprising 2,428 patients with AD and asthma in infancy and childhood, respectively, seven mutations linked to AM have been identified: FLG [1q21.3], AP5B1/OVOL1 [11q13.1], IL4/KIF3A [5q31.1], IKZF3 [17q21], C11orf30/LRRC329, EFHC1[6p12.3], and rs99322 [12q21.3].

CHRONIC INFLAMMATION IN ALLERGY

Allergic inflammation is a specific type of inflammatory response triggered by allergens, characterized by symptoms like itching, sneezing, and nasal congestion. When long-term exposure to allergens leads to persistent inflammation over a prolonged duration, it is defined as chronic allergy.

Mast Cells and Basophils

Mast cells and basophils play an important role in chronic allergic inflammation. Activated mast cells release a cascade of inflammatory mediators that can damage tissues, recruit other immune cells, and contribute to the persistence of inflammation.

Eosinophils and Remodeling

In chronic allergic conditions, particularly asthma and chronic rhinosinusitis with nasal polyps, eosinophils play a significant role in tissue remodeling, leading to altered airway structure and impaired lung function. In chronic conditions, eosinophils are recruited to the site of inflammation and activated eosinophils release cytokines such as transforming growth factor beta 1 (TGF-β1), IL-4, and IL-13 which can directly stimulate epithelial and mesenchymal cells to produce extracellular matrix components like collagen. It can also release enzymes such as major basic protein (MBP) and eosinophil cationic protein (ECP), can damage the extracellular matrix, and promote fibrosis. Eosinophils also contribute to remodeling through the release of reactive oxygen species such as eosinophils peroxidases, thrombotic factors, and other molecules that contribute to tissue damage and remodeling.

Airway Remodeling and Fibrosis

Airway remodeling encompasses structural changes in the airway wall, including epithelial cell alterations, smooth muscle cell hypertrophy and hyperplasia, goblet cell metaplasia, and subepithelial fibrosis. In asthma, airway remodeling is characterized by subepithelial fibrosis, smooth muscle hypertrophy, goblet cell metaplasia, neovascularization, and epithelial alterations. These are primarily driven by IL-13, TGF-β, and leukotrienes which leads to irreversible airflow limitation.

Role of Tregs and Th17 Cells

Th17 and Tregs are both subsets of $CD4^+$ T cells that play opposing roles. Th17 cells produce IL-17, a cytokine that promotes inflammation and tissue damage. Tregs, on the other hand, have an immunosuppressive effect on the activity of other cytokines such as IL-17 and play a vital role in maintaining immune homeostasis. Abrogation of tolerance has been observed wherein Th17 cells disrupt the regulatory mechanisms of Treg cells, leading to a loss of tolerance to allergens and perpetuating chronic allergic inflammation. Some asthma demonstrates predominant neutrophilic inflammation versus those which exert eosinophil predominance, and it is now understood that these changes are happening at a cellular level.

CONCLUSION

Allergic diseases are the result of a complex immunological dialogue between the innate and adaptive systems, profoundly shaped by genetic and environmental factors. The pathophysiology of allergy spans acute and chronic phases with distinct immunologic footprints as observed in IgE-mediated mast cell degranulation, chronic eosinophilic inflammation, and airway remodeling. The epigenetic landscape adds further nuance influencing susceptibility and disease trajectory through epigenetic modulations or gene–environment interactions.

In vitro advances have led to better understanding of underlying mechanisms of allergic diseases. State-of-the-art diagnostic procedures such as component-resolved diagnostics to identify potential allergens, basophil activation tests, and methylation markers can reshape therapeutic strategies. Advanced therapeutics such as monoclonal antibodies (such as omalizumab for IgE, Dupilumab for IL-4Rα), allergen immunotherapy to induce tolerance, and epigenetic modulators offer targeted approaches to managing allergic reactions and potentially inducing long-term remission by modulating the immune response. Various prevention strategies can be implemented such as prenatal maternal diet, early allergen exposure, and avoidance of unnecessary antibiotics in the infancy.

An understanding of the complex allergy pathophysiology coupled with the advanced therapeutics represents a shift from traditional symptomatic treatments toward a more targeted disease-modifying approach for allergic diseases, offering hope for better disease management, long-term outcomes, and improved quality of life.

KEY POINTS

- Allergic diseases result from complex interactions between genetic susceptibility, environmental triggers, and immune dysregulation.
- The updated EACCI 2025 classification expands hypersensitivity beyond the classical four types, incorporating tissue-driven, metabolic, and chemical mechanisms (types V–VII).
- Epigenetics and the microbiome play pivotal roles in modulating immune tolerance and allergy risk, especially in early life.
- The concept of AM is evolving toward atopic multimorbidity, reflecting overlapping and nonlinear disease trajectories.

- Chronic allergic inflammation involves mast cells, basophils, eosinophils, and Th17/Treg imbalance, leading to tissue remodeling and persistent disease.

SUGGESTED READING

1. Calzada D, Singh SS, Torres-González M, et al. Immunological mechanisms in allergic diseases and allergen tolerance. Clin Dev Immunol. 2018;2018:6012053.
2. Ogulur I, Monticelli S, et al. Type 2 immunity in allergic diseases. Cellular & Molecular Immunology. 2025;[Epub ahead of print].
3. Sampson HA. Mechanisms of food allergy: immune pathways and tolerance. J Allergy Clin Immunol. 2018; 141(1):11-7.
4. Wang J, Zhang L, et al. Pathogenesis of allergic diseases and implications for therapeutic interventions. Sig Transduct Target Ther. 2023;8:344.

4 CHAPTER

Epidemiology and Risk Factors of Allergies

Soumyashree Bahalia, Jose Ouseph

INTRODUCTION

Allergies are a growing concern globally, with their development and prevalence influenced by a combination of genetic predisposition and environmental factors. Recognizing these risk factors is crucial for developing personalized prevention strategies and targeted treatments, particularly in areas with increasing incidence. The prevalence of allergic diseases like asthma, atopic dermatitis, allergic rhinitis, and food allergy has been increasing over the last decades. However, the prevalence of allergic diseases may have a plateau in high-income countries in the last decade, while it is still on the rise in low- and middle-income countries.

Data suggests that not all atopic dermatitis and asthma cases are attributable to atopic sensitization. The genetic association studies have prompted the unravelling of barrier dysfunction as a mainstay in the pathologic mechanisms leading to atopic dermatitis and asthma with atopic sensitization secondary to this dysfunction. Research by epidemiological studies, on risk and protective factors for allergic disease, on the basis of genetic susceptibility has been suggestive of the same.

Studies suggest that in developed countries, the prevalence of allergic diseases could affect 10–30% of adults and exceed 40% in children. The reasons for this increase are multifactorial, involving a complex interplay of host (genetic) and environmental factors. The prevalence varies depending on the specific allergy and geographical region, according to the American Academy of Allergy, Asthma & Immunology (AAAAI), with allergic rhinitis affecting between 10 and 30% of the population and drug allergies potentially impacting up to 10% of the world's population.

RISK FACTORS FOR DEVELOPING ALLERGIES

Genetic Predisposition (Heredity)

Genetic predisposition is the most significant host factor, playing a major role in susceptibility. If both parents have allergies, the risk for the child is significantly higher (around 70%), compared to children with one atopic parent (50%) or no atopic parents (9–18%). According to the American College of Allergy Asthma and Immunology, if one of the parents has allergy, there are higher chances that their children will have allergy in their kids. While genetic factors play a crucial role, environmental factors are also essential in the development and manifestation of allergic diseases.

Environmental Allergen Exposure

Allergen exposure can occur by inhalation, ingestion, injection, or contact with the offending antigens.

- *Airborne allergens:* Pollen (trees, grasses, weeds), house dust mites, animal dander, and mold spores are common triggers, especially in respiratory, ocular, and skin allergies.
- *Food allergens:* Specific foods like peanuts, tree nuts, wheat, soy, fish, shellfish, eggs, and milk are frequent triggers, particularly in food allergies.
- *Insect stings:* Bee or wasp stings can cause allergic reactions in some individuals.
- *Contact allergens:* Latex and other substances like nickel can trigger allergic skin reactions.

Air Pollution

Both outdoor and indoor air pollution play a significant role in the development of allergic symptoms. Inhaling polluted air, throughout childhood, is linked to impaired lung function. Notably, 99% of children under 5 years are exposed to particulate matter levels exceeding the World Health Organization (WHO) safety limits, with India experiencing higher concentrations compared to high-income countries.

- Traffic-related air pollution (TRAP), including black carbon from diesel exhaust, nitrogen oxides, sulfur oxides, carbon monoxide, benzene, and particulate matter (PM), has been linked to increased risk of allergic rhinitis and asthma. Pollutants can damage airways, increase allergic sensitization, and worsen symptoms. Studies have shown that children exposed to TRAP in utero and during the first year of life may have a higher risk of developing allergic rhinitis.

- Exposure to indoor allergens like dust mites, mold, and pet dander can significantly contribute to the development and aggravation of allergic symptoms. Specifically, poor indoor air quality resulting from dampness, inadequate ventilation, household emissions, and the use of solid fuels for cooking can increase the risk of allergic disorders.

Additional factors such as mosquito coils, incense sticks, and residing in industrial areas further exacerbate this risk.

Microbial Exposure and the Hygiene Hypothesis

The hygiene hypothesis suggests that reduced exposure to diverse microbes in early life may contribute to the rise in allergic and autoimmune diseases in industrialized nations. This includes exposure to environmental microorganisms found in soil and nature, as well as reduced exposure to certain infections that may prime the immune system toward tolerance. Early versions of the hypothesis focused on infections in general, but later versions emphasize the importance of specific microbes that have co-evolved with humans, sometimes called "old friends".

Rural children exposed to diverse microorganisms in barn dust can shape their immune system possibly reducing allergy risk, the possible mechanism being induction of IgG antibodies to Neu5Gc (glycolylneuraminic acid) which in turn downregulates IL-17 and promotes differentiation of Treg cells. Studies in India have shown reduced allergy risk in children raised in farming environments or with increased microbial exposure.

In contrast, urbanization and associated lifestyle changes may increase allergy risk due to limited exposure to beneficial microbes, indoor environments with poor ventilation, and sedentary habits.

Maternal Factors

Maternal factors during pregnancy can influence the risk for the development of allergic disorders in children. Key findings include the following:

- Maternal consumption of processed foods and added sugars during pregnancy may increase asthma risk in children.
- Vitamin D supplementation to pregnant females has shown to reduce house dust mite sensitization and asthma-related issues in the children.
- Exposure to household cleaning agents during pregnancy increases the risk of non-allergic asthma in children.
- Particulate matter exposure during pregnancy and early childhood is a significant contributor to the development of asthma and airway hyper-responsiveness.
- Maternal tobacco smoke exposure, whether through active smoking or second-hand smoke, increases the risk of asthma in children.
- Children born by cesarean section are more predisposed to developing allergic disorders due to limited exposure to maternal vaginal microbiota at birth.
- Maternal intake of medications, like acetaminophen and antibiotics, also influences the development of allergic disorders in the offspring.
- Apart from the abovementioned factors, a mother's psychological state during pregnancy, including stress, anxiety, and depression, can significantly increase her child's risk of developing allergic disorders like atopic dermatitis, asthma, and allergic rhinitis.

Perinatal Factors

Preterm births, neonatal jaundice, cesarean delivery, and early use of antibiotics are associated with an increased risk of development of allergic diseases.

Postnatal Factors

- Breastfeeding plays a crucial role in shaping the gut microbiome of infants. By promoting a balance between Th1 and Th2 cytokines, it helps to regulate the immune response. Research including systematic reviews and meta-analyses has consistently shown prolonged breastfeeding with a reduced risk of asthma in children.
- In contrast, formula-fed infants are at an increased risk of allergies.
- BCG vaccination can also have a protective effect by induction of Th1 response. The differences in vaccination practices, genetic backgrounds, and environmental exposures between Indian and western populations may lead to variations in disease susceptibility and manifestation.

Climate Change

Longer pollen seasons, increased pollen concentrations, and altered geographical distribution of allergenic plants due to global warming and changes in CO_2 levels can increase the duration and severity of seasonal allergies.

Extreme weather events like thunderstorms and wildfires can also exacerbate allergy symptoms. (Notably, thunderstorms can rupture pollens, releasing allergenic particles into the air and causing asthma exacerbation.)

Lifestyle Factors

- The shift toward western dietary patterns, characterized by increased consumption of ultraprocessed foods rich in unhealthy fats and sugars, lead to obesity, altered gut microbiome, and increased inflammation, potentially increasing the risk for allergies.
- Higher socioeconomic status and increased psychological stress have been linked to allergic disorders.
- Lifestyle changes associated with urbanization and less time spent outdoors along with adaptation of sedentary lifestyles also contribute to the risk.
- Disrupted sleep patterns, poor work–life balance, and irregular circadian rhythms (weakened immune system and increased inflammation) can contribute to a higher risk of developing allergic disorders.

CONCLUSION

The rising global and Indian burden of allergic diseases reflects the complex interplay between genetic susceptibility, environmental exposures, and evolving lifestyle patterns. While heredity remains a strong predictor of atopy, the influence of air pollution, urbanization, microbial deprivation, maternal and perinatal factors, and changing dietary habits is increasingly evident. Identifying modifiable risk factors—such as indoor pollutants, poor ventilation, tobacco smoke, and early-life microbial imbalance—offers opportunities for prevention, early intervention, and tailored counseling. A better understanding of these determinants is essential for designing public-health strategies, guiding clinicians in risk stratification, and ultimately reducing the long-term burden of allergic disorders in children.

KEY POINTS

- There has been an increase in the prevalence of allergic diseases in the middle- and low-income countries over the past decade.
- Complex interplay of genetic and environmental factors contributes to the development of allergic disorders.
- Maternal exposure to pollutants, stress, and unhealthy diet during pregnancy increases allergy risk in children.
- Breastfeeding has a protective effect.
- Adaptation of sedentary lifestyle, inclusion of ultra-processed food in diet, childhood obesity, psychological stress, depression, air pollution, and global warming contribute to increased allergies.
- Poor quality of sleep and disrupted circadian rhythm weaken the immune system, leading to chronic inflammation and atopy.

SUGGESTED READING

1. Eggesbo M, Botten G, Halvorsen R, Magnus P. The prevalence of CMA/CMPI in young children: the validity of parentally perceived reactions in a population-based study. Allergy. 2001;56(5):393-402.
2. Gupta N, Saibal Moitra S, Nagarajan S. Comprehensive Textbook of Allergy: Striking the Right Balance. New Delhi: Jaypee Brothers Medical Publishers Pvt Ltd; 2024.
3. Mahesh PA, Moitra S, Mabalirajan U, Garg M, Malamardi S, Vedanthan PK, et al. Allergic diseases in India – Prevalence, risk factors and current challenges. Clin Exp Allergy. 2023;53(3):276-94.
4. Peters RL, Koplin JJ, Gurrin LC, Dharmage SC, Wake M, Ponsonby AL, et al . The prevalence of food allergy and other allergy diseases in early childhood in population based study. J Allergy Clin Immunol. 2017;140(1):145-153.
5. Zablotsly B , Blade LI, Akinbami LJ. Diagnosed Allergic Conditions in Children Aged 0–17 Years: United States, 2021. NCHS Data Brief. 2023:(459):1-8.

5 CHAPTER

Allergens in the Indian Perspective

Soundarya M

INTRODUCTION

Allergic diseases are increasing worldwide, with India witnessing a rapid rise over the last two decades. While data on allergens are abundant globally, information specific to the Indian subcontinent remains limited. India's diverse geography, climate, and cultural practices influence the spectrum of aeroallergens, food allergens, insect allergens, and occupational allergens unique to this region. Understanding these patterns is essential for accurate diagnosis, prevention, and management of allergic disorders in the Indian context.

The main categories of allergens that are responsible for the myriad of allergic disorders are as follows:

- *Aeroallergens:* House dust mite (HDM), cockroach frass, pollens, pet dander, and molds.
- *Food allergens:* Milk, wheat. soy, nuts, sea food, eggs, and regional allergens like brinjal, chickpeas, and lentils.
- *Insect allergens:* Honeybee, wasp, fire ants, and yellow jackets.
- *Occupational allergens:* Latex, silk, flour/grain dust, fish and bird proteins, chemical compounds like isocyanates, acid anhydrides, etc.

AEROALLERGENS

Inhalant allergens are aeroallergens and are characterized by being light weight, air borne easily, and get inhaled into lower airways.

House Dust Mite

The most common aeroallergen is the HDM worldwide and even in India, although there are regional variations with pollens in different seasons. The warm, humid climate and the preference for urbanized indoor comfort living have led to use of carpeted floors, air conditioning, and softer mattresses and fabrics, all of which are home to the HDM.

House dust mite species most relevant to India are *Dermatophagoides pteronyssinus, Dermatophagoides farinae,* and *Blomia tropicalis,* although there are other subspecies as well including other mite species, i.e., storage mites. To include all these types, they hence have also been labeled as allergenic domestic mites.

Characteristics: The allergen in HDM is the fecal particle of the mite,

- ~30 µm in size
- Stays airborne for a short period of time and settles down
- 33 antigenic epitopes; Der p 1, 2, 23 and Der f 1, 2, 23 are the major allergens. In India, the main allergens that have been identified are the Der p 1, Der f 1, Der p 2, and Der f 2.
- The allergens of the HDM are primarily proteases, lipid-binding proteins, contractile proteins, glycosidases, etc., and can cleave the proteins in the airway epithelium and break the epithelial barrier triggering the Th2 allergic response.
- The clinically significant amount of HDM allergen is >2 µg/g of house dust.

Cockroach

Cockroach is also another clinically relevant allergen in most countries, especially the low- to middle-income countries and densely populated areas. Presence of open food sources, piling of dirty dishes, kitchens with accumulation and spillage of food, garbage bins, and open drains are reservoirs for the cockroach.

The species relevant to India are *Periplanata americana, Blatella germanica,* and *Blatella orientalis.*

- The main allergen is in the cockroach frass (fecal matter) which is a protease antigen, which cleaves the proteins on the airway epithelium and activates a cellular response in the epithelium through the toll-like receptors and C-type lectin receptors.
- The antigenic epitopes are Bla g 1, Bla g 2, Bla g 3, Bla g 4, Bla g 5, Bla g 6, Bla g 7 and Bla g 8 for *B. orientalis* and Per a 1, Per a 3, Per a 6, Per a 7, Per a 9, and Per a10 for *P. americana.*

- The clinically relevant amount of allergen is 2 U/g house dust for Bla g 1 and 8 U/g for Bla g 2.
- Small antigen; 10–20 µg and easily airborne and settles in half an hour.

Pollens

Pollens belong to three main categories—trees, weeds, and grasses. Being a tropical country with diverse climatic zones, pollens that are common here are *Prosopis juliflora, Ricinus communis, Morus, Mallotus, Alnus, Querecus, Cedrus, Argemone, Amaranthus, Chenopodium, Holoptelea, Brassica, Cocos, Cannabis, Parthenium, Cassia,* and grasses. Most of these are perineal plants/trees/ weeds; hence, in many patients not much seasonality is noted in pollen allergy.

- Larger antigens of 20–25 –m size and settle in upper and larger airways contributing majorly to allergic rhinitis and rhinoconjunctivitis
- The antigenic epitopes belong to profilin, lipid transfer protein, besides others, and these act as NADPH oxidases and proteases which damage the epithelium and cause epithelial permeability, resulting in mucosal edema and congestion.
- Maintenance of detailed pollen calendars, which is region-wise, helps in identifying days when symptoms will flare.

Molds

Molds are ubiquitous and thrive in damp, humid areas. The common molds in India are *Aspergillus fumigatus* and *Aspergillus flavus* along with *Helminthosporium, Alternaria nigrospora, Penicillium,* and *Cladosporium.*

- Out of these, the most relevant antigenic epitopes among the indoor fungal environment are Asp f 1 (Mitogillin), Alt a 1 (Unknown protein), Cla h 6 (Enolase), Cla h 8 (Mannitol dehydrogenase), Pen ch 13 (Serine protease), and Pen ch 18 (Serine protease).
- <5 µm in size (average 2.55.8 µm) and get easily inhaled into lower airways where the germination of these spores can trigger the Th2 and Th17 pathways
- The mold antigens are of varied types and concentrations varied with seasons. Highest mold concentrations were seen in autumn and winter months in India.
- Mold concentration of >250,000 spores/m^3 signifies heavy mold growth.
- Any mold concentration of more than 1,000 sporesm^3 can affect human health.

Pet Dander

Pets in India are commonly dogs, cats, rabbits, and rodents. Exposure to their flaky skin cells, saliva, urine, and fur can trigger aeroallergies.

- Size ranges between 1 and 20 µm.
- The dog antigen Can f 1 is the heavier antigen and settles after a short airborne period.
- The cat antigen Fel d 1 is a light antigen, can remain airborne for days and carried around with wind, and attaches to carpets and upholstered furniture. This takes months to degrade (24 weeks).
- The rodent antigen Mus m 1 is urinary protein which can cause epigenetic changes toward asthma predisposition.
- In most countries, while there was evidence of pet sensitization, the symptomatology was not as evident, probably due to the protective effects of pets when in pregnancy and the first year of life.

FOOD ALLERGENS

The main food allergens are milk, egg, soy, wheat, shellfish, and nuts (tree nuts and peanuts) prevalent nearly in all countries although regional differences may be present. In India, food allergies have been much less prevalent and this has been attributed to the traditional practices with inclusion of different cooking practices. Numerous studies have shown higher rates of food sensitization in India, however, with much lower rates of actual food allergy. Certain regional studies in India have shown that legumes have another emerging allergen along with prawns, peas, and banana. As a part of the EUROPREVALL study, in India brinjal and chickpea were also found as potential allergens, despite a high rate of food sensitization to multiple food allergens.

Traditional cooking practices where food is boiled, fermented, and steamed as well as given in conjunction with carbohydrates seem to have a role in reducing the allergenic potential of foods and may hence explain the complex nature of food allergens and their interactions with other foods as the reason for reduced food allergies in India.

Milk

- The milk allergen contains more than 20 protein fractions. The major allergens in milk are casein and whey containing alpha lactalbumin and beta lactaglobulin. The main heat-labile proteins are

lactalbumin and lactaglobulin, while casein proteins are heat stable.
- Milk still remains the most common protein causing food allergy in India and is one of the common causes of atopic dermatitis flare.

Egg

The most important allergenic components of egg are the ovomucoid (Gal d 1), ovalbumin (Gal d 2), ovotransferrin (Gal d 3), and lysozyme (Gal d 4). These proteins are mostly heat labile, except ovomucoid and ovotransferrin which are heat stable. Similarly, alpha livetins (Gal d 5) and vitellins are the allergens found in egg yolk and can cause allergic reactions. Egg allergy in India is not as common as world over, but is however on the rise as a part of the urbanized lifestyles and cultures adopted nowadays.

Wheat

Wheat allergy is more prevalent in north India, and the occurrence of celiac disease as a form of non-IgE wheat allergy is more prevalent. The wheat allergen contains albumins, globulins, gliadins, and glutenins. Out of these, most wheat allergies are due to gliadins and glutenins and ω5gliadin has now been found to play a role in wheat-dependent exercise-induced anaphylaxis.

Soy

Soy protein has allergenic components primarily from the 7S fraction and the 11S fraction of the soya bean globulins. The epitopes are Gly m Bd, Gly m 4, 5, 6, and 8. Of these, gly m 4 is a pathogenesis-related protein and is more associated with anaphylaxis and death. There is significant cross reactivity between soy, peanut, and birch allergens.

Nuts

Peanut allergy is not common in India with a low prevalence of only 0.03% in the population. The allergenic epitopes of peanut belong to seven main families of which Ara h 1 and Ara h 2 are the high molecular weight proteins and rest low molecular weight (Ara h 3, 4, 5, 6, 7, 8, 9, 10, 11, 12, 13). Cross reactivity exists between the peanut and other tree nuts, soy, lentils, and birch. In India, the low incidence of peanut allergy is attributed to the cooking processes (boiling) and early introduction of peanut in infancy.

Shellfish

Shellfish allergy is more common than nuts or soy in India with a prevalence of 4 to 5% among adults. The main allergenic components are the tropomyosin (Pen m 1), arginine kinase (Pen m 2), myosin light chain (Pen m 3), troponin (Cra c 6), triosephosphate isomerase (Cra c 8) and sarcoplasmic calcium binding protein (Pen m 4). These are common between prawns, shrimp, crab, lobster and cross react highly withmolluscs and to an extent with mites, cockroaches and parasites.

A. *Brinjal:* Brinjal/Eggplant allergy has been found to be prevalent in India with a wide variation based on local cultural practices, ranging from 0.8 to 11%. The main allergenic proteins are polyphenol oxidases and profilins. They are mainly heat stable glycoproteins and are found in the pulp, skin, seeds and even in raw and cooked versions. The main allergenic epitope is Sola m 1 can cause oral allergy syndrome and is found concentrated in seeds.
B. *Lentils:* Lentils are a broad group of pulses which can be allergenic, though uncommon, with a prevalence of 1% (some studies indicate upto 5.5%). The main allergenic proteins are common to the group and are vicilins (Len c 1) which is responsible for majority (>80%) of the allergic reactions. Len c 2 is a biotinylated protein and Len c 3 is a lipid transfer protein which can also contribute to lentil allergy. Cross reactivity to legumes, chickpeas and peas can be seen with lentils. In recent literature, non-priority legumes like beans, peas, lupines, fenugreek, cow pea, pigeon pea and chickpeas have been noted as emerging allergens.
C. *Chickpeas:* Chickpeas are another family within legumes and allergy in the Indian subpopulation to chickpeas was noted in literature. Vicilins, albumins, PR 10 proteins and legumin are the allergenic proteins in chickpea. Cross reactivity with lentils, peanut and other legumes has been seen. Cic a 1 is a minor allergenic epitope in chickpea but causes clinical symptoms.

INSECT ALLERGENS

The main insect allergenic species in India are Apidae, Bombidae (bees), Vespidae (wasps) and Formicidae (Ants).

1. *Apidae (Apis mellifera):* These are the honey bees and one of the commonest insect venom allergens in India (15). These are mainly stinging insects

and their venom contains high molecular weight antigens mainly phospholipases A1/A2 that trigger the Th2hypersensitivity (T I) pathway and even cause anaphylaxis. Other components of the venom are the CCD which are allergenic and can also activate the type III and type IV pathway.

2. *Bombidae:* These are the group of bumblebees who are not as common as honey bees but nevertheless have venom. The allergens here too are primarily contain a mixture of proteases, phospholipases (PLA2) hyaluronidase and arginine kinase, all which similarly activate the Th2 pathway.
3. *Vespidae:* The Vespidae family seen in India and South East Asia comprises of the group of stinging insects like the waspsieVespa velutina (yellow legged Asian hornet), Vespa tropica (Indian tropical wasp) and hornets like the Asian giant hornet (Vespa mandarinia), the Oriental hornet (Vespa orientalis), the lesser banded hornet (Vespa affinis) as well as the paper wasps like the yellow paper wasp (Polistes versicolor) and the Indian Paper Wasp (Ropalida marginata). These group of insects sting in defense of their colonies and the antigens are a complex mix of histamine, serotonin, phospholipase and hyaluronidase which induce an intense local reaction.

   There is known cross reactivity between the Vespidae and Apidae/Bombidae venomand the sting reactions can evolve into anaphylaxis in successive stings.
4. *Formicidae:* these are the group of fire ants among which the commonest is the Red imported fire ant (Solenopsis invicta). Other species seen in India are black imported fire ant (Solenopsis richteri) along with *Pachycondyla* spp. (Ponerinae). The ant venom is also a complex composition with formic acid, biogenic amines, neurotoxic peptides, proteins, free amines and hydrocarbons and can cause paralytic, hemolytic, cytolytic, proinflammatory reactions as well as anaphylaxis and severe pain. Ant venom also contains several hydrolases, oxidoreductases, proteases, Kunitz-like polypeptides, and inhibitor cysteine knot (ICK)-like (knottin) neurotoxins and insect defensins.

   In India, very few articles and reviews are on diverse ant species and reactions and only case reports are available with the details of the complex cocktail in the ant venom and its varied consequences.

OCCUPATIONAL ALLERGENS

The occupational allergens most relevant to India are:

1. *Latex allergy:* Latex allergy can present as mild allergic contact dermatitis and can even be as severe as anaphylaxis. Exposure is through contact with articles containing natural rubber latex like balloons, toys, gloves, etc. Latex is derived from natural rubber which is from the tree Hevea brasiliensis and Hev b 1 and Hev b 3 are the major allergenic proteins. Hevein and β1,3 glucanases are the other allergenic proteins. Cross reactivity with banana, avocado, kiwi and tomato has been noted. There is no known allergy to the pollens of the Hevea brasiliensis tree and this is noted only with the proteins in the tree sap. The prevalence in India has not been detailed well in literature but in the variable articles, the incidence was found to be as high as 9.1–10% among health care workers. The regular use of powdered latex gloves exposes the user to inhalation of aerosolized latex antigens and is implicated in respiratory allergies and anaphylaxis.
2. *Silk allergy:* In India, there is an abundance of usage of silk garments and sarees, from many states. The main silk producing states are Karnataka, Andhra Pradesh, Tamil Nadu, Assam and West Bengal. Silk allergy is an occupational allergy due to exposure to the silk antigen and occurs mainly in workers of silk factories/filatures. Silk is produced from the silk worm Bombyx mori cocoon, pupae and larvae mainly during the silk harvesting. During the processing, the workers are exposed to high molecular proteins like Sericin and Fibroin as inhalants and this causes occupational asthma, allergic rhinitis, conjunctivitis and dermatitis. The prevalence of silk sensitization was as high as 35% in studies done on these workers. Due to the inhalational route of exposure, allergy and sensitization to silk has also been reported from non factory workers living in the same geographical area with a prevalence of nearly 20%.

The major allergens of hymenoptera family and occupational allergy is as summarized in **Table 1**.

CONCLUSION

India's unique climate, geography, cultural diversity, and food practices shape a distinct allergen profile that differs significantly from Western data. Knowledge of prevalent aeroallergens such as HDM, cockroach antigens, pollens,

TABLE 1: Insect and occupational allergens.

Category	Common species/source	Major allergens	Clinical features
Insects	Honeybee, Wasp, Fire ant	PLA2, phospholipase, hyaluronidase, venom peptides	Local/systemic reactions, anaphylaxis
Latex	Hevea brasiliensis proteins (Hev b 1, 3)	Hevein, β-1,3 glucanases	Contact urticaria, anaphylaxis
Silk	Sericin, Fibroin	High MW proteins	Asthma, dermatitis in silk workers

molds, and animal dander, along with region-specific food allergens like legumes, chickpea, lentils, brinjal, and seafood, is central to accurate diagnosis and management. Understanding allergen characteristics, cross-reactivity, and the modifying effect of Indian cooking practices helps clinicians avoid overdiagnosis and unnecessary food restrictions. Developing robust Indian allergen panels, regional pollen calendars, and standardized testing will enhance precision in allergy care. Ultimately, a contextualized approach empowers clinicians to deliver evidence-based, culturally aligned, and patient-specific allergy management.

KEY POINTS

- Allergens in India show *regional variation* due to climate, geography, and cultural practices.
- HDM, *cockroach, and pollens* remain the leading aeroallergens, while molds peak during monsoon and winter.
- *Food allergy prevalence is lower in India* than in the West, possibly due to traditional cooking methods, though legumes and brinjal are unique regional allergens.
- *Insect venoms (bees, wasps, ants) and occupational allergens (latex, silk)* are important but under-reported in Indian literature.
- A *national allergen registry and region-wise pollen/mold calendars* are urgently needed for improved diagnosis and patient management.

SUGGESTED READING

1. Anuja R, Midhun M. Food allergen sensitivity in atopy. IP Indian Journal of Immunology and Respiratory Medicine 2023;8:24-7.
2. Arruda LK, Barbosa MC, Santos AB, Moreno AS, Chapman MD, Pomés A. Recombinant allergens for diagnosis of cockroach allergy. Curr Allergy Asthma Rep. 2014;14(4):428.
3. Babu BN, Venkatesh YP. Clinico-Immunological Analysis of Eggplant (Solanum melongena) Allergy Indicates Preponderance of Allergens in the Peel. World Allergy Organ J. 2009;2(9):192-200.
4. Bhagwat K. Levels of indoor allergens in the homes of allergic patients from India Allergy. 2018;73(Suppl 105):173
5. Briceno D, Hendriks L, Breedveld A, Savelkoul HFJ, Jansen A, Teodorowicz M, Ruinemans-Koerts J. Soy Gly m 8 sIgE Has Limited Value in the Diagnosis of Soy Allergy in Peanut Ara h 2-Sensitized Adults. Int Arch Allergy Immunol. 2023;184(8):767-75.
6. Chowdary VS. Environmental and Occupational Respiratory Disease – 1030: Role of fungi (molds) in allergic airway disease – an analysis in South Indian Otolaryngology Center. World Allergy Organ J. 2013;6(Suppl 1):P29.
7. Cockroach exposure and its allergy sensitization in asthma patients. Monaldi Arch Chest Dis. [Internet]. 2021 May 11 [cited 2025 Aug. 17];91(3). Available from: https://www.monaldi-archives.org/macd/article/view/1685
8. Gaur, S. N. An Indian perspective on dust mites. Indian Journal of Allergy, Asthma and Immunology. 33(1):p 14-18, Jan–Jun 2019.
9. Gowda G, Shivalingaiah AH, Vijayeendra AM, Sarkar N, Nagaraj C, Masthi NR. Sensitization to silk allergen among workers of silk filatures in India: a comparative study. Asia Pac Allergy. 2016;6(2):90-3.
10. Hosoki K, Boldogh I, Sur S. Innate responses to pollen allergens. Curr Opin Allergy Clin Immunol. 2015 Feb;15(1):79-88.
11. Jusufovic E. Molds as a cause of asthma and exacerbations. J Lung Pulm Respir Res. 2022;9(4):94-98.
12. Kumar, Raj1, Kumar, Manoj, Mavi, Anil Kumar. Cockroach allergy in respiratory allergic patients. Indian Journal of Allergy, Asthma and Immunology. 2022;36(2):63-4.
13. Kumar R, Kumar M, Bisht I, Singh K. Prevalence of aeroallergens in patients of bronchial asthma and/or allergic rhinitis in India based on skin prick test reactivity. Indian Journal of Allergy, Asthma and Immunology. 2017; 31(2): 45-55.
14. Lopata AL, Kleine-Tebbe J, Kamath SD. Allergens and molecular diagnostics of shellfish allergy: Part 22 of the Series Molecular Allergology. Allergo J Int. 2016;25(7):210-18.
15. Mahesh PA, Kaleem Ullah M, Parthasarathi A. Allergic sensitization to foods in India and other Low-Middle-income countries. Clin Exp Allergy. 2023;53(7):739-50.
16. Ruëff F, Bauer A, Becker S, Brehler R, Brockow K, Chaker AM, et al. Diagnosis and treatment of Hymenoptera

venom allergy: S2k Guideline of the German Society of Allergology and Clinical Immunology (DGAKI) in collaboration with the Arbeitsgemeinschaft für Berufs- und Umweltdermatologie e.V. (ABD), the Medical Association of German Allergologists (AeDA), the German Society of Dermatology (DDG), the German Society of Oto-Rhino-Laryngology, Head and Neck Surgery (DGHNOKC), the German Society of Pediatrics and Adolescent Medicine (DGKJ), the Society for Pediatric Allergy and Environmental Medicine (GPA), German Respiratory Society (DGP), and the Austrian Society for Allergy and Immunology (ÖGAI). Allergol Select. 2023 Oct 2;7:154-90.

17. Sharma R, Deval R, Priyadarshi V, Gaur SN, Singh VP, Singh AB. Indoor fungal concentration in the homes of allergic/asthmatic children in Delhi, India. Allergy Rhinol (Providence). 2011;2(1):21-32. Erratum in: Allergy Rhinol (Providence). 2011;2(2):e62. Devala, Ravi [corrected to Deval, Ravi].
18. Simran S, Upadhyay RK. Toxic and Immune Allergic Responses of Ant Venom Toxins: A Review. Int J Pharm Pharm Sci. 2021;13(10;23-30.
19. Singh AB, Kumar P. Aeroallergens in clinical practice of allergy in India. An overview. Ann Agric Environ Med. 2003;10(2):131-6.
20. Sridhar, Jandhyala; Ray, VSM, Rahul. Prevalence and Associated Factors of Latex-Related Symptoms and Sensitization at a Multispecialty Hospital: A Cross-Sectional Study. Journal of Marine Medical Society. 2018;20(2):122-6.
21. Sánchez P, Vélez-Del-Burgo A, Suñén E, Martínez J, Postigo I. Fungal Allergen and Mold Allergy Diagnosis: Role and Relevance of Alternaria alternata Alt a 1 Protein Family. J Fungi (Basel). 2022;8(3):277.
22. Wangorsch A, Kulkarni A, Jamin A, Spiric J, Bräcker J, Brockmeyer J, et al. Identification and Characterization of IgE-Reactive Proteins and a New Allergen (Cic a 1.01) from Chickpea (Cicer arietinum). Mol Nutr Food Res. 2020;64(19):e2000560.
23. Zahradnik E, Nöllenheidt C, Sander I, Beine A, Lehnert M, Hoffmeyer F, Raulf M. Animal exposure, sensitization, and allergic symptoms in first-year veterinary medicine students. Allergol Select. 2024;8:51-63.

2 SECTION

Diagnostic Approach

Section Editors: Narayan Prasad Modi, Mohit Poddar

6 CHAPTER

Clinical History and Examination

Arif Ahmed M

INTRODUCTION

Allergic diseases are becoming increasingly prevalent worldwide, driven by environmental changes and growing awareness due to improved education and advanced diagnostic techniques. However, diagnosing allergies is often deceptive, as highlighted by Sherlock Holmes: "There is nothing more deceptive than the obvious fact."

A thorough clinical history acts as a critical investigative tool, often more revealing than any test alone. Like a detective piecing together evidence, a meticulous history helps us trace allergens and identify the pattern of disease evolution, enabling targeted diagnosis and management.

This chapter outlines a structured approach to history taking and physical examination in pediatric allergies, with a focus on recognizing subtle clues and avoiding common pitfalls.

HISTORY TAKING

The history should start right from the antenatal period.

Antenatal: The maternal diet has been found to have a role in the development of allergy. The place of birth too plays a role. It has been found that Indian descent children have a higher incidence in the west as compared to those born in India. The environment could be the complicating factor in children of similar genes.

Delivery: Allergies have been found to have a higher incidence in cesarean section babies as compared to a normal delivery.

Breastfeeding: The incidence of allergic diseases is lower in atopic children who have been exclusively breast fed as compared to those who were bottle fed. This does not hold true for nonatopic babies.

Weaning: The weaning diet and time are very important. The leap study showed that an infant susceptible to peanut allergy had a lower incidence when introduced peanut at an earlier age.

Family history of allergy is the single most important factor predisposing a child to development of an allergic disease. There is no gender selectivity in it. There are high chances of allergic rhinitis (AR) and food allergy as mentioned:

- 50% with one parent having atopy
- 66% with both parents having atopy
- 85% children have similar allergy like parents

Past Medical History

Since allergy follows a typical march in most cases, it is essential that the history should specifically look for the following from birth onward.

Skin changes: Skin changes in the form of dry skin are the earliest changes. Signs of palmar hyperlinearity provide clues to an underlying filaggrin gene. Atopic dermatitis (AD) starts within the first few months of life. Eczema which starts in adolescence is less likely to be AD.

The distribution varies with age. In infants, the face and in older children the flexural surfaces are affected. The details of medication should also be included to give relief, which include steroids and immunomodulators.

Urticarial rash may come on much later in children and could be due to a food allergy.

Wheezing: This usually starts in the second year of life. There is a need to evaluate whether the wheezing was persistent, transient, or intermittent type. The therapy needed such as bronchodilators and steroids for relief will give a clue to the phenotyping.

Rhinitis: Time of onset and treatment needed along with soft signs of allergy such as mouth breathing, snoring, teeth grinding, and behavioral abnormalities.

If any of the above was present in infancy or toddler age group, then the particular symptoms might follow into adulthood. Allergy never goes away but changes its form from one presentation to another.

Treatment History

The drugs and devices used and the therapeutic response to the treatment are to be elicited. If there was no significant response to the correct drugs, then there is a need to enquire whether the devices were taken as per the correct technique. Very often, nose sprays are not taken as per the correct technique, inhaled steroids are used without a spacer, and the timing of the antihistamine may not have a proper relationship to food consumption.

In our country, there are formulations of Montelukast and antihistamine which make the drugs ineffective.

Environmental History

A detailed environmental history to find the irritants and the allergens is an absolute must in any respiratory allergy.

Triggers for AR are as follows:
- Aerobiological (tested by skin or by blood testing)
- Dust mite 60%
- Cockroach 17.5%
- Fungi/Pollens 7.5%
- Pets 5%

The irritants can cause symptoms similar to allergy in patients having an underlying allergic disease to the above aerobiologicals or to any individual having an underlying defect in the upper airway system, especially the nose. The irritants cannot be tested by skin or a blood test. Any laboratory that tests for any of the below irritants is misleading the patients, and their reports should be discarded. This is to reiterate the fact that we are allergic to a living substance and not to chemicals:
- Cigarette smoke
- Mosquito coil
- Other smokes
- Formaldehyde, benzene
- Volatile organic compounds and perfumes, deodorants, etc.

Development History

It has become an essential part of the history because many children with allergies may present with hyperactivity due to improper sleep and features suggestive of autism due to repeated middle ear effusion.

The above is a basic history. The approach may need to be detailed and classified as per the allergy and the system affected. We analyze below a structured approach for different allergies.

Allergic Rhinitis

The four major cardinal symptoms of AR are:
1. Sneezing
2. Itching (nasal)
3. Rhinorrhea
4. Congestion

Allergic rhinitis is more than just a simple sneeze. It needs to be considered in the context of a systemic allergic disease. The range of symptoms may include the following:
- Cough
- Sneezing
- Nasal pruritus
- Nasal congestion
- Sore throats—recurrent infections
- Halitosis
- Respiratory distress—infant
- Hypernasality
- Behavioral problems

Hence, a detailed history should try to elicit all of the above symptoms in the patient. An AR may not have the classical four symptoms sometimes; hence, the above subtle presentations need to be elicited.

Allergic rhinitis may often be accompanied by comorbid disorders. These are:
- Conjunctivitis
- Pharyngitis
- Sinusitis
- Asthma
- Eczema
- Otitis media
- Lymphoid hypertrophy/obstructive sleep apnea
- Speech impairment
- Failure to thrive
- Reduced quality of life
- Lacrimation
- Headache
- Ear fullness/otalgia
- Palatal pruritic
- Itching eyes
- Fatigue
- Depression
- Cognitive impairment
- Sleep disturbances

History Taking: Important questions to be asked?
- Is there a family history of allergy?
- What are the major symptoms?
- How long have your symptoms been persisting?
- When do you get symptoms more?
    - Diurnal/seasonal Variations
    - Does your child snore or breathe through mouth?

EXAMINATION

In children, examination of the nose can be better done by lifting their tip of the nose with the thumb to visualize the nasal mucosa, septum, and inferior turbinate **(Fig. 1)**. The head needs to be stabilized with the palm of the same hand. Children will be very scared if we use nasal speculum, so we should put a finger into the nose.

The inferior turbinate needs to be visualized for hypertrophy and color changes such as a bluish or reddish hue. Also, look for any deviation of nasal septum. If there is any discharge, note the color, nature, and smell and whether it is bilateral.

- Inspection—general appearance
- Nasal mucosa
  - Polyps may present
  - Turbinate hypertrophy
- Mouth
  - Cobble stoning of oropharynx
  - Lymphoid hypertrophy of posterior pharyngeal wall
- Ear—middle ear pathology
- Neck—lymphadenopathy
- Skin—atopic dermatitis
- Allergic shiners—lower eyelid venous stasis
- Allergic salute—rubbing nose in an upward direction **(Fig. 2)**
- Dennie's lines—creases in the lower eyelid (Mueller's muscle spasm)
- Allergic lashes—long, silky full eyelashes
- Allergic crease—nose may have a lateral crease
- Allergic gape—constant mouth breathing, frequent snoring **(Fig. 3)**
- Darier's line—a horizontal crease above the tip of nose
- Listen to the sounds
  - Clearing of throat
  - Sniffling
  - Palatoglossal sound to address itchy palate
  - Hypernasality (voice tone)
- *Wheezing:* The presence of wheezing is to be recorded on auscultation.

  The following will rule out an allergy and may require an ENT referral:
  - Unilateral symptoms are unlikely to be an allergy and more a local pathology.
  - Nasal obstruction with or without symptoms

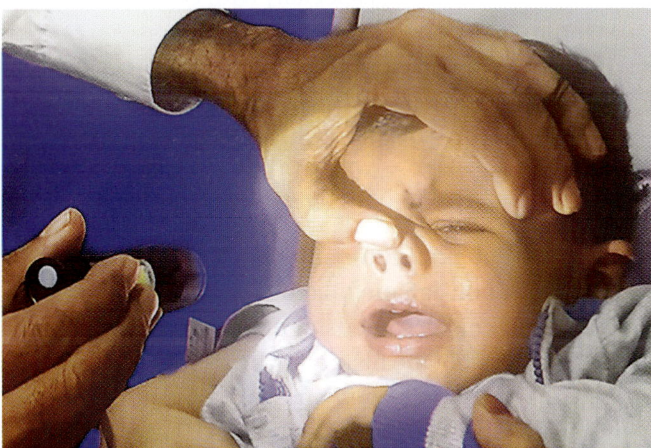

Fig. 1: Anterior nasal examination by elevating the nasal tip.
Source: Parthasarathy A, NAIR MKC, Dharmapalan D. IAP Color Atlas of Pediatrics, 3rd edition. New Delhi: Jaypee Brothers Medical Publishers; 2024.

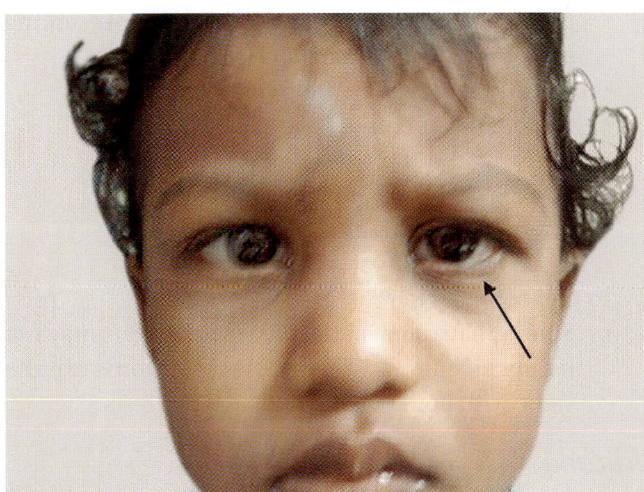

Fig. 2: Allergic shiners.
Source: Parthasarathy A, NAIR MKC, Dharmapalan D. IAP Color Atlas of Pediatrics, 3rd edition. New Delhi: Jaypee Brothers Medical Publishers; 2024.

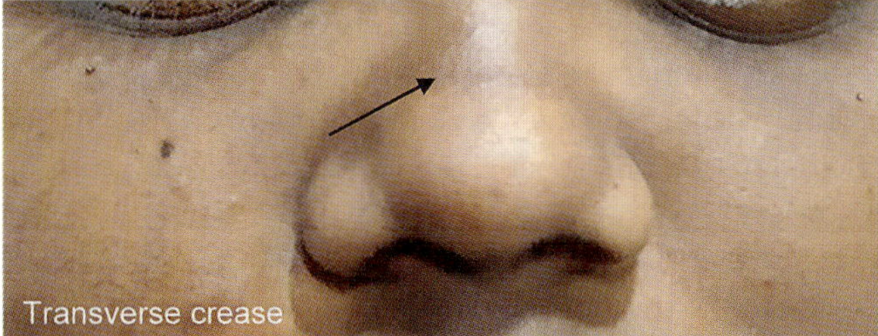

Fig. 3: Allergic transverse crease on the nose secondary to allergic salute.
Source: Parthasarathy A, NAIR MKC, Dharmapalan D. IAP Color Atlas of Pediatrics, 3rd edition. New Delhi: Jaypee Brothers Medical Publishers; 2024.

- Mucopurulent rhinorrhea would suggest an infection. However, an AR can sometimes get secondarily infected.
- Posterior rhinorrhea (postnasal drip) with thick mucus and/or no anterior rhinorrhea is less likely to be allergy.
- Pain, recurrent epistaxis, and anosmia are ominous signs suggesting a pathology.

Asthma

The history and examination are very similar to those of AR and would be helpful.

Allergic Conjunctivitis

The history should be two-fold:

1. Find the severity of the diseases. These would include the following:
   - Periocular itching (the most common presenting symptom), recurrent itching (hallmark)
   - Sensitivity to light or photophobia
   - Hyperemia or redness of eye
   - Excessive tearing
   - Foreign body sensation in the affected eye
   - Chemosis (swelling)
   - Visual loss in very severe cases
2. To find aeroallergen
   - Studies have shown that the aeroallergens may not be positive in all VKC and the symptoms are the same with both positive and negative tests.

Urticaria

Although the examination is a spot diagnosis, the history is very essential. First, there is a need to differentiate urticaria into acute (less than 6 weeks) and chronic.

Acute urticaria has a definite etiology and could be due to infections, infestations, drugs, and adverse food reactions. Allergy as a cause of chronic urticaria is very rare. Very often, the etiology may not be found and labeled as idiopathic. However, a detailed history needs to be elicited to rule out hepatic, renal, thyroid, or autoimmune disorders.

On examination, there are raised skin lesions always associated with itching. The red raised patches will be of various shapes and sizes, isolated, or may coalesce with each other and present all over the body.

Sometimes, there may be no rashes but in cholinergic urticaria these rashes can get elicited by pressure, stroking, temperature changes, and ice cubes.

A rare but important disease which may be confused with allergy is hereditary angioedema (HAE). Its characteristic feature is angioedema without any skin rashes.

Atopic Dermatitis

Both AD and contact dermatitis are spot diagnosis with no tests to prove except a biopsy.

The history should be exclusively focused on finding the aggravating factors.

Examination: The physician needs to run down the volar surface of his palm along the skin to feel the dryness of skin which is a precursor of AD.

The skin is thickened, and whitish yellow areas are the characterize features of chronic AD.

In older children, flexural surfaces are involved. This consists of the forearm and back of the knees.

Papular urticaria characterized by chronic or recurrent papules could be a precursor of AD.

Food Allergy

Almost 20% of individuals in the population believe that they have adverse reactions to foods. Not all these reactions are food allergies, as they are not immune-mediated. Many patients tend to limit their diet based on perceived adverse reactions to foods/additive.

Hence, the following group would need a detailed evaluation:

- Persisting or intermittent symptoms without any other known reason, especially with concurrent atopic symptoms
- Persons experiencing allergic symptoms (itch, angioedema, urticaria, wheezing, and gastroesophageal responses) in association with food exposure

Approach

History

It is very essential to differentiate an IgE-mediated food allergy from a non-IgE meditated food allergy.

Hence, the history needs to be meticulous. The most important aspect of the history is chronology.

Did the reaction occur on every consumption and whether cooking had any impact? Activities and drug consumption simultaneously will give important clues. The foodstuff consumed was fresh and processed or contained colorants. These have an impact on the histamine content which could cause a reaction.

Symptoms and signs: The symptoms of food allergy can be localized or systemic. It could be a just a mild urticaria or a severe reaction like anaphylaxis.

The reaction is usually always generalized except in oral allergy syndrome where it is typically local and limited to oral and perioral regions.

Urticaria is the most prevalent symptom of a food allergy. It may or may not be accompanied with angioedema which is caused by microleakage from blood vessel. The typical rash occurs within minutes to maximum 4 hours of food consumption and may disappear within 24 hours if the food is not consumed.

Chronic urticaria as a cause of food allergy is very rare. Recurrent urticaria may be a cause of food allergy.

Respiratory symptoms alone without other systemic changes are uncommon. They are more common as standalone if the allergen was inhaled.

Gastrointestinal symptoms are very common and consist of vomiting, loose motions, distension, flatulence, and in infants may be limited to only colic symptoms. Food protein-induced enterocolitis syndrome (FPIES) can present as severe dehydration and without systemic symptoms.

Anaphylaxis is the most dangerous and severe form of reaction due to food or sometimes drug allergy.

Drug Allergy

It is very common in practice for patients to attribute their rashes and other adverse effects to a particular drug prescribed by the physician. Hence, the physician should be able to differentiate the two main type of adverse effects as shown in **Table 1**.

Once the physician is sure that the drug effect is not type A, then he should subject the patient to a detailed questionnaire as mentioned below.

TABLE 1: Types of adverse effects of drugs.

Type A side effect	*Type B side effect*
Predictable	Not predictable
Along expected lines and strictly dose dependent	Not dose dependent and unexpected
Symptoms include diarrhea after amoxicillin or gastrointestinal bleeding as in NSAID like aspirin	These are the ones which can turn out to be serious enough to cause death
Occurrence is as high as 80% of all side reactions of all drugs included	Usually are uncommon

Questionnaire for Drug Allergies

The patient should have the below-mentioned information ready before entering the physician's chamber:

- The time of onset of symptoms from the time of consumption of the drug. It has to be as specific as possible.
- The duration of the symptoms.
- The timing of medications, any increase in medications, or stoppage of the medications are to be informed.
- Treatment taken for the symptoms and its effect
- Past drug reactions
- Similar-type symptoms without taking the drug
- Do you have asthma, nasal allergies, food allergy, or other allergies?
- Family history of drug allergies
- Always take pictures of any condition, such as a rash/swelling, to show your doctor.

(Winning Over Allergies: Myths and Facts by Hay House Publications)

The above history may give a lot of clues to the etiology because in drug hypersensitivity very few drugs can be evaluated by prick testing. A provocation test albeit risky is the gold standard.

Insect Bite

In the pediatric agc group, stinging insect bite can contribute to skin allergies presentation, especially urticaria. Sometimes, it can lead to severe manifestations such as respiratory difficulties, hypotension, and anaphylaxis.

The local reactions are restricted to cutaneous manifestations limited to <10 cm in diameter along with itching, redness, and edema.

Anaphylaxis

After a severe allergic reaction without a known cause to identify a trigger, a detailed history is very important. WDEIA, i.e., wheat-dependent exercise-induced anaphylaxis, may be normal on normal routine testing. A detailed history of increased activity, even as subtle as climbing stairs or having a bath, may be the key to the diagnosis.

COUNSELING

After a detailed history and examination, a diagnosis with the possible allergen suspected should be explained to the parents or the patient. Allergy is a chronic disorder, and some diagnosis, especially asthma, may create apprehension in the parents. Thus, time is an essence to convince the patient for further testing which would only confirm our clinical evaluation.

CONCLUSION

A meticulous clinical history and targeted physical examination remain the cornerstone of allergy diagnosis and often provide more diagnostic clarity than any single laboratory test. Recognizing the temporal evolution of allergies, identifying environmental triggers, and assessing symptom patterns across organ systems allow clinicians to distinguish true allergic disease from mimickers. Careful evaluation of comorbidities, subtle clinical signs, treatment responses, and environmental exposures helps build a comprehensive clinical picture. As advanced diagnostics become available, their interpretation continues to rely heavily on a well-structured history and examination. Strengthening these fundamental clinical skills is essential for accurate diagnosis, rational testing, and effective long-term management of pediatric allergic disorders.

KEY POINTS

- *History is central:* Start from antenatal history, delivery mode, breastfeeding, family history, development, past medical treatment, environmental exposure, and triggers.
- *Key allergy triggers:*
  - Aerobiological (dust mites, cockroach, pollens)
  - Irritants (cigarette smoke, perfumes, mosquito coils)—not testable by laboratories
- *Red flags ruling out allergy:* Unilateral symptoms, mucopurulent discharge, anosmia, recurrent epistaxis
- *Important clinical signs:* Allergic shiners, Dennie's lines, allergic salute, palatal pruritus, hypernasality.
- *Specific allergy syndromes:*
  - *Systemic juvenile idiopathic arthritis (JIA):* IL-6 driven fever
  - *Food allergy:* Acute urticaria or anaphylaxis following food intake
  - *Drug allergy:* Distinguish type A versus type B reactions; provocation test is gold standard
  - *Anaphylaxis:* May be triggered by exercise (WDEIA)
- *Counseling is vital:* Allergy is chronic; clear communication with families builds confidence in further diagnostic steps.

SUGGESTED READING

1. American Academy of Allergy, Asthma & Immunology (AAAAI) Practice Parameters.
2. Franklin Adkinson Jr N, Bochner BS, Wesley Burks A, Busse WW, Holgate ST. Middleton's Allergy: Principles and Practice (8th edition). Philadelphia: Elsevier; 2013.
3. EAACI Food Allergy and Anaphylaxis Guidelines 2021. Muraro A, Worm M, Alviani C, Cardona V, DunnGalvin V, Heise Garvey L, et al. EAACI guidelines: Anaphylaxis (2021 update)European Academy of Allergy and Clinical Immunology (EAACI). Allergy. 2022;77(2):357-77.
4. NICE Clinical Guideline CG95 – Allergic Rhinitis: Diagnosis and Management National Institute for Health and Care Excellence (NICE), UK, 2017.

7 CHAPTER

In Vitro Allergy Diagnostics

Karthik Nagaraju, Mohit Poddar

INTRODUCTION

Allergy diagnosis forms the cornerstone in the management of allergic diseases. Clinicians rely on a comprehensive approach, beginning with a detailed history and physical examination, but laboratory tests have become indispensable for confirmation and characterization of immune responses. Among these, invitro allergy tests—from a patient's serum—play a vital role in defining IgE-mediated sensitization when in vivo tests such as skin prick testing (SPT) are contraindicated, impractical, or equivocal. In vitro tests eliminate risks associated with direct allergen exposure, such as systemic reactions, and are unaffected by medications such antihistamines or corticosteroids, which can suppress skin test responses **(Table 1)**. The precise identification of culprit allergens through these laboratory methods optimizes management, avoidance strategies, and when indicated, consideration of allergen-specific immunotherapy. Modern in vitro techniques have evolved from simple total IgE assessments to sophisticated assays measuring specific immunoglobulin E (sIgE) to allergen extracts or components, and even cellular assays evaluating cellular responses, reflecting the paradigm shift toward precision medicine in allergy.

TABLE 1: When to choose in vitro over in vivo tests.

Criteria	*Prefer in vitro*	*Prefer in vivo (Skin test)*
Widespread skin disease, dermographism	✓	
Unable to stop antihistamines	✓	
High anaphylaxis risk with skin testing	✓	
Patient with needle phobia (blood draw difficult)		✓
Testing rare/unavailable allergens	✓	
Cost and rapid availability		✓
Immediate result required		✓

IMPORTANCE OF ALLERGY DIAGNOSIS

A precise allergy diagnosis guides targeted treatment, prevents unnecessary avoidance and anxiety, and reduces morbidity associated with allergic diseases.

OVERVIEW OF ALLERGY MECHANISM

Allergic diseases are immune-mediated and fall overwhelmingly under type 1 hypersensitivity reactions, driven by IgE antibodies, and type 4 hypersensitivity (T-cell mediated), relevant in some drug and contact allergies.

- *Type 1 (immediate/IgE-mediated):* Classic hay fever, asthma, food allergy; in vitro tests for sIgE are gold standard.
- *Type 4 (delayed/T cell-mediated):* Some drug reactions, contact dermatitis; in vitro methods are evolving, like lymphocyte transformation tests (LTT).

In vitro tests are highly useful in type 1 reactions and are expanding in relevance to select type 4 scenarios.

HISTORY OF IN VITRO TESTS

- *1960s:* Discovery of IgE, launch of radio-allergosorbent test (RAST)
- *1990s:* Shift to enzyme-linked immunoassays (ELISA), ImmunoCAP [fluorescent enzyme immuno assay (FEIA)]
- *2000s:* Advent of component-resolved diagnostics (CRD), multiplex testing, basophil activation test (BAT).

TYPES OF IN VITRO TESTS

Total Serum IgE

Total serum IgE quantifies the overall concentration of IgE immunoglobulin in the blood, expressed in international units per milliliter (IU/mL). The test is typically performed using enzyme-linked immunoassays or other automated immunoassay platforms. Age-specific reference ranges are important, as IgE levels are lowest in infancy, gradually increasing through childhood and adolescence, and stabilizing in

TABLE 2: Reference ranges (varies with method).

Age group	*Reference range (IU/mL)*
Infants	0–15
Children	1–60
Adults	0–100

adults **(Table 2)**. However, total IgE is a nonspecific marker of atopy: Elevated levels may suggest atopic tendency but are *neither sensitive nor specific* for any allergic condition. High values can also be seen in parasitic infections, certain immunodeficiencies, or even healthy individuals. Conversely, a normal concentration does not exclude clinically relevant allergies, as some allergic patients may have normal total IgE. Thus, total serum IgE has a limited role in diagnosis; it is best used as an adjunct in selected cases, such as severe, difficult-to-classify disease presentations in children, or in screening for conditions like hyper-IgE syndromes. Total IgE should not be used as the sole diagnostic test for allergy nor as a substitute for clinical correlation and allergen-specific testing. Its main strength lies in forming an initial impression of atopic status, identifying grossly elevated levels in atypical cases, and as a baseline for broader immunological investigations.

- *Role:* Screening; useful to suggest atopy but lacks specificity
- *Limitations:* Not diagnostic; raised in infections, parasitosis, some immunodeficiencies
- *Recommendations:* Do not use as a sole criterion for allergy diagnosis.

Specific IgE

Specific IgE testing is the backbone of in vitro diagnosis of type 1 (IgE-mediated) allergic diseases. This testing quantifies the presence of IgE antibodies directed against individual allergens in blood, providing objective evidence of sensitization. While SPT is often considered the first-line method, measurement of serum allergen-specific IgE provides a complementary and sometimes superior alternative in certain clinical scenarios. sIgE testing bridges the gap between clinical suspicion and confirmation of sensitization, yet interpretation requires careful integration with history and physical examination. Sensitization does not equate to clinical allergy, and judicious use is critical to avoid overdiagnosis and unnecessary avoidance measures.

Principle of sIgE Testing

sIgE testing is based on the principle of *immunoassay testing*. Allergen molecules are immobilized on a solid phase and bind to a patient's serum sIgE, which is then detected by labeled anti-IgE antibodies using enzymatic, fluorometric, or chemiluminescent reactions.

Methods of sIgE Testing

Common commercial platforms:

- *ImmunoCAP (Thermo Fisher):* Allergen coupled to hydrophilic polymer, detection via fluorescent substrate. Gold standard. Highly sensitive and quantitative
- *IMMULITE (Siemens):* Allergen linked to biotinylated polymers, chemiluminescent detection via adamantyl-dioxetane substrate. Widely used, variable standardization
- *Hytec-288 ELISA (Hycor):* Allergen on activated cellulose; colorimetric detection with nitrophenyl phosphate

Each method employs standardized, highly sensitive calibration using World Health Organization (WHO) total IgE standards. Assays are typically automated and designed to minimize cross-reactivity and interference.

Indications for Ordering sIgE

- When skin testing is contraindicated (extensive eczema, dermographism, urticaria, antihistamine use)
- When the risk of systemic reactions during SPT is high (e.g., suspected anaphylaxis to food, venom, drug)
- When patients or caregivers are unwilling to undergo skin testing
- In infants or very young children where skin reactivity is poor
- To quantify allergen-specific IgE for prognosis and risk stratification **(Table 3)**
- As part of a structured diagnostic pathway [e.g., before oral food challenges (OFCs)].

Pearl of Wisdom

Choose sIgE testing based on clinical features, suspected allergen, and patient history. Avoid indiscriminate panels, as they carry high false-positive rates.

Grading

Results are expressed as kUA/L. Quantitative range: 0.1–100 kUA/L.

TABLE 3: Grading based on sIgE values (ImmunoCAP).

Grade	IgE level (kUA/L)	Interpretation
0	<0.35	Negative or undetectable
1	0.35–0.7	Weak positive (low likelihood)
2	0.7–3.5	Positive (possible)
3	3.5–17.5	Moderate/high (more likely)
4	17.5–50.0	Strong/extremely likely
5	50–100.0	Strong/extremely likely
6	>100	Strong/extremely likely

TABLE 4: sIgE cutoffs for specific food allergens.

Food allergen	sIgE level (kUA/L)	Clinical implication
Egg (children)	>2 (if <2 years), >7 (if >2 years)	Likely clinical allergy
Cow's milk	>5 (if <2 years), >15 (if >2 years)	High probability of clinical allergy
Peanut	>14	Strongly predictive of systemic reaction
Fish	>20	Likely clinical allergy
Wheat	>20	High probability of reactivity

Interpretation of Sige Results

- *sIgE, sensitization, and clinical allergy:*
    - *Positive sIgE:* Sensitization, but only clinical history determines allergy
    - Useful in immunotherapy decision
    - *False positives:* Cross-reactive carbohydrate determinants (CCDs), profilins or other pan-allergens—common on nonstandardized ELISA (Enzyme-Linked Immunosorbent Assay) tests
    - *False negatives:* Very young infants, low IgE producers or testing outside allergen season
- *Predictive thresholds:* Several studies have identified sIgE cutoffs with >95% positive predictive value (PPV) for certain food allergies **(Table 4)**.
- *Monitoring trends:*
    - Falling sIgE over time suggests natural tolerance development (e.g., milk, egg).
    - Rising or persistently high levels suggest persistent allergy (e.g., peanut, tree nuts, shellfish).
    - *Risk stratification:* Higher sIgE titers are associated with an increased likelihood of clinical reactivity and more severe reactions.
    - There is no strict linear correlation between IgE levels and severity.

Advantages of sIgE Testing

- *Safe:* No risk of systemic reactions as in skin testing
- *Practical:* Can be performed on stored serum; useful in infants and during antihistamine therapy
- *Quantitative:* Allows tracking of allergen sensitization over time
- *Standardized:* ImmunoCAP and other FEIA methods are validated
- *Wide allergen repertoire:* Availability of hundreds of allergen extracts and components.

Limitations of sIgE Testing

- *Sensitization ≠ Allergy:* Positive result without symptoms may lead to overdiagnosis.
- *Cross-reactivity:* Pan-allergens and CCDs cause false positivity.
- *Cost:* Higher than SPT
- *Turnaround time:* Longer than bedside SPT
- *Availability:* May be limited in resource-constrained settings
- *Assay variability:* Results from different platforms are not interchangeable.
- Nonvalidated ELISA techniques are not recommended for interpretation
- *Predictive thresholds vary:* No universal cutoff; pediatric specific validation is needed.

Recommendations

- Interpret sIgE in the context of clinical history.
- sIgE testing should be guided by focused, allergy-oriented history, including exposure, symptoms and known tolerance.
- Avoid testing to allergens not linked to symptoms or environment.
- Analytical technique must be specified when using published cutoffs.
- Avoid panel-based testing; prefer single allergen tests to reduce false positives.
- Use serial measurements for monitoring resolution in certain food allergies, e.g., milk, egg, and wheat allergy.
- In polysensitized patients, consider CRD to refine interpretation.
- In diagnostic uncertainty, or to assess readiness for reintroduction, oral food challenge remains the gold standard.

Component-resolved Diagnosis

It is well known that antigen proteins contain specific epitopes or components which can be allergenic or nonallergenic. These epitopes are capable of stimulating specific IgE individually and thus can elicit a clinical reaction on exposure. CRD is a state-of-the-art study of the specific epitopes or allergenic molecules and their specific IgE. CRD helps to gain further insight into the relationship of causative allergens with clinical diagnosis of allergy and to differentiate cross-reactivity from clinical sensitization, estimation of risk and severity, as well as guide precision-based strategies such as allergen immunotherapy (AIT) or food avoidance. CRD is also known as molecular allergology or precision allergy molecular diagnostics applications (PAMD@).

Principle of CRD

Allergen extracts are composed of a mix of protein components which are capable of individual immune responses **(Fig. 1)**. Immune response to allergenic components varies depending on several characteristics including heat or digestion resistance, structural similarity to closely related proteins, etc. **(Table 5)**. CRD utilizes recombinant or purified proteins to detect these component-specific IgE. In addition to detecting allergic components, it also helps identify nonallergenic components such as cross reactive carbohydrate determinants (CCDs) which contribute to false positives on extract-based testing **(Table 6)**.

Further, based on population prevalence, allergen components are classified as major and minor allergens.

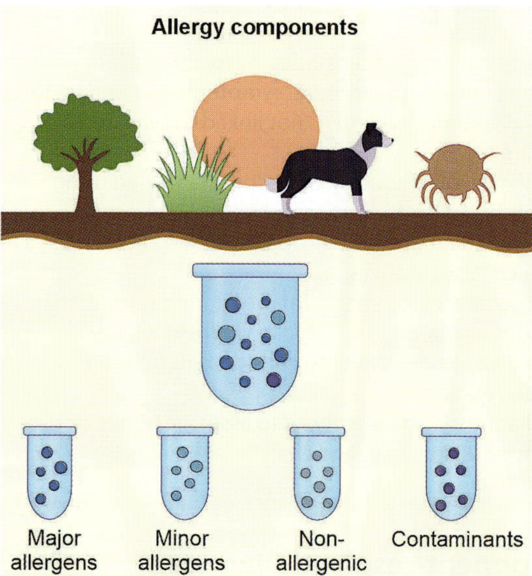

Fig. 1: Composition of whole allergen extracts and their separation into purified components. Examples of nonallergenic components include CCD (cross-reactive carbohydrate determinants).

Major allergens are those which bind to >50% of IgE from the serum of clinically allergic patients. *Examples include:* Der p 1 and Der p 2 components of house dust mite (*Dermatophagoides pteronyssinus*) and Api m 1

TABLE 5: Examples of component proteins and reactions based on protein characteristics.

Characteristic	*Example*	*Reaction*
Heat/digestion stability	• 2S/7S albumins Peanut (Ara h 2) • Casein (Bos d 8) • Omega-5 Gliadin (Tri a 19)	• Severe systemic reactions • Severe systemic reactions • FDEIA
Epitope similarity (cross-reactivity)	• Bet v 1 homologue (birch tree, peanut, apple, soy) • Profilin (tree, grass, fruits, vegetables, latex) • nsLTP (wheat, tomato, peach, apple, peanut, soy)	• Pollen related AR, Oral allergy symptoms to fresh fruits • Pollen-related AR, mild OAS • Bizarre, severe systemic reactions

(AR: allergic rhinitis; FDEIA: food-dependent exercise-induced anaphylaxis; nsLTP: nonspecific lipid transfer protein; OAS: oral allergy syndrome)

TABLE 6: Advantages of CRD over extract-based testing.

Aspect	*Extract-based testing*	*CRD (molecular testing)*
Specificity	Crude extracts contain multiple proteins, nonaller-genic components, batch variability	High specificity; purified or recombinant allergen molecules
Cross-reactivity	Cannot distinguish genuine sensitization from cross reactivity	Identifies true primary sensitizer vs. cross-reactivity (e.g., profilin, Bet v 1 homologue)
Risk assessment	Limited predictive value	Certain components predict severe systemic reactions (storage proteins, nsLTP, etc.)
Therapy guidance	Poor predictor of response if driven by cross reactivity	Enables precise AIT selection (e.g., house dust mite components Der p 1, Der p 2)
Dietary avoidance	Risk of unnecessary broad avoidance	Tailored avoidance based on clinically relevant sensitizers

of honeybee. Major allergens are responsible for true clinical allergy. Minor allergens are proteins which bind to <50% of IgE from the sera of clinically allergic patients. *Example:* Der p 10 and Der p 5 of *D. pteronyssinus*. Major allergens are a sign of true allergen sensitization. This helps in differentiating true sensitization from cross-reactivity.

Techniques in CRD

- *Singleplex assays:*
  - Detect IgE against one component at a time
  - *Most widely used platform:* ImmunoCAP (Thermo Fisher)
  - High sensitivity, quantitative results
  - Suitable for testing a small number of specific components guided by history
- *Multiplex assays:*
  - Detect IgE to dozens and even hundreds of components at a time
  - *Available platforms:* ImmunoCAP ISAC (Thermo Fisher), ALEX (MADx diagnostics)
  - Requires small serum volume, useful in children
  - Provides broad sensitization profiles, particularly cross-reactivity
  - Semiquantitative

Role in Allergy Diagnosis (Table 7)

Risk stratification:
  - Storage protein sensitization identifies risk of systemic reactions [Ara h 1, Bos d 8 (Casein), Gal d 1 (Ovomucoid)]
  - Predicts positive OFC, guides testing
- *Treatment decisions:*
  - Tailor AIT by confirming true sensitization to major allergens (Der p 1, Der p 2, Phl p 1, Ves v 1)
  - Avoid unnecessary immunotherapy when cross-reactivity predominates
- *Counseling and lifestyle guidance:*
  - Reduces unnecessary food avoidance
  - Improves clarity in polysensitized patients

Limitations of CRD

- *Availability and cost:* Limited availability; expensive compared to extract-based testing
- *Complex interpretation:* Requires specialist knowledge; risk of misinterpretation if taken in isolation
- *Sensitivity:* Not all defined allergens have defined components; negative CRD does not rule out allergy
- *Standardization:* Singleplex (quantitative) and multiarray or multiplex tests (semiquantitative) are not comparable
- *Overuse risk:* Ordering broad panels without history leads to irrelevant findings and adds to patient's confusion.
- *Not gold standard:* Direct organ challenges are the gold standard to prove clinical allergy.

Recommendations
- Use CRD as a complement, not as replacement: Interpret with clinical history, physical findings
- *Indications where CRD adds superior value:*
  - Polysensitized patients
  - Food allergy risk assessment
  - Pollen-food syndrome clarification
  - Venom allergy (distinguish between bee and wasp)
  - Considering allergen immunotherapy
- *Avoid overuse:* Do not order CRD as a screening tool without suggestive history
- *Interpret results in context:* Detection of cross-reactive molecules (profilins, CCDs) does not always translate into clinical allergy

Basophil Activation Test

Basophils along with mast cells are important cells involved in the immediate-type hypersensitivity reactions (type 1 hypersensitivity). They express high affinity IgE receptors (FCεRI) which upon activation by allergen binding leads to basophil or mast cell degranulation, mediator release, and subsequent clinical reaction. Compared to mast cells which are tissue based, basophils are acccessible due to their predominance in circulating blood.

Principle of BAT

Basophil activation test is an ex vivo test. Circulating basophils are separated and identified using flow cytometry. Specific markers of basophil activation include CD63 and CD203c. Upon exposure to allergen, specific IgE cross linking occurs which leads to an increase in upregulation and expression of CD63 and CD203c **(Fig. 2)**. Thus, activated basophils are identified along with the concentration and dose of allergen exposed. Thus, it replaces real-time exposure of provocation tests and mitigates complications and risks.

TABLE 7: Major component families and clinical relevance.

Protein family	*Examples (source)*	*Stability (heat/digestion)*	*Typical clinical reaction*	*Notes*
PR-10 proteins (pathogenesis-related protein family 10) *Or* Bet v 1 homologues	Bet v 1 (birch), Mal d 1 (apple), Cor a 1 (hazelnut), Gly m 4 (soy), Ara h 8 (peanut)	Heat- and digestion-labile	Oral allergy syndrome (OAS), mild local reactions	Strong cross-reactivity with birch pollen; usually mild symptoms
Profilins	Bet v 2 (birch), Phl p 12 (grass), Hev b 8 (latex)	Labile	OAS, mild local reactions	Pan-allergens across pollens and foods; rarely cause systemic symptoms
Polcalcins (calcium-binding proteins)	Bet v 4 (birch), Phl p 7 (grass)	Labile	OAS or mild rhinoconjunctivitis	Highly cross-reactive, rarely clinically significant
Storage proteins (globulins, cupins, vicilins, legumins)	Ara h 1, 2, 3 (peanut); Cor a 9, 14 (hazelnut); Jug r 1, 2 (walnut); Gly m 5, 6 (soy)	Heat- and digestion-stable	Severe systemic reactions, anaphylaxis	Strong predictors of persistent and severe food allergy
Nonspecific lipid transfer proteins (nsLTPs)	Pru p 3 (peach), Ara h 9 (peanut), Cor a 8 (hazelnut), Mal d 3 (apple)	Highly stable	Systemic reactions, anaphylaxis	Prevalent in Mediterranean regions; associated with "LTP syndrome"
Tropomyosins	Der p 10 (HDM), Pen a 1 (shrimp), Bla g 7 (cockroach)	Stable	Respiratory allergy, food allergy, systemic reactions	Cross-reactivity between mite, crustaceans, and insects
Serum albumins	Fel d 2 (cat), Can f 3 (dog), Bos d 6 (bovine)	Labile	Rarely systemic; sometimes OAS; "pork–cat syndrome"	Cross-reactivity across mammals due to conserved albumin
Caseins	Bos d 8 (cow's milk)	Heat-stable	Persistent milk allergy, systemic reactions	Marker of severe, persistent allergy
Ovomucoid	Gal d 1 (egg)	Heat-stable	Severe egg allergy, systemic reactions	Predictor of persistent egg allergy

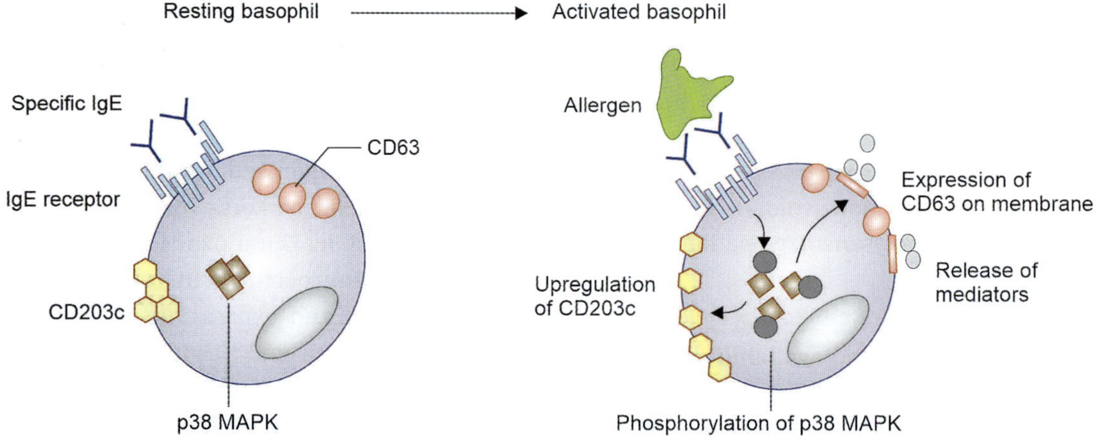

Fig. 2: Principle of basophil activation test (BAT).

Uses

- *Diagnosis:* Particularly in IgE-mediated allergies
    - Food allergy
    - Drug allergy
    - Venom hypersensitivity
    - Allergic rhinitis
    - Allergic asthma
    - Occupational allergy
    - Chronic spontaneous urticaria
- *Determine eligibility for allergen-specific immunotherapy:*
    - Oral immunotherapy for food allergy
    - Anti-IgE therapy
    - Other immunomodulatory treatments
- *Monitoring treatment response:*
    - Response to AIT
    - Food allergy—natural tolerance induction

Role in Allergy Diagnosis

- *Establish diagnosis:* Quick and reliable
- Identify allergen thresholds
- Unable to stop antihistamines
- Unwilling or unfit to perform provocation testing or oral food challenge (OFC)
- No allergen source for skin or sIgE testing
- Discordant history and skin or sIgE test
- Prior to provocation testing

Limitations

- Research tool
- Availability limited
- Expensive and labor intensive
- Short life of basophil activity—immediate processing needed
- Lack of standardized allergen extracts
- Lack of standard protocols for interpretation

Recommendations
- Mimics the provocation test or OFC, risks
- Avoids complications of challenge testing
- Excellent tool to identify allergen threshold and response to therapy
- *Future roles:* As a biomarker of allergy diagnosis, treatment response as well as predict OFC outcomes

Serum Tryptase

- *Marker:* Confirms anaphylaxis, screens for mastocytosis (not a diagnostic test)
- In the setting of anaphylaxis, serum sample for tryptase should be collected within 2 hours of reaction. Normal serum tryptase levels are <11 mg/mL.
- Values >20 mg/mL should raise suspicion of recent mastocyte activation.
- Sustained elevated values (>4 weeks) should raise possibility of systemic mastocytosis.

EMERGING/RESEARCH TOOLS

- *LTT:* It measures proliferating lymphocytes on exposure to suspected allergen. It is useful in type 4 drug hypersensitivity, particularly in drug-related delayed hypersensitivity reactions. It is currently available as a research tool in limited centers only.
- *Histamine-release test:* Similar to BAT, this test measures degranulation of eosinophils or mast cells with release of histamine. Limited availability, research use
- *Specific IgG4 levels:* IgG4 antibodies are produced by Treg cells suggestive of switching to Th2 to Th1 response. They are typically inert antibodies and are indicative of tolerance development. They are used as a research tool in identifying adequate allergen exposure for patients on AIT. Rising IgG4 levels suggest a possible induction of allergen tolerance.

CONCLUSION

In vitro allergy diagnostics complement clinical assessment and skin testing by providing objective evidence of IgE-mediated sensitization while avoiding risks linked to direct allergen exposure. Modern assays—from total and specific IgE to CRD and cellular tests—have expanded diagnostic precision, enabling improved risk assessment and individualized management. However, interpretation must always be contextualized within a well-taken history, as sensitization does not equate to clinical allergy. Thoughtful selection of tests, avoidance of indiscriminate panels, awareness of assay limitations, and correlation with clinical findings are essential. When used judiciously, in vitro methods significantly enhance diagnostic accuracy and support tailored therapeutic decisions, including AIT and food reintroduction strategies.

KEY POINTS

- *In vitro tests* confirm IgE-mediated sensitization, especially where skin tests are contraindicated or impractical.
- They are *safer* than in vivo testing as they do not expose patients to allergens directly.

- They are useful when patients are on medications (antihistamines/corticosteroids) that suppress skin test responses.
- They use focused, history-driven test selection; avoid indiscriminate panel-based testing.
- They incorporate serial measurements in monitoring resolution of allergy, especially food allergies.
- They complement laboratory findings with OFCs when appropriate; they remain the gold standard.
- CRD is especially beneficial in polysensitized patients, food allergy risk assessment, pollen-food syndrome, venom allergy, and prior to immunotherapy.

SUGGESTED READING

1. A WAO—ARIA—GA2LEN consensus document on molecular-based allergy diagnosis (PAMD@): Update 2020. World Allergy Organ J. 2020;13(2):100091.
2. Ansotegui IJ, Melioli G, Canonica GW, Caraballo L, Villa E, Ebisawa M, et al. IgE allergy diagnostics and other relevant tests in allergy, a World Allergy Organization position paper. World Allergy Organ J. 2020;13(2):100080.
3. Hoffmann HJ, Santos AF, Mayorga C, Nopp A, Eberlein B, Ferrer M, et al. The clinical utility of basophil activation testing in diagnosis and monitoring of allergic disease. Allergy. 2015;70:1393-405.
4. Santos AF, Alpan O, Hoffmann H-J. Basophil activation test: Mechanisms and considerations for use in clinical trials and clinical practice. Allergy. 2021;76:2420-32.
5. Santos AF, Riggioni C, Agache I, Akdis CZ, Akdis M, Alvarez-Perea A, et al. EAACI guidelines on the diagnosis of IgE-mediated food allergy. Allergy. 2023;78:3057-76.

8 CHAPTER In Vivo Tests in Allergic Diseases

Narayan Prasad Modi, Sanjay Kumar Sahu

INTRODUCTION

Allergic disorders are a major cause of both acute and chronic morbidity in children globally, and their incidence is notably rising. Increasing urbanization, environmental pollution, climatic changes, dietary modifications, and early-life microbial exposures have all been implicated in this upsurge. The most prevalent pediatric allergic diseases include allergic rhinitis, bronchial asthma, atopic dermatitis, urticaria, food allergies, and allergic contact dermatitis (ACD). Proper diagnosis is the bedrock of effective allergy management and is critical to prevent disease progression, complications, or unnecessary interventions.

Among diagnostic modalities, in vivo allergy tests provide a real-time assessment of the immune system's response to specific allergens introduced via the skin. These tests include the skin prick test (SPT), intradermal test (IDT), and patch test (PT) in the diagnosis of allergic diseases. Each method assesses different types of hypersensitivity reactions and is chosen based on the suspected allergic condition. The interpretation of these tests requires a comprehensive understanding of immunopathophysiology, patient age, regional allergen profiles, and clinical context.

This chapter describes the principles, methodology, interpretation, and clinical utility of in vivo allergy tests in children, with particular emphasis on the Indian scenario, where environmental factors and allergen exposures vary significantly across regions.

SKIN PRICK TEST

Historical Background

The origins of skin testing can be traced back to the early 20th century. Charles Blackley first described pollen allergy and performed early rudimentary testing in the 1800s, but it was Dr Clemens von Pirquet who linked clinical allergy to immune hypersensitivity. Standardization and commercial availability of allergen extracts made SPT a routine clinical tool by the middle of the last century. Over time, the procedure has been refined and validated for clinical use.

Pathophysiology and Immunologic Basis

The SPT identifies type I hypersensitivity, which involves a rapid IgE-mediated immune response. Upon re-exposure to a specific allergen, cross-linking of allergen-specific IgE antibodies bound to high-affinity IgE receptors (FcεRI) on mast cells leads to degranulation and release of histamine, leukotrienes, prostaglandins, etc. These mediators cause localized vasodilation, increased vascular permeability, and sensory nerve stimulation, resulting in the characteristic wheal and flare reaction.

Sensitization versus Allergy

The SPT detects sensitization, which is the presence of allergen-specific IgE bound to mast cells. However, sensitization does not always equate to clinical allergy. A positive test indicates that the immune system has produced IgE against the allergen, but only when accompanied by relevant symptoms on exposure, it confirms clinical allergy. Hence, clinical history is critical for interpretation. For example, a child may have a positive SPT to peanut without any history of reaction—this denotes sensitization but not allergy. On the contrary, a child can have allergy symptoms without SPT being positive.

Indications of Skin Prick Test

The SPT is considered the "gold standard" test for identifying IgE-mediated allergic diseases. It is the first-line test in children with:

- *Allergic rhinitis* (seasonal or perennial)
- *Asthma*, especially allergen induced or triggered
- *Atopic dermatitis*, to identify contributingaeroallergen
- *Food allergy*, when IgE-mediated mechanisms are suspected
- *Venom hypersensitivity*, particularly bee and wasp stings

Contraindications of Skin Prick Test

The SPT is contraindicated in generalized eczema, urticaria, severe dermographism, or children at high risk for anaphylaxis.

Types of Skin Prick Test

- *Prick technique:* An allergen drop is placed on intact skin and pricked with a lancet epicutaneously.
- *Puncture method:* Similar to prick but penetrates slightly deeper; often interchangeable
- *Scratch test:* Older method, allergen is applied to a superficial abrasion made by a lancet; less standardized and not recommended due to a higher risk of infection.

Procedure and Technique

The SPT is a safe and painless procedure and can be done in children as young as 6 months. In practice, however, it is more commonly performed after 2 years of age due to better skin reactivity and child cooperation. For infants and toddlers, testing is often limited to high-yield allergens. However, skin reactivity declines after 60 years.

Pre-test Instructions

- Antihistamines, systemic corticosteroids, and some other medications should be avoided before testing **(Table 1)**.
- Avoid topical steroids on test site for 3 days.
- Ensure that the child is clinically stable and not experiencing acute exacerbation.
- Explain the procedure to parents and child to minimize anxiety.

TABLE 1: Drugs to be avoided before skin prick test (SPT).

Drug/class	*Recommendation before SPT*
Antihistamines (cetirizine, levocetirizine, loratadine, hydroxyzine)	Stop 3–7 days prior
Tricyclic antidepressants (e.g., doxepin)	Stop 1–2 weeks prior
Systemic corticosteroids	May suppress response if used in high doses
Topical corticosteroids	Avoid on test site at least 3 days prior
Montelukast and omalizumab	May attenuate responses over time, though not usually stopped for SPT

- Consent form should be obtained from the guardian/parent.

Selection of Allergens for Skin Prick Test

A focused, detailed allergy history lays the foundation for the selection of allergens to be tested. The selection majorly depends on the patient's age, clinical symptoms, environmental exposure, and likely triggering factors. It is not essential to test a large number of allergens; instead, focusing on a limited number of clinically relevant allergens is often more meaningful.

Allergen Categories

Allergen exposure varies with geography, climate, and lifestyle. Allergens used in SPT fall into three main categories: Aeroallergens, food allergens, and stinging insect venoms.

Aeroallergens are subdivided into:

- *Indoor allergens:* House dust mites, cockroaches, pet dander (cats and dogs), and indoor molds
- *Outdoor allergens:* Tree, grass, and weed pollens, as well as outdoor mold spores.

Among these, house dust mites, cockroach allergens, and animal dander are common triggers of allergic asthma and should be tested when an allergic cause is suspected, as this aids in both diagnosis and treatment planning.

Food allergens are divided into:

- *Class 1:* Primary protein antigens
- *Class 2:* Plant-derived allergens that typically cause symptoms in sensitized individuals.

Insect allergen extracts typically contain venom from stinging insects like those in the Hymenoptera family (e.g., bees, wasps). For other insects like ants, only whole-body extracts are usually available.

Preparation and Storage of Allergen Extracts

The source of allergen used for SPT and immunotherapy is soaked in a buffered saline or glycerinated solution under controlled conditions to extract proteins that are standardized, sterile, and free from preservatives. Potency is adjusted and expressed in bioequivalent allergy units (BAU) or protein nitrogen units (PNU), ensuring consistency batch-to-batch. Extracts must be stored according to manufacturer guidelines—typically at 2–8°C, protected from light. Improper storage leads to denaturation of proteins and reduced potency. Vials should be labeled with expiration dates and opened bottles should be replaced regularly to maintain accuracy.

Positive and Negative Controls

Controls are critical for validating test results:

- *Positive control:* Histamine dihydrochloride (usually 10 mg/mL) should elicit a wheal of at least 3 mm in diameter and 3 mm larger than the negative saline control to confirm validity of the test.
- *Negative control:* Signifies baseline skin reactivity. Glycerinated saline or diluent should elicit no reaction or a wheal <3 mm. Any reaction >3 mm may indicate dermatographism or irritant response.

Lancets and Pricking Devices Used for Skin Prick Test

Lancets must be sterile, single-use, and designed for consistent skin penetration (approximately 1 mm depth). The choice of device significantly impacts the accuracy and comfort of the test. Common types include the following:

- *Single-use metal lancets:* Flat or pointed tips designed for manual skin prick. Inexpensive and widely used in resource-limited settings **(Fig. 1)**
- *Plastic disposable lancets:* Blunt-tipped and safer, with consistent penetration. Often used in pediatric patients **(Fig. 2)**
- *Multitest devices (e.g., Multi-Test II, Quintest):* Can test multiple allergens simultaneously; ideal for high-throughput clinics
- *Duotip-Test®:* Dual-pronged lancet with reduced discomfort; suitable for children.
- *Hollister-Stier device:* Spring-loaded lancet ensuring standard depth and pressure, improving reproducibility.

Reusable lancets should never be used due to the risk of infection and inconsistent results. Selection of a suitable pricking device should balance precision, safety, and patient comfort, especially in pediatric settings.

- *Test site:* The mid and upper back are about 33% more reactive compared to the lower back, and the back overall is 53% more reactive than the forearm. For testing on the forearm, the site is typically selected around 5 cm above the wrist and 3 cm below the antecubital fossa. The volar aspect of the left forearm is most commonly used due to ease of access and good reactivity. In infants or when forearm is not suitable, the upper back may be used.
- *Application:* Place allergen droplets 2 cm apart; puncture gently superficially (epidermis) at around 45° with sterile lancets so that it does not bleed **(Figs. 3A and B)**.
- *Distance between two pricks:* A minimum distance of 2 cm should be maintained between adjacent test sites to prevent nonspecific enhancement caused by nearby axon reflexes and to avoid the merging of wheals resulting from strong local reactions.
- *Observation:* Read positive and negative controls after 10 and 15 minutes respectively; measure wheal diameter in millimeters. A positive reaction is indicated by the formation of a wheal at the site of the skin prick. The largest diameter of the wheal is measured, and the reaction is recorded in millimeters **(Fig. 4)**. If a pseudopod—an irregular projection extending beyond

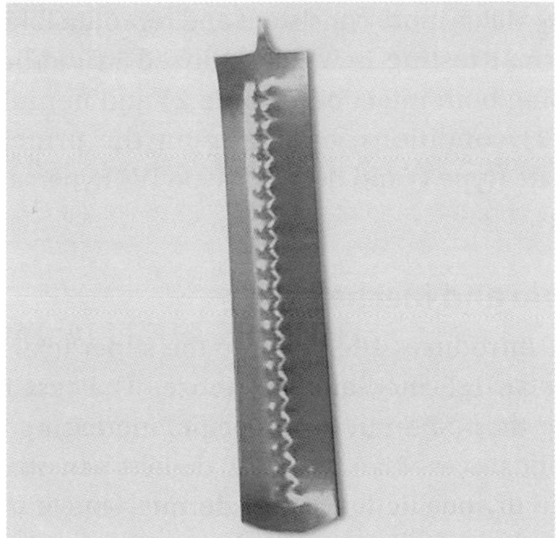

Fig. 1: Commercially available single-use metal lancet.

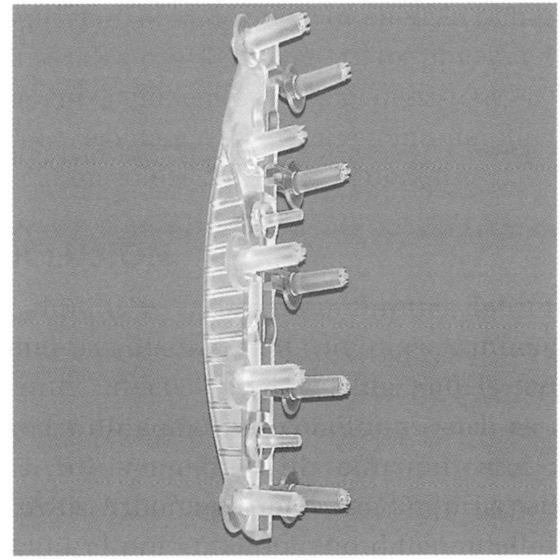

Fig. 2: Commercially available multitest plastic disposable lancet.

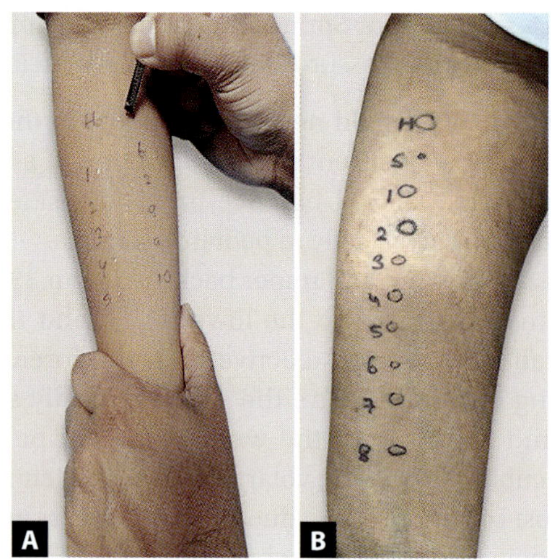

Figs. 3A and B: Skin prick test (SPT) being performed.

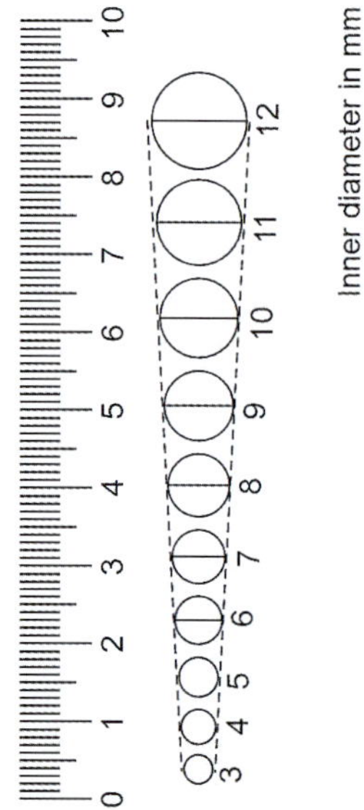

Fig. 4: Scale to measure wheal size in skin prick test (SPT).

the typical circular shape—is present, it should be noted separately (has higher clinical significance).

- *Interpretation:* A wheal measuring ≥3 mm larger than the negative control in response to an allergen is regarded as a positive indicator of hypersensitivity. A wheal size exceeding 8 mm correlates with a high positive predictive value.

In cases where standardized allergen extracts are not available, the *prick-prick test* may be employed, especially for evaluating fresh food allergens. In this technique, a sterile lancet is first pricked into the fresh food (such as banana, apple, or guava) and then immediately used to prick the patient's skin. This method helps identify true food allergies when commercial extracts are unreliable or unavailable, which is particularly relevant in the dietary context.

Limitations and Pitfalls

- *False positives:*
    - Dermographism (exaggerated skin reactivity)
    - Improper technique or contaminated lancets
    - High allergen concentration or irritant preservatives
    - Intradermal/subcutaneous puncture
- *False negatives:*
    - Recent antihistamine use
    - Improper storage or expired allergen extracts
    - Anergy due to immunosuppression or severe eczema
    - Poor technique with insufficient skin penetration

Advantages

- Immediate results (within 15–20 minutes)
- Cost-effective
- High sensitivity and specificity in the hands of trained personnel
- Well accepted by older children when conducted in a friendly environment.

INTRADERMAL TEST

Intradermal testing involves the use of a hypodermic syringe and needle to inject a small volume (0.02–0.05 mL) of allergen extract into the dermis, creating a raised bleb approximately 3 mm in diameter. This method is more sensitive than skin prick or puncture tests, and it generally yields more consistent and reproducible results. Intradermal testing is widely utilized in medicine for diagnosing both infectious **(Table 2)** and noninfectious **(Table 3)** conditions, operating on the principles of immediate (type I) and delayed (type IV) hypersensitivity reactions.

Principle and Mechanism

The IDT introduces allergen into the superficial dermis, eliciting an IgE-mediated response. The test is more sensitive than SPT but less specific, increasing the risk of false positives. Like SPT, IDT detects sensitization—presence of specific IgE in the dermis—but it does not confirm clinical allergy in isolation. Due to its higher sensitivity, IDT may detect low-level sensitization even

TABLE 2: Intradermal tests: Indications for infectious conditions.

Intradermal test	*Disease*
Bacterial infections	
Tuberculin test (Mantoux test)	Tuberculosis
Lepromin test	Leprosy
Frei's test	Lymphogranuloma venereum
Ito Reenstierna test	Chancroid
Foshay test	Bartonellosis
Dick's test	Scarlet fever
Anthraxin test	Human anthrax
Fungal infections	
Candidin test	Candidiasis
Trichophytin test	Dermatophytosis due to *Trichophyton* spp.
Coccidioidin test	Coccidioidomycosis
Histoplasmin test	Histoplasmosis
Parasitic infections	
Montenegro test	Leishmaniasis
Onchocerciasis skin test	Onchocerciasis (river blindness)

TABLE 3: Intradermal tests: Indications for noninfectious diseases.

Intradermal test	*Remarks*
Intradermal test in acute urticaria	Detects type I hypersensitivity to drugs or allergens
Autologous serum skin test	Diagnosis of autoimmune urticaria
Kveim–Siltzbach test	Detects sarcoid antigen; supports sarcoidosis diagnosis
Pathergy test	Nonspecific hypersensitivity in pyoderma gangrenosum, Behçet's disease
Autoerythrocyte sensitization test	Diagnosis of autoerythrocyte sensitization or Gardner–Diamond syndrome
Pilocarpine test	Assesses nerve integrity; detects hypohidrosis in leprosy
Histamine test	Assesses nerve integrity; detects neural deficit in leprosy

in nonallergic individuals. Therefore, it should only be interpreted alongside a detailed clinical history. A positive IDT in an asymptomatic patient should not be mistaken for allergy.

Indications

- Venom allergy when SPT is negative but history is suggestive

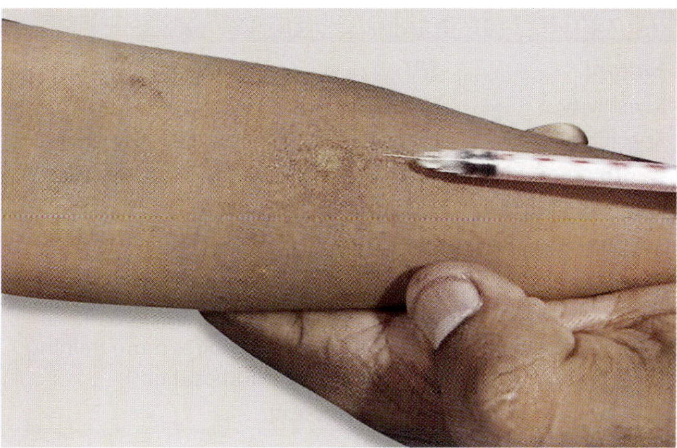

Fig. 5: Intradermal test.

- Beta-lactam allergy evaluation
- Perioperative drug allergy workup
- Select cases of latex allergy.

Technique

- Inject 0.02–0.05 mL diluted allergen intradermally.
- A bleb of 3 mm is expected **(Fig. 5)**.

Interpretation

The ideal time to assess the test reaction varies based on the pharmacological substance administered and the specific type of immune response being evaluated. For IDTs aimed at detecting type I hypersensitivity reaction, reading is taken after 20–30 minutes and for delayed-type hypersensitivity (DTH), readings are typically taken at 48 hours, though they may be assessed as early as 12 hours or as late as 4 days' post injection. A positive test is indicated by a ≥3 mm increase in wheal from baseline but when interpreting type IV hypersensitivity reactions, the measurement of induration is considered more significant than the presence of erythema.

Pediatric Relevance

The IDT is used cautiously in children due to increased pain and risk of systemic reaction. It must be conducted in a monitored environment by experienced staff.

Pitfalls

- High rate of false positives
- Greater risk of systemic reactions than SPT
- Requires skill and experience.

The differences between SPT and IDT are enumerated in **Table 4**.

TABLE 4: Comparison of SPT versus IDT.

Feature	*SPT*	*IDT*
Sensitivity	Moderate	High
Specificity	High	Lower
Pain/discomfort	Minimal	Moderate to significant
Risk of anaphylaxis	Very low	Higher
Suitable in children	Yes	With caution
Indications	First-line for most allergens	Reserved for select scenarios
Cost and logistics	Low, simple	Requires more training and caution

(IDT: intradermal test; SPT: skin prick test)

DRUG PROVOCATION TEST

The drug provocation test (DPT) is considered the gold standard to confirm or exclude drug hypersensitivity when skin testing is inconclusive or not validated. It involves administering the suspected drug in increasing doses under controlled conditions.

Indications

- Suspected beta-lactam allergy with negative skin tests
- Nonsteroidal anti-inflammatory drug (NSAID) hypersensitivity evaluation
- To confirm tolerance to alternative drugs

Procedure

- Performed in a hospital setting with resuscitation facilities
- Begin with 1/100th or 1/10th of therapeutic dose
- Gradually increase to full dose under observation

Contraindications

- History of severe anaphylaxis
- Uncontrolled asthma or cardiovascular disease
- Pregnancy

Clinical Relevance

Though used selectively, DPT plays a crucial role in reintroducing essential antibiotics in children falsely labeled as allergic, thereby reducing antibiotic resistance and optimizing therapy.

NASAL PROVOCATION TEST

The nasal provocation test (NPT) is a diagnostic procedure in which the nasal mucosa is exposed to a specific allergen under controlled conditions to reproduce allergic symptoms such as sneezing, rhinorrhea, nasal obstruction, and itching. It is primarily used to confirm allergic rhinitis, especially in cases with inconclusive history or conflicting skin and serological test results.

Indications

- Confirmation of allergic rhinitis diagnosis, especially in multisensitized patients
- Resolving discrepancies between clinical history and skin/serological test results
- Assessing degree of sensitivity to specific allergens
- Evaluating efficacy and safety of rhinitis treatments
- Monitoring response to specific immunotherapy
- Etiological study of occupational allergic respiratory diseases

Contraindications

- Uncontrolled asthma or severe chronic obstructive pulmonary disease (COPD)
- Significant nasal obstruction or septal perforation
- Recent nasal surgery (within 6–8 weeks)
- Recent respiratory infection (within 4 weeks)
- Pregnancy

Methodology

- *Preparation:* Avoid drugs that modify nasal response (e.g., antihistamines, corticosteroids) before the test; patient should be asymptomatic
- *Allergen application:* Usually bilateral; applied via micropipette, nasal spray, or impregnated disk to inferior turbinate
- *Dosing:* Start with low concentration (e.g., 1:1,000 of SPT concentration) and increase stepwise
- *Monitoring:* Symptom scoring plus objective nasal obstruction assessment (acoustic rhinometry, rhinomanometry, or nasal peak inspiratory flow).

Assessment Criteria for Positivity

- Symptom score increase ≥5 points
- *Acoustic rhinometry:* ≥25% reduction in minimal cross-sectional area or nasal volume (2–6 cm from nostril)
- *Rhinomanometry:* ≥100% increase in total nasal airway resistance
- *Nasal peak inspiratory flow:* ≥40% reduction

Applications

- Research on pathophysiology of nasal allergic responses
- Drug efficacy studies
- Occupational allergy diagnosis

PATCH TEST

Immunologic Basis

The PT evaluates type IV DTH reactions, also known as cell-mediated immunity. These reactions are mediated by antigen-specific T lymphocytes. On initial exposure, metals such as nickel, fragrances, preservatives or drugs bind to skin proteins to form hapten–protein complexes, which are processed by Langerhans cells and presented to naïve T cells in the regional lymph nodes.

Upon re-exposure, memory T cells in the dermis recognize the allergen and become activated. They release cytokines like interferon γ (IFN-γ), tumor necrosis factor α (TNF-α), and interleukin 17 (IL-17), leading to skin inflammation and recruitment of immune cells. This results in the characteristic delayed erythematous and vesicular reaction, typically observed 48–72 hours after allergen application.

Because this mechanism is distinct from the IgE-mediated type I hypersensitivity reactions seen in SPT and IDT, patch testing is particularly valuable for diagnosing ACD and other delayed hypersensitivity disorders. It is essential in diagnosing ACD.

Sensitization versus Allergy in Patch Testing

Patch testing identifies delayed-type sensitization. A positive PT means that the immune system has been sensitized to a substance through prior exposure. However, clinical correlation is essential, as not all sensitizations cause symptoms. For example, a child may react to nickel in the test but not develop dermatitis unless exposed through skin contact. Hence, interpretation must be symptom-driven.

Indications (Table 5)

- Chronic or recurrent dermatitis not responsive to treatment
- Suspected ACD due to cosmetics, metals, rubber, topical drugs
- Aggravation of atopic dermatitis by topical products
- Occupational dermatitis

TABLE 5: International Contact Dermatitis Research Group (ICDRG) criteria for patch test interpretation.

Grade	Reaction description
Negative (–)	No visible reaction
Doubtful (±)	Faint erythema only; no infiltration
Weak positive (+)	Erythema, infiltration, possibly papules
Strong positive (++)	Erythema, infiltration, papules, and vesicles
Extreme (+++)	Intense erythema, infiltration, coalescing vesicles, bullae, or ulceration

Components of Patch Test

A typical PT system includes the following key components:

- *Allergen preparations:* Predosed, standardized allergens series (Indian Standard Series, TRUE Test) in a vehicle (usually petrolatum or aqueous base). Examples include nickel sulfate, fragrance mix, parthenium, neomycin, and potassium dichromate.
- *Chambers:* Small aluminum or plastic discs (e.g., Finn chambers) designed to hold allergens and apply them to the skin under occlusion
- *Adhesive strips:* Hypoallergenic tape to secure the chambers onto the upper back for 48 hours
- *Control substances:* Sometimes included to identify irritant reactions or baseline skin reactivity
- *Scoring and grading chart:* Based on International Contact Dermatitis Research Group (ICDRG) criteria for standardized interpretation **(Table 5)**.

These components ensure safe, reproducible, and interpretable testing for DTH reactions.

Procedure

- Apply standard allergens (typically 20–30 allergens) on discs mounted on hypoallergenic tape.
- Affix to the child's back or thigh in smaller children **(Fig. 6)**.
- Leave occluded for 48 hours.
- First reading at 48 hours and second at 72 or 96 hours.

False Positives and False Negatives in Patch Testing

False positives may occur due to:

- Irritant reactions rather than true allergic responses
- Occlusion-induced irritation, especially with certain vehicles (e.g., aqueous base)

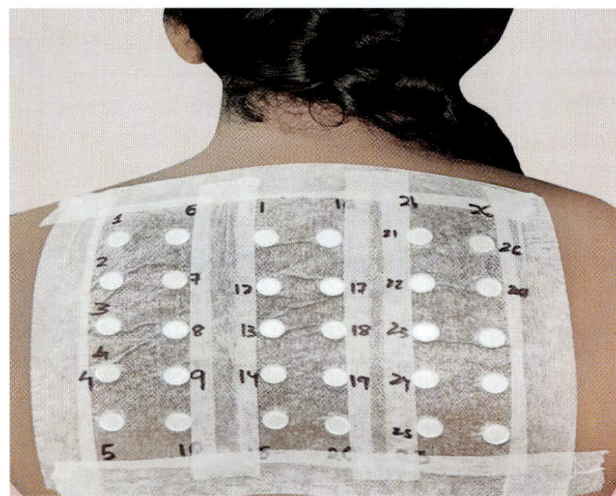

Fig. 6: Patch test.

- High concentrations or impurities in allergen preparations
- Testing over damaged or inflamed skin

False negatives may occur due to:
- Use of degraded or improperly stored allergens
- Testing in immunosuppressed individuals (e.g., on corticosteroids)
- Short exposure time or premature removal of patches
- Testing outside the flare phase of dermatitis
- Low concentration of allergen or poor penetration.

Proper patient preparation, technique, and interpretation are essential to minimize these errors.

Cross-sensitivity in Patch Testing

Cross-sensitivity refers to an immune response triggered by a substance that shares structural or functional similarities with another allergen to which the patient is already sensitized. In patch testing, this phenomenon may result in multiple positive reactions that are not due to separate sensitizations but shared antigenic determinants.

Examples include:
- Fragrance mix and balsam of Peru
- Neomycin and other aminoglycosides
- Paraphenylenediamine (PPD) and hair dyes or textile dyes
- Thiuram mix and carbamates.

Cross-sensitivities must be interpreted cautiously and correlated with clinical relevance. PT results should be contextualized with the patient's exposure history and symptom profile to avoid unnecessary allergen avoidance or mislabeling.

TABLE 6: Common allergens in India (Indian Standard Series).

Sr. No.	*Patch test allergen*
1.	Vaseline (control)
2.	Perubalsam
3.	Formaldehyde
4.	Mercaptobenzothiazole
5.	Potassium dichromate
6.	Nickel sulfate
7.	Cobalt sulfate
8.	Colophony
9.	Epoxy resins
10.	Parabens mix
11.	Paraphenylenediamine
12.	Parthenium
13.	Neomycin sulfate
14.	Benzocaine
15.	Wool alcohols
16.	Chlorocresol
17.	Fragrance mix
18.	Thiuram mix
19.	Nitrofurazone
20.	Black rubber mix

Clinical Relevance

Children increasingly experience contact dermatitis due to:
- Exposure to metals (jewellery, school accessories)
- Cosmetics (lip balms, nail polish)
- Topical antibiotics and steroids.

Patch testing, though underutilized in children, is safe and reliable. It helps identify avoidable allergens and prevent recurrences. Common allergens used are enumerated in **Table 6**.

Contraindications

- Extensive eczema, dermatitis, or broken skin over the test area
- Active dermatologic infections or recent severe sunburn at the test site
- Uncontrolled asthma or severe systemic allergic disease
- Recent anaphylaxis or high risk for systemic reactions (for SPT/IDT)
- Use of immunosuppressive therapy or systemic corticosteroids in high doses
- Pregnancy (for IDT and drug provocation)

TABLE 7: Choosing the right test.

Clinical situation	*Preferred test*
Allergic rhinitis or asthma	SPT
Chronic eczema/possible ACD	PT
Venom/drug allergy	SPT → IDT (if needed)
Food allergy	SPT ± oral food challenge

(ACD: allergic contact dermatitis; IDT: intradermal test; PT: patch test; SPT: skin prick test)

- Inability to follow-up (particularly important in patch testing).

Limitations

- Requires multiple visits
- Not suitable during active flare-ups or in high humidity seasons
- May induce flare in underlying eczema.

Special Considerations

- Use pediatric-friendly chambers.
- Allergen relevance must be established in clinical context.
- Educate caregivers about avoidance strategies.

The relevance of these tests in probable clinical scenarios is enumerated in **Table 7**.

COADEX SYSTEM APPROACH

The *COADEX system* is a structured approach for interpreting allergy test results by correlating them with *C*linical history, *O*nset of symptoms, *A*llergen exposure, *D*uration of symptoms, *E*xclusion of differential diagnoses, and e*X*acerbating/relieving factors. It ensures that test results are clinically relevant, reducing misdiagnosis from mere sensitization.

QUENCHING

Quenching refers to the suppression or masking of allergic reactions during in vivo testing due to various internal or external factors. It is especially relevant in patients undergoing testing while on antihistamines, corticosteroids, or other immunomodulatory agents. Quenching can result in false-negative results by inhibiting mast cell degranulation or dampening T-cell responses. To minimize quenching, medications should be withheld for appropriate durations prior to testing, and testing should be deferred during active infections or systemic inflammation.

CONCLUSION

In vivo allergy testing—SPT, IDT, and PT—forms an essential pillar of pediatric allergy diagnosis. In India where access to advanced in vitro diagnostics may be limited and environmental exposures are highly variable, these tests offer a practical, cost-effective, and reliable means to establish allergic sensitizations and guide evidence-based treatment.

A tailored approach based on clinical history, regional exposures, and child-specific factors ensures the most judicious use of in vivo testing. Pediatricians, allergists, and general practitioners must be familiar with these tools, integrating them into routine practice to improve diagnostic accuracy and long-term outcome in childhood allergy.

KEY POINTS

- *SPT, IDT, and PT are complementary tools* for diagnosing allergic diseases, targeting different hypersensitivity mechanisms.
- *SPT is the first-line test in children*—it is safe, minimally invasive, and highly informative for IgE-mediated allergy.
- *IDT offers higher sensitivity but lower specificity*, with greater risk of systemic reactions; it is reserved for selected cases such as venom and drug allergy.
- *Patch testing is essential for delayed hypersensitivity*, particularly ACD and chronic eczema.
- *Accurate interpretation requires clinical correlation*—history, exposure, and context (e.g., COADEX approach)—to distinguish sensitization from true allergy.
- Region-specific allergens and careful pre-test preparation (avoiding interfering drugs) are critical for reliability in the Indian pediatric population.

SUGGESTED READING

1. Bernstein IL, Li JT, Bernstein DI, Hamilton R, Spector SL, Tan R, et al. Allergy diagnostic testing: An updated practice parameter. Ann Allergy Asthma Immunol. 2008;100(3 Suppl 3):S1-148.
2. Bousquet J, Heinzerling L, Bachert C, Papadopoulos NG, Bousquet PJ, Burney PG, et al. Practical guide to skin prick tests in allergy to aeroallergens. Allergy. 2012;67(1):18-24.
3. Gupta N, Agarwal P, Sachdev A, Gupta D. Allergy testing – An overview. Indian Pediatr. 2019;56:951-7.
4. Sharma VK, Chakrabarti A. Common contact sensitizers in India. In: Contact Dermatitis. New York: Springer; 2007. pp. 471-83.

9 CHAPTER

Functional and Advanced Diagnostic Tools in Pediatric Allergy

Hima Mathews P

INTRODUCTION

In the new era of precision medicine, objective assessment of the airway function plays a crucial role in pediatric allergy. New advancements in the allergy diagnosis provide valuable information on upper and lower airway structure and function, airway pathologies, and measures to assess the effectiveness of medical and surgical intervention. Common procedures include direct nasal endoscopy (DNE), rhinometry and rhinomanometry, spirometry, peak expiratory flow rate (PEFR) measurement, impulse oscillometry (IOS), and FeNO measurement. Understanding these diagnostic modalities is essential for accurate diagnosis and management of respiratory allergies in children.

DIRECT NASAL ENDOSCOPY

Nasal endoscopy is a minimally invasive diagnostic tool, which helps in direct and magnified visualization of the nose, paranasal sinuses (PNS), and nasopharynx. It utilizes a thin, flexible, or rigid tube with a light source and camera to visualize the internal structures of the nose and sinuses. The endoscope is gently inserted into the nostrils, allowing real-time examination of the nasal mucosa, turbinates, septum, and sinus openings on the attached monitor.

Indications of nasal endoscopy include the following:

- Diagnose diseases of nose and PNS.
- Identify the source of bleeding in epistaxis.
- Assess the medical and surgical treatment response in diseases of nose and PNS.
- Take biopsy from nose and nasopharynx.

Indications for DNE in allergic rhinitis (AR):

- DNE helps to confirm the diagnosis of AR by visualizing signs of allergic inflammation like mucosa, especially in cases of diagnostic uncertainty.
- It aids in detecting complications like nasal polyps or chronic sinusitis early.
- DNE provides insights to make personalized treatment plans—both medical and surgical.
- It helps to assess the treatment response and monitor the progress by direct visualization of the degree of inflammation of nasal mucosa.
- It helps to determine the necessity of surgical intervention like sinus surgeries.

Direct Nasal Endoscopy Procedure and Technique

The nasal cavity is decongested with gauze soaked with xylometazoline and a topical anesthetic agent xylocaine for 5 minutes before introducing the endoscope. The endoscope is gently inserted into a nostril, allowing examination of the nasal cavity, sinuses, and nasopharynx, including the mucosa, presence of polyps **(Figs. 1A and B)**, secretions, or any other abnormalities **(Fig. 2)**.

- *First pass (inferior pass):* The endoscope is introduced along the floor of the nasal cavity toward the nasopharynx. The first structure seen will be the inferior meatus and opening of the nasolacrimal duct. Then it is advanced posteriorly to examine the nasopharynx including the openings of the Eustachian tubes and fossa of Rosenmuller.
- *Second pass:* The scope is passed between the middle and inferior turbinates which allows for detailed inspection of the middle meatus, sphenoethmoid recess, ostia of sphenoid sinus, and superior turbinate. While withdrawing, the scope is laterally rotated to see infundibulum, uncinate process, and bulla ethmoidalis.
- *Third pass:* This pass focuses on areas like the olfactory cleft and any lesions or polyps present in that region.

Even though generally safe, potential complications of DNE include adverse reactions to anesthetic or decongestant, pain or discomfort, epistaxis, and vasovagal episodes.

Key learning points:

- DNE is a valuable tool in diagnosing and managing AR.
- It provides a detailed view of the nasal passages and sinuses, aiding in accurate diagnosis, complication

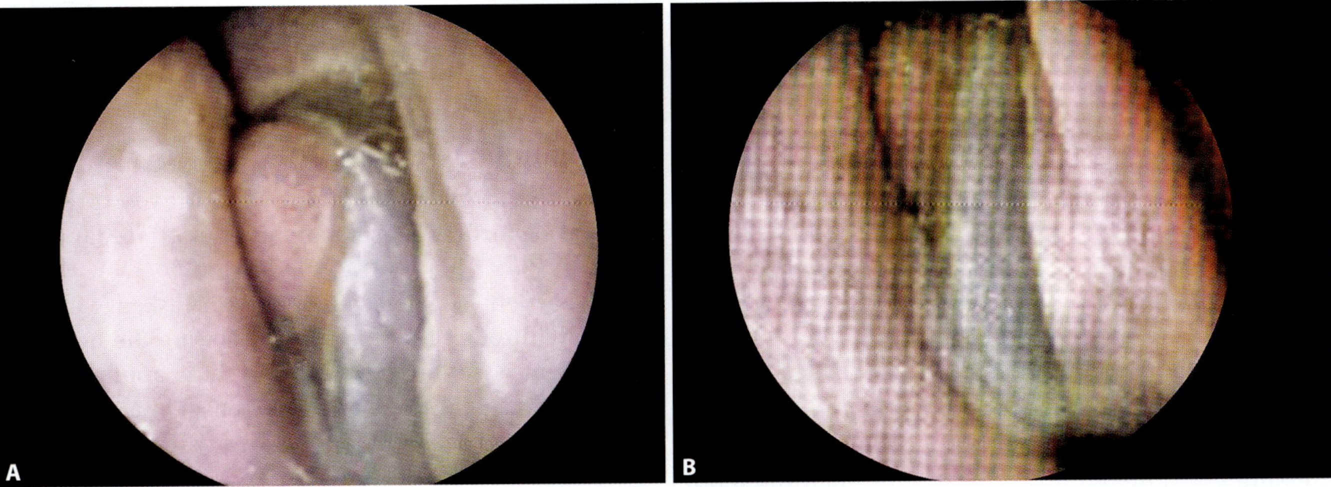

Figs. 1A and B: Direct nasal endoscopy (DNE) showing nasal polyp.

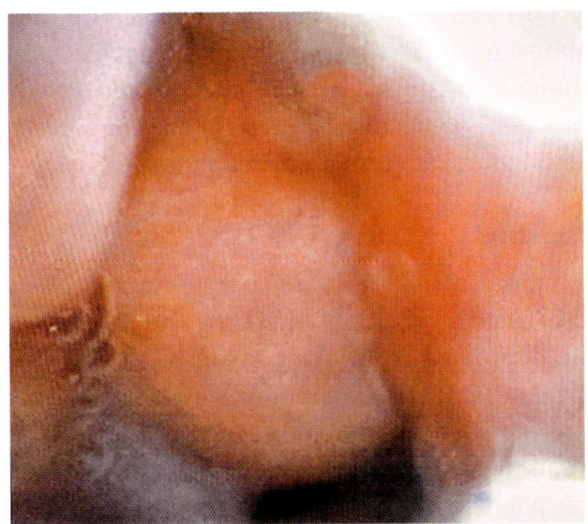

Fig. 2: Direct nasal endoscopy (DNE) showing grade 4 adenoid hypertrophy.

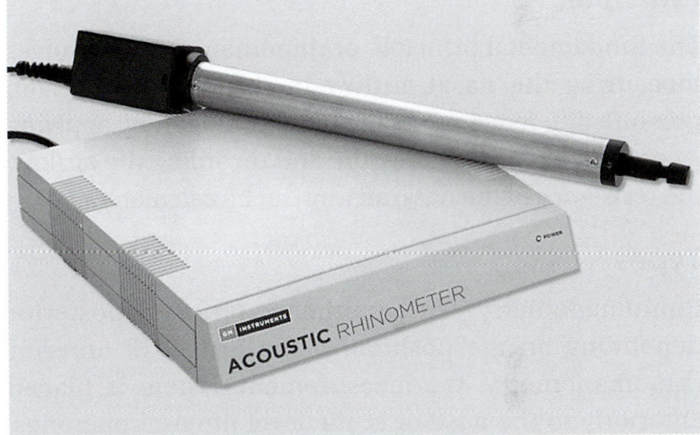

Fig. 3: Acoustic rhinometer.

detection, and personalized treatment, which improves patient outcomes.

RHINOMETRY

Rhinometry is an objective assessment method used to evaluate nasal airflow and patency. It encompasses various techniques, including rhinomanometry, acoustic rhinometry, and optical rhinometry **(Fig. 3)**.

It measures the geometry of the nasal cavity, including cross-sectional area and volume. Acoustic rhinometry uses acoustic waves to map the nasal passages, and the reflected sound waves are analyzed to find out the dimensions of the nasal cavity. The time delay of these reflections indicates the distance from the nostril, while the magnitude of the reflections reveals the cross-sectional area at that point. Finally, an area-distance graph is generated, often with a characteristic "W" shape, providing a topographic map of the nasal passage.

Role of acoustic rhinometry in assessing nasal obstruction:

- From the area-distance graph, the area of constrictions can be identified.
- It can differentiate between structural anomalies and mucosal inflammation.
- It can be used in monitoring the treatment response.

Limitations:

- Being a static measurement not suitable to identify dynamic changes in nasal airflow
- Nasal congestion can affect the accuracy of recording.

- Require highly skilled operator
- Not suitable for primary diagnosis of AR

Key points:
- Acoustic rhinometry is a noninvasive tool to assess nasal obstruction.
- Role of acoustic rhinometry is limited in diagnosing AR.
- It has a role in research being a safe noninvasive procedure.

RHINOMANOMETRY IN ALLERGIC RHINITIS

Rhinomanometry is a diagnostic tool used to measure the airflow and nasal airway resistance. It measures the pressure encountered by air passing through the nasal cavity using an equipment which measure airflow and resistance while breathing.

Principle

The fundamental principle of rhinomanometry involves measuring the nasal airflow in response to a given pressure difference across the nasal passages. By applying a constant or variable pressure and recording the airflow, the resistance of the nasal airway can be calculated.

Types

Rhinomanometry can be either anterior or posterior depending on the position of the probe. In anterior rhinomanometry, the measurement system is placed anteriorly to the nose or at the level of nasal openings. Posterior rhinomanometry requires placement of an intraoral device to detect choanal pressure. Both methods can be active or passive depending on whether the patient is spontaneously or holding breath with a predetermined flow is allowed to pass through nose.

Role of Rhinomanometry

1. Rhinomanometry provides quantitative data on nasal airway resistance, and hence the degree of nasal obstruction caused by allergic inflammation can be assessed.
2. It allows clinicians to measure the severity of nasal airflow limitation which correlates with the disease severity.
3. It can be used to assess the treatment response.
4. It helps distinguish between allergic-related nasal obstruction and other causes such as structural abnormalities (e.g., deviated septum).
5. It can be used in research studies including the nasal function and pathophysiology in AR and other nasal disorders.

Equipment and Procedure

A rhinomanometry machine includes a pressure transducer, airflow sensor, computer interface, and face mask.

The patient is seated comfortably and asked to breathe normally through the nose. After clearing the nose, the equipment is calibrated. A face mask is applied to the patient with a tight seal. A pressure sensor or a specialized mask is placed at the nostril or used with a nasal insert to measure intranasal pressure. A flow sensor, such as a pneumotachograph, measures airflow. The patient breathes normally or performs controlled breathing. The device records the pressure difference inside the nasal cavity and the airflow simultaneously. The software calculates nasal resistance by dividing the pressure difference by airflow during inhalation and exhalation. The process is typically repeated to ensure consistency, and readings are documented for analysis **(Fig. 4)**.

Limitations

- The nasal resistance vales can be unreliable as the nasal cycle is constantly changing and dynamic.
- The degree of nasal obstruction perceived may not correlate with the rhinomanometric values.
- Active anterior rhinomanometry is difficult to perform in complete nasal obstruction.
- The machine is not freely available and hence restricted mainly to research purposes.

Key Points

- Rhinomanometry serves as a tool for objectively assessing nasal patency and airflow resistance in AR.
- It requires a complex and high maintenance equipment; hence, it is suitable mainly for research purposes.

SPIROMETRY

Spirometry is a simple test which measures lung volume changes during forced breathing maneuvers with graphical display along with the numerical values, which gives an estimation of lung function, and it is a good tool for the diagnosis of airway obstruction and follow-up for asthma and chronic obstructive pulmonary disease (COPD).

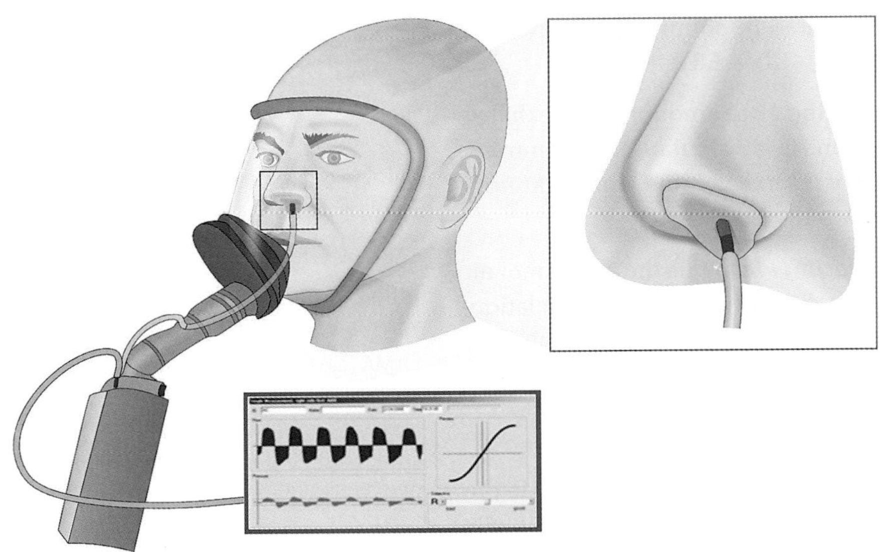

Fig. 4: Technique of performing rhinomanometry.

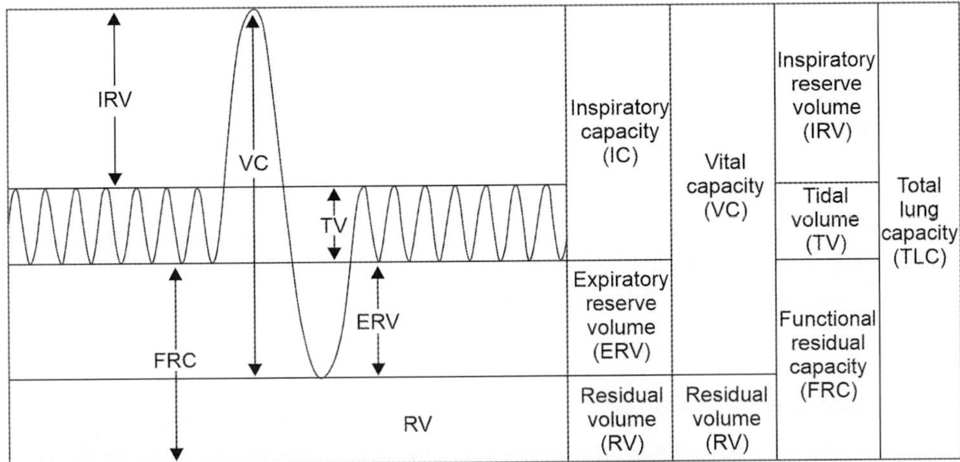

Fig. 5: Normal lung volumes and capacities.

Lung volume is divided according to normal physiologic function, and each subdivision is called a volume, whereas any combination of two or more volumes is called a capacity.

Lung Volumes (Fig. 5)

Tidal volume (TV): The volume of air inhaled or exhaled during each respiratory cycle

Expiratory reserve volume (ERV): It is the volume of air that can be exhaled forcibly after exhalation of normal tidal volume.

Inspiratory reserve volume (IRV): It is the amount of air that can be forcibly inhaled after a normal tidal volume. IRV is usually kept in reserve but is used during deep breathing.

Residual volume (RV): The volume of air remaining in the lungs after a maximal exhalation

Lung Capacities (Fig. 5)

Inspiratory capacity (IC): It is the maximum volume of air that can be inhaled following a resting state. It is calculated from the sum of inspiratory reserve volume and tidal volume. IC = IRV + TV.

Total lung capacity (TLC): It is the maximum volume of air the lungs can accommodate or sum of all volume compartments or volume of air in lungs after maximum inspiration. TLC is calculated by summation of the four primary lung volumes . TV + IRV + ERV + RV.

Vital capacity (VC): It is the total amount of air exhaled after maximal inhalation. It is calculated by summing tidal volume, inspiratory reserve volume, and expiratory reserve volume. VC = TV + IRV + ERV.

Functional residual capacity (FRC): It is the amount of air remaining in the lungs at the end of a normal exhalation. It is calculated by adding together residual and expiratory reserve volumes. FRC = RV + ERV.

Spirometric Measures

Forced expiratory volume in 1 second (FEV_1): FEV_1 is the volume of air in liters that can be forcefully and maximally exhaled in the first second after a maximal inspiration. It is the volume of air that is exhaled in the first second of the forced vital capacity (FVC).

FVC: Volume of air in liters that can be forcefully and maximally exhaled after a maximal inspiration

FEV_1/FVC ratio: This ratio is used to differentiate an obstructive from a restrictive pattern. In obstructive disorders, FEV_1 decreases more significantly than FVC; hence, the ratio will be decreased and in restrictive disorders, the ratio is either normal or increased as the drop in FVC is either proportional to or more marked than the drop in FEV_1. It decreases with age; it is higher in children up to 0.9 and 0.7 in adults due to a decrease in elastic recoil of the lungs that occurs with aging.

Forced expiratory flow at 25 and 75% of the pulmonary volume ($FEF_{25\text{-}75\%}$): It is the mean forced expiratory flow (FEF) during the middle half of the FVC and measures average flow rates on the FVC segment and includes flow from medium-to-small airways. $FEF_{25\text{-}75\%}$ is supposed to be the most sensitive indicator of airflow in peripheral airways where primary airflow obstruction originates, and it is reduced in early bronchial impairment, which is associated with small airway disease.

Peak expiratory flow (PEF): It is the maximum flow (in L/s) of air during a forceful exhalation, which occurs immediately after the start of the exhalation and is effort-dependent. It can be also measured with a peak flow meter.

Checklist to avoid before a spirometry test:

- Check the medications list **(Table 1)**
- Smoking within 1 hour (to avoid bronchoconstriction)
- Consuming alcohol within 4 hours and other intoxicants within 8 hours before testing (as it can affect coordination, comprehension, and physical ability)
- Performing vigorous exercise within 1 hour (to avoid exercise-induced bronchospasm)
- Wearing restrictive clothing as it may prevent proper chest expansion
- Eating a large meal within 2 hours

TABLE 1: Withholding time of bronchodilators prior to spirometry.

Bronchodilator medication	*Withholding time (hours)*
SABA (e.g., albuterol or salbutamol)	4–6
SAMA (e.g., ipratropium bromide)	12
LABA (e.g., formoterol or salmeterol)	24
Ultra-LABA (e.g., indacaterol, vilanterol, or olodaterol)	36
LAMA (e.g., tiotropium, umeclidinium, aclidinium, or glycopyrronium)	36–48

(LABA: long-acting beta-agonist; LAMA: long-acting muscarinic antagonist; SABA: short-acting beta-agonist; SAMA: short-acting muscarinic antagonist)

Common Indications of Pediatric Spirometry

- Chronic cough
- Persistent wheezing
- Diagnosis and prognostication of asthma
- For assessing the control of asthma and disease activity of cystic fibrosis in children
- Preoperative spirometry is found to be helpful in assessing the postoperative lung status of the pediatric population
- Assessing the pediatric lung function, in transfusion-dependent thalassemia major and sickle cell anemia, connective tissue disorders, and chest wall deformities
- Effective tool for assessing the lung health of school going children

Contraindications

Although there is no absolute contraindication for spirometry, the following conditions are considered relative contraindications. If any of the following has occurred recently, then it may be better to wait until the patient has fully recovered before carrying out spirometry.

- *Cardiovascular:* Unstable cardiovascular status, recent myocardial infarction or pulmonary embolism,

uncontrolled systemic or pulmonary hypertension, significant arrythmias, cough syncope
- *Raised intracranial or intraocular pressure:* Cerebral aneurysms, recent concussion injury, recent eye surgery (1 week), or recent brain surgery (4 weeks)
- *Raised thoracic and abdominal pressure:* Hemoptysis of unknown origin, pneumothorax, recent thoracic or abdominal surgeries
- Sinus/middle ear infection or recent surgery, transmissible respiratory infections
- Any acute disorders affecting test performance, such as nausea or vomiting

Steps in Performing Spirometry

- Equipment performance criteria/equipment validation/quality control
- Prepare the child and ask history, recent illness, and medications.
- Check for contraindications. Enter the patient's demographics accurately, as well as age, gender, height, weight, and race.
- Explain the test. Instruct and demonstrate the test to the subject.
- *Sit upright:* Standing position and sitting up straight without leaning forward with no restrictions is the preferred posture.
- Feet should be flat on floor with legs uncrossed to avoid the use of abdominal muscles
- *Avoid tight-fitting clothing:* Tight clothes can give falsely lower volumes, i.e., restrictive pictures on spirometry. While exhaling maximally, patients can become light-headed and faint; hence, a chair with arms is preferred.

Technique

Before performing the forced expiration, normal tidal breaths can be taken initially followed by a deep breath taken with or without a mouthpiece, followed by a quick, full inspiration; that is, blast air out as hard and fast as possible and for as long as possible, followed by deep inspiration, measuring expiratory and inspiratory flow **(Figs. 6 to 9)**.

While performing spirometry in children:

- Explain the procedure to the child in a simple way and allow the child to have one or two practice trials in a relaxed fashion.
- Reemphasize by exaggerated demonstration rather than words on how to do it correctly with a positive reinforcement technique.
- Different interactive programs like games and animated incentives in software designed to encourage rapid and prolonged expiration help in pediatric spirometry.
- The study should be brief, lasting no more than 15 minutes, and if the patient cries during the study, there should be no further attempt, and the test should be done later only.
- Repeat for a minimum of three maneuvers.
- Check for acceptability **(Table 2)**, usability **(Table 2)**, and repeatability **(Box 1)** and perform more maneuvers as necessary.
- Check for bronchodilator responsiveness.
- Interpret the graph and values and assess the defect.

End of Forced Expiration Acceptability Criteria

Children as well as those with restrictive lung disease cannot expire long enough to achieve a plateau due to high elastic recoil and in that scenario, the measure of whether end of forced expiration (EOFE) has been reached is for the patient to repeatedly achieve the same FVC **(Flowchart 1)**.

- The best two measurements must fulfil the repeatability criteria.
- If the criteria are not met, more attempts are required.
- As performing forced exhalations is extremely tiring, a maximum of eight maneuvers are kept as an upper limit and beyond that point it is unlikely to obtain better values.
- Forced expiration can cause bronchoconstriction, so there must be ≥30 seconds in between the maneuvers. Asthmatics may require several minutes in between.

Factors Affecting Spirometry Values

- *Age:* Lung function generally increases with age up to ~25 years, then declines with increasing age afterward.
- *Sex:* Prepubescent males and females generally have the same lung function, but post puberty, the growth of the thorax is greater in males, giving marked differences in lung volumes.
- *Height:* The taller the person, the bigger the lungs.
- *Weight:* Weight affects lung function in that increasing weight causes increasing lung function until obesity is reached, after which it has the opposite effect.
- Ethnic origin
- *Smoking:* This can cause a more rapid decline in lung function compared with nonsmokers over time. It should not be adjusted for in predicted equations, since any reduction is abnormal.

TABLE 2: Acceptability and usability criteria (new ATS guidelines).

	Required for acceptability		Required for usability	
Acceptability and usability criterion	***FEV_1***	***FVC***	***FEV_1***	***FVC***
Must have BEV ≤5% of FVC or 0.100 L, whichever is greater	Yes	Yes	Yes	Yes
Must have no evidence of a faulty zero-flow setting	Yes	Yes	Yes	Yes
Must have no cough in the first second of expiration*	Yes	No	Yes	No
Must have no glottic closure in the first second of expiration*	Yes	Yes	Yes	Yes
Must have no glottic closure after 1 second of expiration	No	Yes	No	No
Must achieve one of these three EOFE indicators: 1. Expiratory plateau (≤0.025 L in the last 1 second of expiration) 2. Expiratory time ≥15 seconds 3. FVC is within the repeatability tolerance of or is greater than the largest prior observed FVC†*	No	Yes	No	No
Must have no evidence of obstructed mouthpiece or spirometer	Yes	Yes	No	No
Must have no evidence of a leak	Yes	Yes	No	No
If the maximal inspiration after EOFE is greater than FVC, then FIVC – FVC must be ≤0.100 L or 5% of FVC, whichever is greater‡	Yes	Yes	No	No

(BEV: back-extrapolated volume; EOFE: end of forced expiration; FEV_1: forced expiratory volume in 1 second; FIVC: forced inspiratory vital capacity; FVC: forced vital capacity)

*For children aged 6 years or younger, must have at least 0.75 seconds of expiration without glottic closure or cough for acceptable or usable measurement of $FEV_{0.75}$.

†Occurs when the patient cannot expire long enough to achieve a plateau (e.g., children with high elastic recoil or patients with restrictive lung disease) or when the patient inspires or comes off the mouthpiece before a plateau. For within-maneuver acceptability, the FVC must be greater than or within the repeatability tolerance of the largest FVC observed before this maneuver within the current prebronchodilator or the current post-bronchodilator testing set.

‡Although the performance of a maximal forced inspiration is strongly recommended, its absence does not preclude a maneuver from being judged acceptable, unless extrathoracic obstruction is specifically being investigated.

BOX 1: Repeatability criteria of spirometry (applied to acceptable FVC and FEV_1 values).

- *Age >6 years:* The difference between the two largest FVC values must be ≤0.150 L, and the difference between the two largest FEV_1 values must be ≤0.150 L
- *Age ≤6 years:* The difference between the two largest FVC values must be ≤0.100 L or 10% of the highest value, whichever is greater, and the difference between the two largest FEV_1 values must be ≤0.100 L or 10% of the highest value, whichever is greater

Flowchart 1: End of forced expiration (EOFE) acceptability criteria for forced vital capacity (FVC).

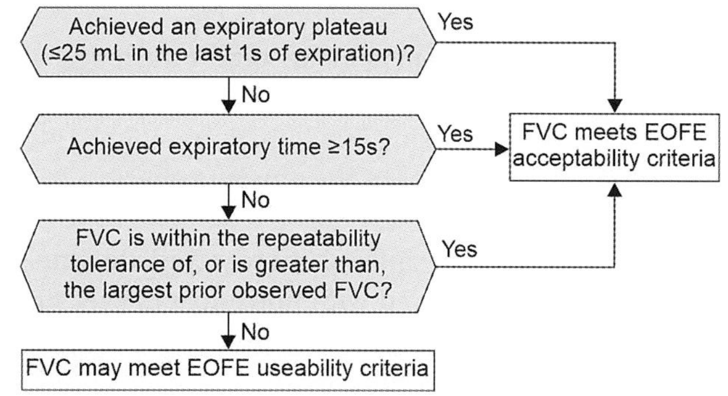

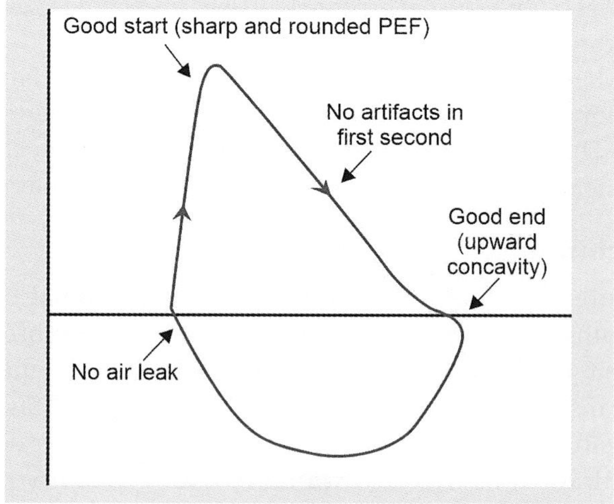

Fig. 6: Normal flow–volume loop. (PEF: peak expiratory flow)

Interpreting Spirometry

A normal spirometry test is characterized by FVC, FEV_1, and FEV_1/FVC, all within the normal range, even though spirometry values in the normal range cannot completely rule out lung disease, especially if the pretest probability

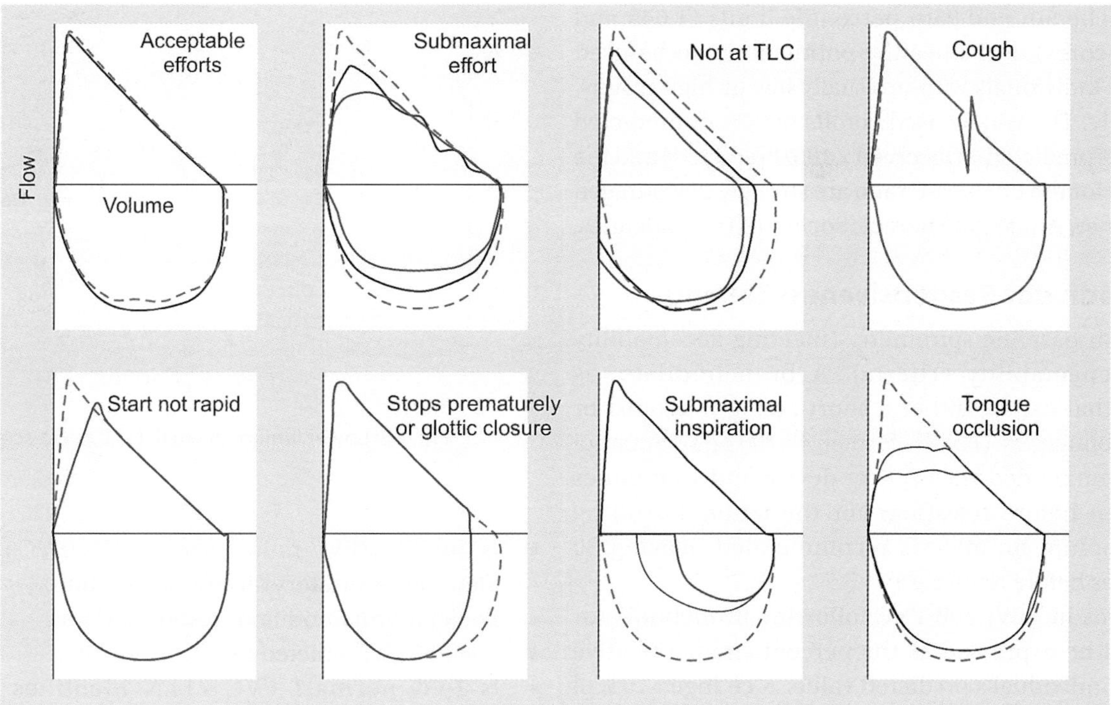

Fig. 7: Examples of unacceptable flow–volume spirometry loops.

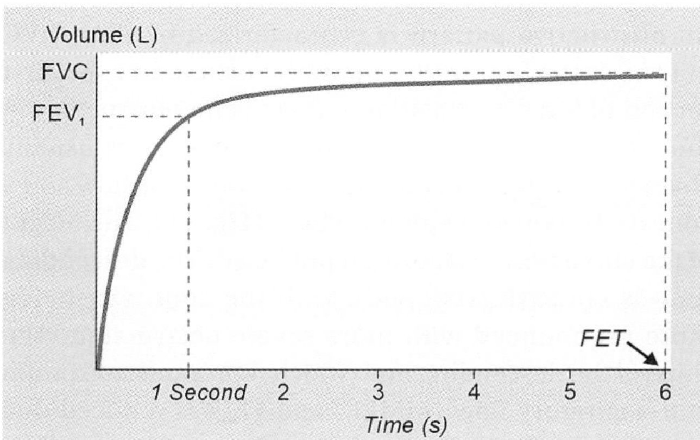

Fig. 8: Normal volume–time curve. (FET: forced expiratory time; FEV_1: forced expiratory volume in 1 second; FVC: forced vital capacity)

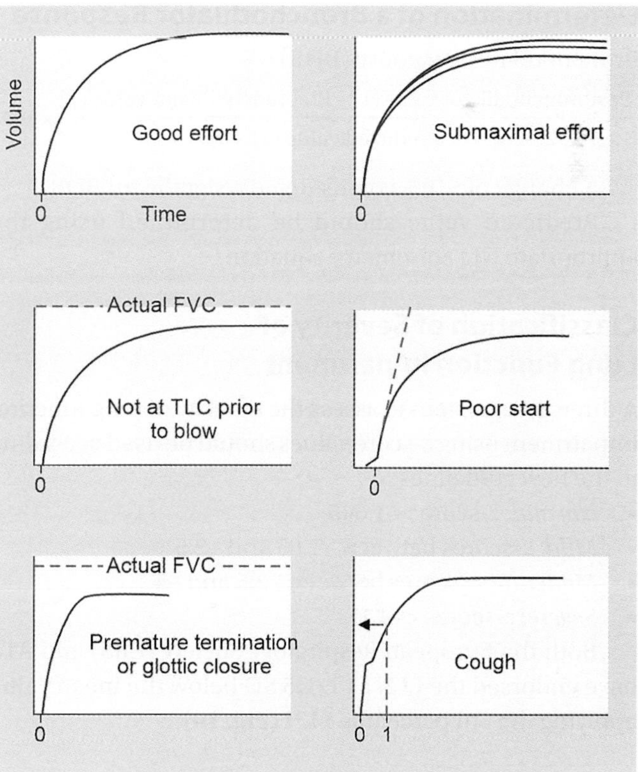

Fig. 9: Examples of unacceptable volume–time curve. (FVC: forced vital capacity; TLC: total lung capacity)

of disease is elevated and if the recorded values are near the lower limit of normal (LLN). A normal spirometry test cannot rule out asthma since many asthmatics spend most of their time with normal lung function.

The Global Lung Function Initiative (GLI) reference equations are available for spirometry which are internally consistent, providing a single suite of pulmonary function test (PFT) equations which will avoid discordant results between PFTs and potential misclassification. Limits of

Normal—The 5th and 95th percentile limits (1.645 and +1.645 *z*-scores) of the healthy population can be used to identify individuals with unusually low or high results, respectively. The widely used cutoffs of 80% of predicted for FEV_1 (% predicted = Observed × 100/Predicted) and the 0.70 cutoff for the FEV_1/FVC ratio are strongly discouraged as per the new American Thoracic Society (ATS) guidelines.

Bronchodilator Responsiveness Testing

- Perform baseline spirometry (meeting acceptability and repeatability criteria). A bronchodilator is given that can be either a short-acting β-agonist or anticholinergics. (For the former, 4 ×100 µg salbutamol is recommended via a spacer device and 15 minutes is given before retesting. For the latter, 4 × 40 µg ipratropium bromide is recommended, leaving 30 minutes before retesting.)
- Changes in FEV_1 and FVC following bronchodilator should be expressed as the percent change relative to the individual's predicted value. A change >10% of the predicted value in FEV_1 or FVC indicates a positive response.

Determination of a Bronchodilator Response

Bronchodilator Response (BDR) =

$$\frac{\text{Postbronchodilator value (1)} - \text{Prebronchodilator value (1)}}{\text{Predicted value (1)}} \times 100$$

A change of >10% is considered a significant BDR.

Predicted value should be determined using the appropriate GLI spirometry equation.

Classification of Severity of Lung Function Impairment

A three-level system to assess the severity of lung function impairment using *z*-score values should be used according to the new guidelines:

- *Normal: z*-score >–1.645
- *Mild: z*-scores between –1.65 and –2.5
- *Moderate: z*-scores between –2.5 and –4
- *Severe: z*-scores <–4.1

Both the European Respiratory Society (ERS) and ATS have endorsed the LLN as 1.645 SD below the mean value applying the 5th percentile LLN **(Fig. 10)**.

Identifying Abnormal Ventilatory Patterns

- Is the shape of the flow–volume curve normal?

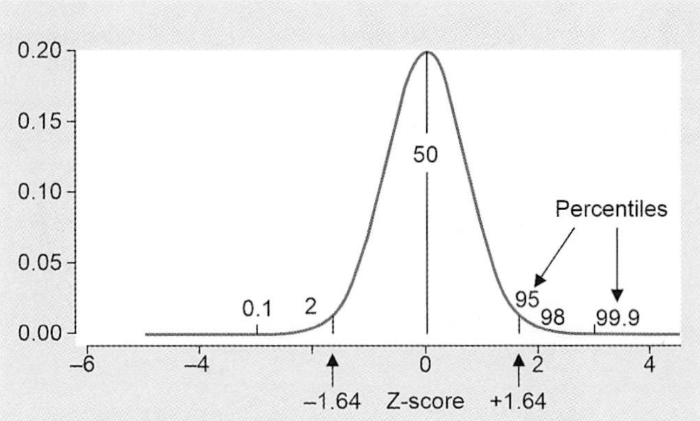

Fig. 10: Lower limit of normal (LLN) and *z*-score.

- Is the FEV_1/FVC ratio normal? FEV_1/FVC ratio <LLN identifies expiratory airflow obstruction.
- Look for bronchodilator responsiveness.
- Use FEV_1% predicted to assess severity.
- Is FVC normal? FVC <LLN identifies potential restriction.

Obstructive Pattern

An obstructive pattern is characterized by FEV_1/FVC <LLN. Most of the FVC should be exhaled in the first second of forced exhalation if there is no obstruction in the airways. Obstructive spirometry pattern is usually characterized by FEV_1 and shows a lower peak flow and a concave (scooped) expiratory loop **(Fig. 11)**. The height of the curve (PEF) is less than predicted. The descending limb is concave (scooped), with the concavity being more pronounced with more severe obstruction. The slope of the descending limb which represents maximum mid-expiratory flow (MMEF) and FEFs is reduced due to airflow limitation at low lung volumes. There will be significant bronchodilator responsiveness **(Figs. 12 and 13)**.

Restrictive Pattern

A restrictive pattern is characterized by FVC and FEV_1 below the LLN. Spirometry may suggest restrictive lung disease, and the restriction must be confirmed by measuring lung volumes and documenting a TLC value. The descending limb of the flow–volume (FV) curve will be steep. Restrictive impairment is classically characterized by a reduction in TLC below the LLN (5th percentile). FVC is reduced, FEV_1/FVC is normal or increased, and the

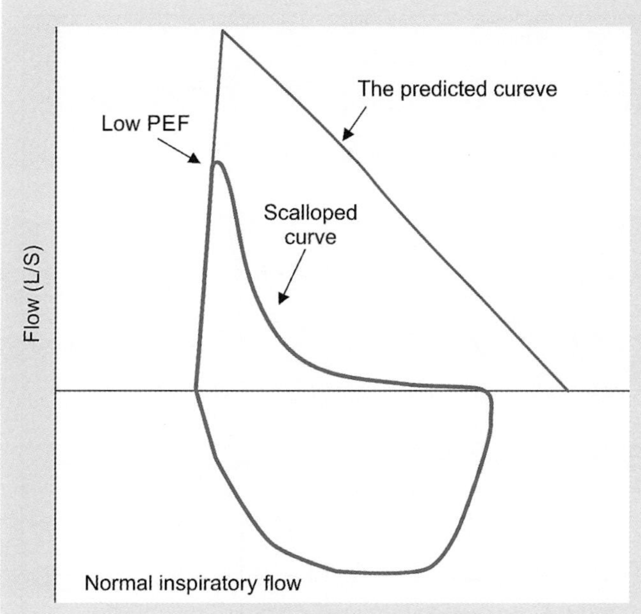

Fig. 11: Flow–volume loop showing an obstructive pattern. (PEF: peak expiratory flow).

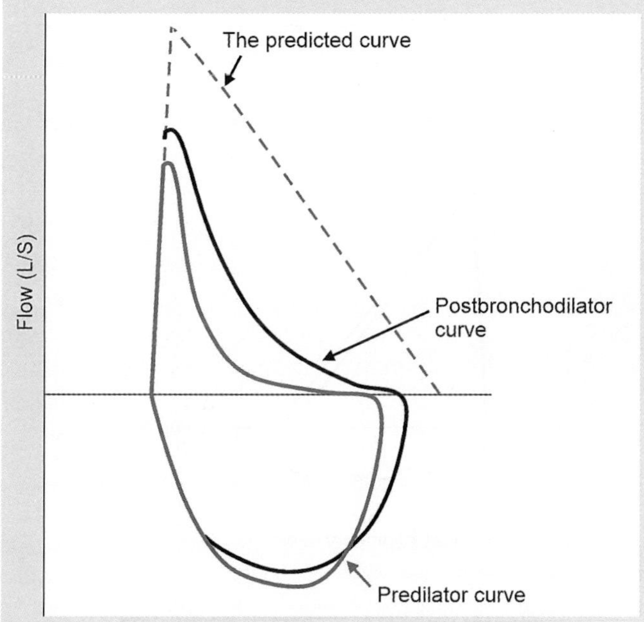

Fig. 12: Flow–volume loop showing significant bronchodilator responsiveness.

flow-volume curve shows a convex pattern (reflecting high elastic recoil). A high PEF with normal FEV_1 may be seen in early interstitial lung disease (ILD) before restriction limits FVC **(Figs. 14 and 15)**.

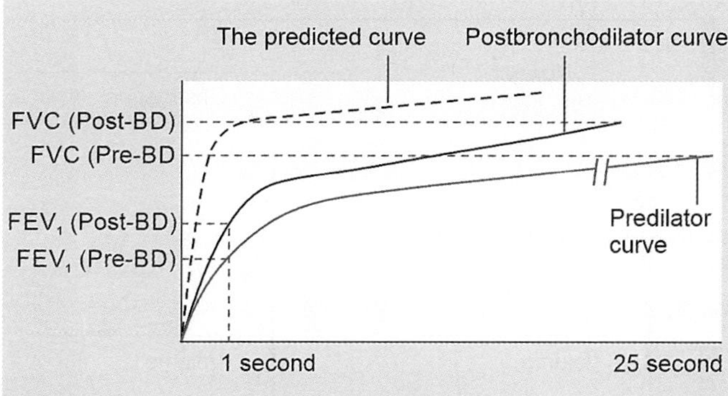

Fig. 13: Volume–time curve showing significant bronchodilator responsiveness. (FEV_1: forced expiratory volume in 1 second; FVC: forced vital capacity)

Spirometry in Upper Airway Obstruction

Variable Extrathoracic Obstruction

In variable extrathoracic obstruction, airway obstruction takes place during inspiration due to the negative pressure inside the airways (larynx, pharynx, and extrathoracic portion of trachea), and hence flow is reduced (flattened curve) during the inspiratory limb of the FV loop. The obstruction must be mobile or dynamic to follow this pattern **(Fig. 16)**.

Variable Intrathoracic Obstruction

In variable intrathoracic obstruction, the obstruction will be more pronounced during expiration. The expiratory component of the FV loop in intrathoracic upper airway obstruction is deformed throughout its entire length, starting right from the PEF **(Fig. 17)**.

Fixed Upper Airway Obstruction

Fixed upper airway obstruction (above or below the sternal notch) does not change with inspiration or expiration, and as a result, both the inspiratory and the expiratory components of the FV loop are flattened **(Fig. 18)**.

GINA Guidelines 2025 on Asthma Diagnosis in Children Using Spirometry

- *Postbronchodilator responsiveness (reversibility) test:* Increase in baseline FEV_1 from ≥12% predicted
- *Positive exercise challenge test:* Fall in baseline FEV_1 of >12% predicted with standardized exercise challenge
- *Excessive variation in lung function between the visits:* Variation in FEV_1 of ≥12% between visits
- *Increase in lung function after weeks of inhaled corticosteroid (ICS) containing treatment:* Increase in baseline FEV_1 from ≥12% predicted

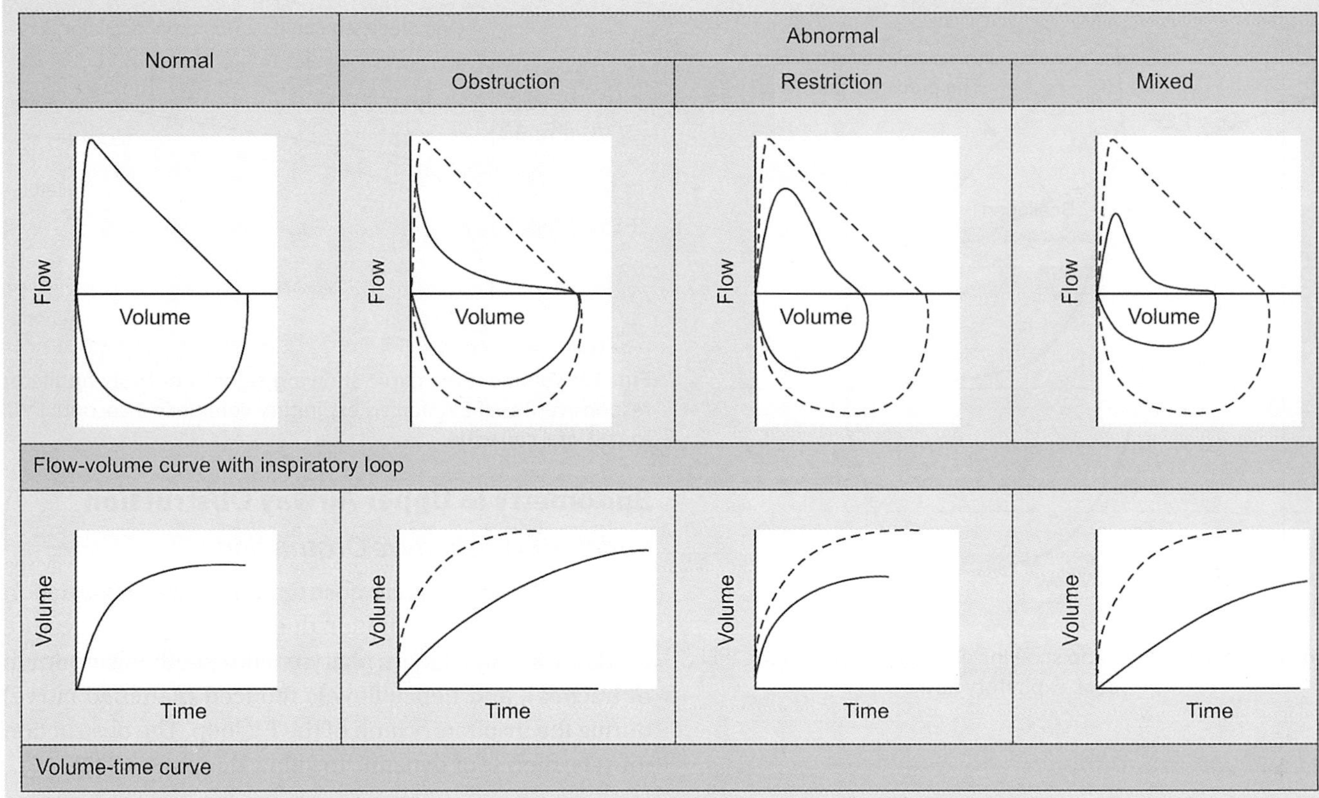

Fig. 14: Abnormal ventilatory patterns on spirometry curve.

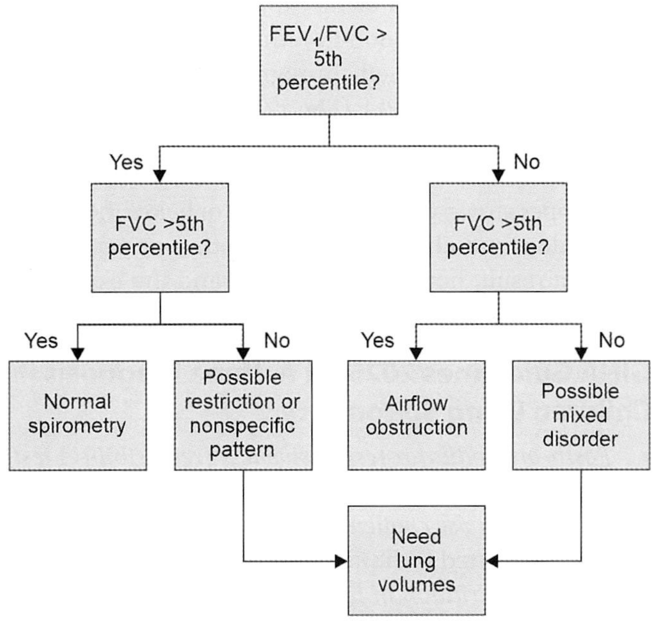

Fig. 15: Approach to interpretation of spirometry. (FEV_1: forced expiratory volume in 1 second; FVC: forced vital capacity)

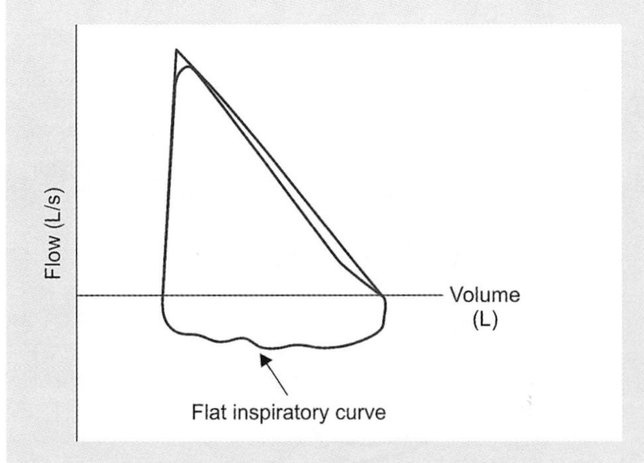

Fig. 16: Variable extrathoracic obstruction.

Key Points

- Spirometry is an important tool in diagnosing obstructive airway disease in children.
- A well-trained technician with a positive reinforcement technique can attain a good spirometry result even from the age of 5 years.

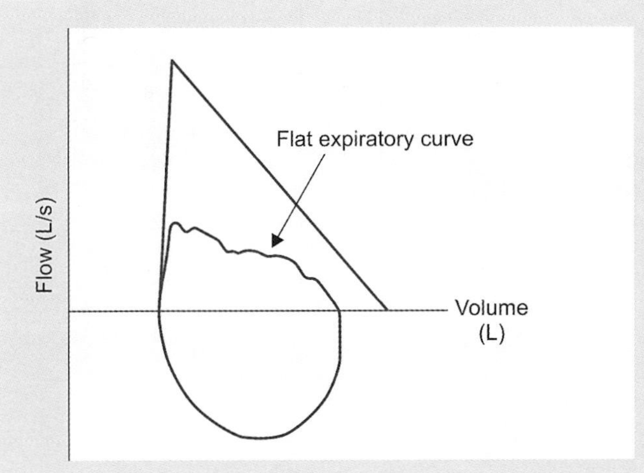

Fig. 17: Variable Intrathoracic Obstruction.

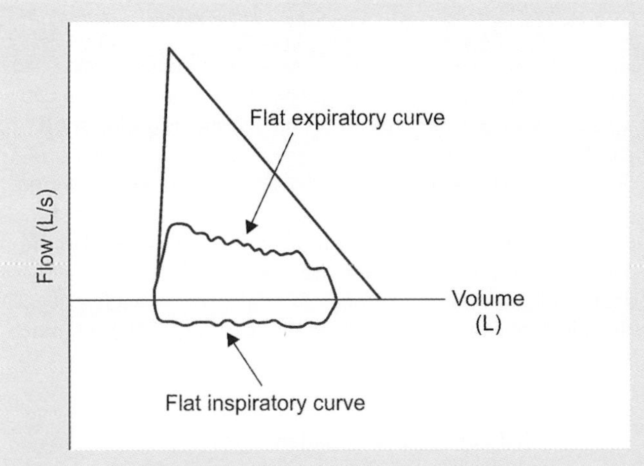

Fig. 18: Fixed upper airway obstruction.

- As per the new ATS guidelines, it should be interpreted in comparison with the LLN values and use of absolute numbers is discouraged.
- Spirometry should be interpreted only based on the history and clinical examination.

PEAK EXPIRATORY FLOW RATE

Peak expiratory flow rate is the highest flow achieved from a maximal forced expiratory maneuver started without hesitation from a position of maximal lung inflation. Maximum flow rate generated during a forceful exhalation, beginning from the level of full inspiration, is called peak expiratory flow rate. Peak flow meter **(Fig. 19)** is a portable hand-held simple flow gauge device with consistent standards of reproducibility and precision. PEFR recording is a simple outpatient procedure to identify airway obstruction and predict impending asthma exacerbation and is also an indicator of the severity of disease. PEFR reflects the caliber of the large or proximal airways, with diameter >2 mm, and it is conventionally measured in liters per minute and, PEFR may not be a good tool for the peripheral small airways.

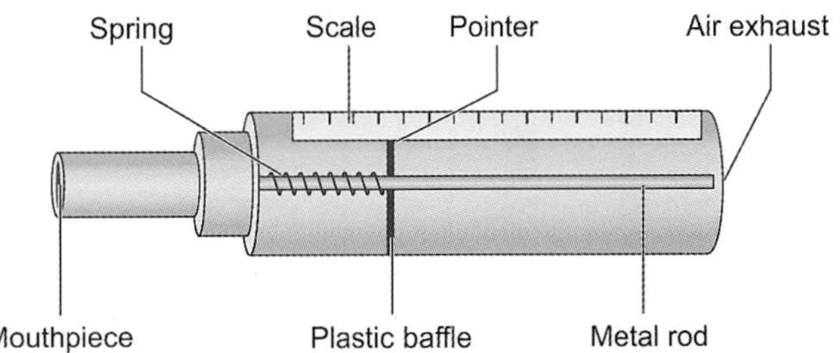

Fig. 19: Parts of a peak flow meter.

BOX 2: Steps in performing peak expiratory flow rate (PEFR).

- Standing or sitting straight is preferred and the same posture should be maintained while repeating the PEFR daily
- Slide the marker down and set at the bottom of the scale
- Fit the mouthpiece correctly
- Take a deep breath in and hold
- Place the mouthpiece in the mouth with tight seal of lips around it
- Blow out as hard and fast as possible
- Remove the device and note the number
- Repeat the same steps two more times resetting the marker to zero each time with proper relaxation between the attempts and peak flow is the highest of these three readings

How to Perform Peak Expiratory Flow Rate

Peak flow rate requires patient cooperation and with appropriate training, it can be performed in children over 5 years of age whereas it will be difficult in small children and those who lack coordination or have difficulty in understanding the instructions **(Box 2 and Fig. 20)**.

Errors in Performing Peak Expiratory Flow Rate

- Failure to achieve maximum inspiration
- Delay in blowing into the meter after maximal inhalation
- Teeth or tongue obstructing the mouthpiece
- Cough during exhalation
- Mouthpiece leaks

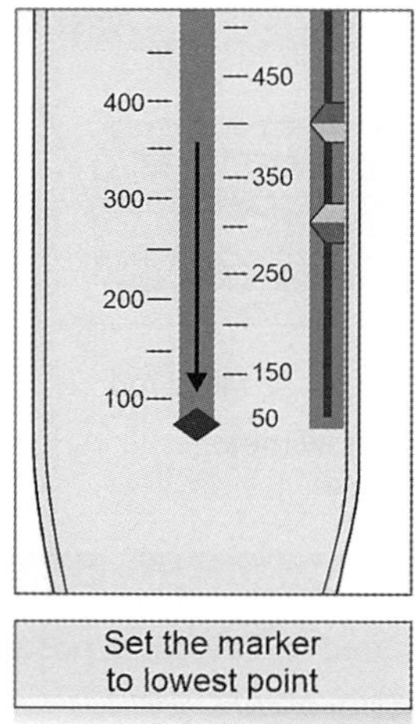

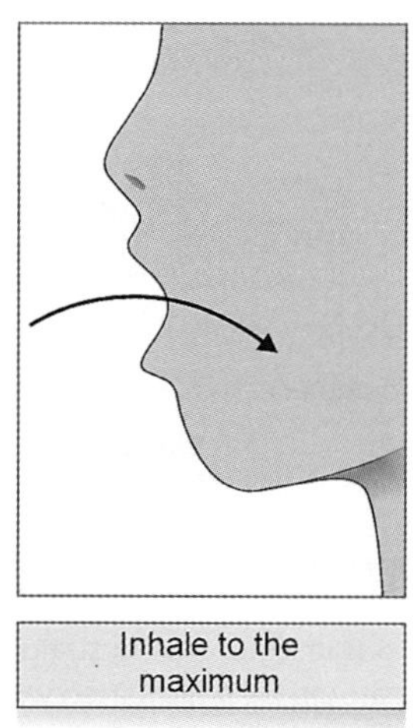

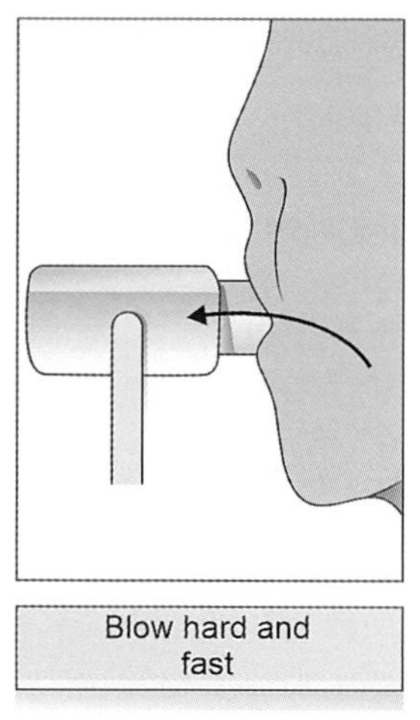

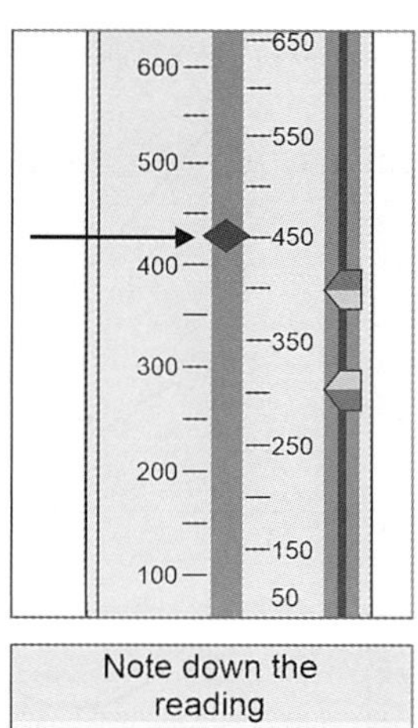

Fig. 20: Steps in performing peak expiratory flow rate (PEFR).

Role of Peak Flow Meter in Practice

- To diagnose asthma if spirometry is not available or not able to perform
- To predict the impending exacerbation in asthma
- To identify the triggers
- As a follow-up tool in asthma
- To diagnose occupational asthma

Interpretation of Peak Expiratory Flow Rate

The reference range for PEFR varies even though more than 80% of the reference value can be considered as normal. PEFR should be ideally interpreted in the pediatric age group in comparison with a patient's best reading. Personal best reading should ideally be recorded over a period of 2 weeks and should be revised regularly as the child grows. If the personal best value is not known, normograms or calculators can be used. If it is significantly below their predicted value, it may reflect background poor control, and the child may be presenting with very significant airway obstruction even with a small fall from their personal best **(Box 3)**.

In asthma action plan, PEFR helps to identify early bronchospasm and reduction in airflow **(Fig. 21)**. Regular use of peak flow will help to prevent severe exacerbation.

Peak Expiratory Flow Rate and Spirometry

FEV_1 is the amount of air forcibly exhaled during the forced maneuver and recorded as part of spirometry. Both PEFR and FEV_1 are used to quantify the degree of obstruction, and correlation between PEFR and FEV_1 is controversial.

BOX 3: Steps in finding the personal best peak expiratory flow (PEF).

- The "personal best" peak flow is the highest number you can perform over a 2-week period when asthma is under good control
- Perform peak flow testing twice a day for 2 weeks following the correct steps
- It has to be done at the same time in the morning and in the early evening using the same device
- It should be preferably done before taking any inhalers
- To calculate the patient's PEF as a percentage of the reference value or best ever reading:

$$\frac{\text{PEF recording}}{\text{Reference value or patient's best}} \times 100$$

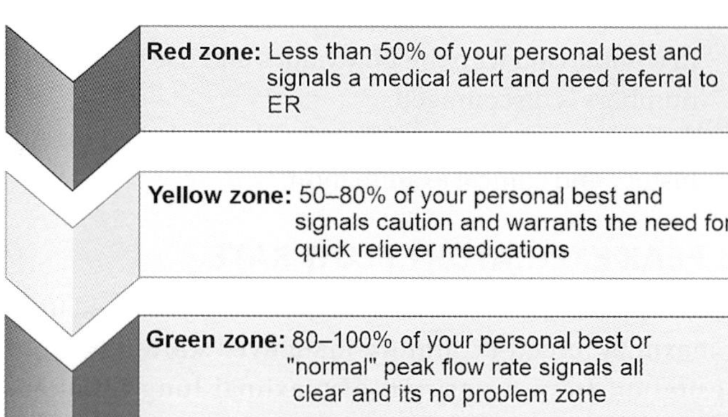

Fig. 21: Different color zones according to peak expiratory flow rate (PEFR) value.

PEFR is widely available and easy to perform. It may not accurately detect the severity of airway obstruction and spirometry can be abnormal even with normal PEFR.

Factors Affecting the Peak Expiratory Flow Rate

- *Anthropometry:* Standing height is the single best predictor in children also having almost a linear relationship with weight, body surface area, and chest expansibility.
- *Age and sex:* PEFR decreases with age from 30–40 years onward after an increase in the pediatric and adolescent age groups. The association is linear in females and curvilinear in males.
- *Ethnicity:* Predicted normal values vary according to population.
- *Environmental factors:* Particulate air pollution and environmental smoke cause a decline in PEFR in children.
- *Respiratory tracts and chest wall abnormalities:* Thoracic cage deformity and respiratory tract infection can affect the PEFR adversely.
- *Malnutrition:* As the growth of the large airways is affected with acute and chronic malnutrition, it can cause reduction in PEFR also.
- *Diurnal variation:* Diurnal variation of 20% or more in PEFR is a good indicator of asthma.

Significance of Peak Expiratory Flow Rate

When a reliable spirometry could not be performed in a child, PEFR can aid in documenting airway obstruction. It is highly recommended to document airway obstruction and to confirm the asthma diagnosis before starting treatment.

Criteria which would suggest variable expiratory flow limitation include (GINA 2025):

- *BDR:* Increase in baseline PEF ≥15% in children and PEF ≥20% in adults (4 × 100 μg salbutamol and retesting after 15 minutes OR anticholinergics 4 × 40 μg ipratropium bromide and retesting after 30 minutes).
- *Increase in lung function after 4 weeks of treatment:* Increase in baseline PEF ≥15%in children and PEF ≥20% in adults
- *Positive bronchial challenge test:* Fall in PEF >15% in children and >20% in adults predicted after a standardized exercise challenge
- *Excessive variation in lung function between the visits:* Variation in PEF ≥15% in children and PEF ≥20% in adults between visits
- *Excessive variability in twice-daily PEF over 2 weeks:* Average daily diurnal PEF variability. 13% in children and >10% in adults

Diurnal variation of PEFR indicates sensitivity of airways. Diurnal variability is calculated from twice-daily readings as the daily amplitude percent mean, i.e., highest reading of the day – lowest reading/mean of both values × 100; then the average of each day's value is calculated over 1–2 weeks.

Role of Peak Expiratory Flow Rate in Monitoring the Asthma Treatment

Recordings above 70% of personal best are an indicator of reducing the drug dosage and below 70% are an indicator of starting or increasing the dose. Average PEFR continues to increase and diurnal PEFR variability decreases for about 3 months after the initiation of treatment. Excessive variation in PEFR recordings (20–30%) suggests suboptimal asthma control and increases the risk of exacerbations. If there is a change >15% after the use of a bronchodilator, in a child on treatment for asthma, it indicates a suboptimal control.

Low PEFR can help in identifying triggers causing worsening of asthma symptoms (especially when the exposure to allergen outside home). Long-term home monitoring of PEFR can be suggested for poorly controlled asthma and those having low perception of worsening of asthma symptoms. Written asthma action plan specifying short-term treatment changes including PEFR values based on their personal best along with symptoms helps the parents to identify and take the necessary step to prevent ER visits.

Key Learning Points

- PEFR is a good tool to detect variable expiratory airflow limitation if spirometry is unavailable or not able to perform.
- It has to be included in the asthma action plan, to assess the severity of the asthma episode and monitoring response to therapy.
- PEFR may underestimate the degree of obstruction, especially the smaller airways.
- PEFR should not be considered as a replacement to spirometry and the value cannot be compared with FEV_1.

TABLE 3: Three isoforms of NO and its function.

Type	Location	Function
Endothelial NOS/eNOS	Vascular endothelial cells	• Vasodilation • Vasoprotection • Atherosclerosis prevention
Inducible NOS/ iNOS	Macrophages	Nonspecific immune defense Mediation of inflammation Septic shock
Neuronal NOS/ nNOS	Neuronal tissue	Synaptic plasticity Blood pressure regulation

(eNOS: endothelial nitric oxide synthase; iNOS: inducible nitric oxide synthase; NOS: nitric oxide synthase)

FeNO

A biomarker is a defined characteristic of a normal or pathogenic biologic process. It should be able to distinguish between health and disease, future risk, and response to treatment. Nitric oxide (NO) is a gaseous molecule that has a central role in signaling pathways involved in numerous physiological processes. Endogenous NO is enzymatically generated from L-arginine by a distinct family of NO synthase (NOS). Three isoforms of NO exist **(Table 3)**. The inducible type of NO synthase (iNOS) generates large quantities of NO when upregulated by inflammatory cytokines and inhibited by glucocorticoids.

Role of Nitric Oxide in Lungs

Nitric oxide promotes vascular and bronchial tone (dilate both vessel and airways). It facilitates coordinated beating of ciliated epithelial vessel. It is a neurotransmitter in the bronchial wall and is detected in the exhaled gas as the fractional exhaled NO which varies in health and disease.

FeNO as a Biomarker in Asthma

Asthma is a chronic inflammatory disease, characterized by reversible airway obstruction and bronchial hyper-responsiveness. Endogenous NO is derived from the iNOS present in airway cells including macrophages, neutrophils, and epithelial, endothelial, and vascular smooth muscle cells. It is produced in response to airway inflammation, with iNOS expression induced by proinflammatory cytokines including tumor necrosis factor-α, interleukin-1b, and interleukin-6. Increased levels of FeNO in asthma are regarded as indirect markers of airway hyper-responsiveness and eosinophilic inflammation and are also associated with exacerbations and disease severity. FeNO levels correlate with bronchial reactivity, sputum, and bronchoalveolar lavage (BAL) eosinophilia. Measurement of FeNO concentration in exhaled air is a safe, economical, easy, and noninvasive method.

Measurement Devices

There are three types of measurement devices:
1. *Chemiluminescence analyzers*: Considered the gold standard for FeNO measurement, these devices are highly sensitive and specific for NO.
2. *Electrochemical sensors*: These are incorporated into portable, handheld devices, making them more suitable for routine clinical use and potentially even home monitoring.,
3. *Laser-based technology*: Newer techniques like photoacoustic spectroscopy (PAS) and quartz-enhanced PAS (QEPAS) use laser light to detect NO.

Preparation for Procedure

- Avoid taking food for at least 1 hour before the test.
- Avoid use of nitrate-rich food like beetroot, spinach, lettuce, etc., 3 hours before the procedure.
- No alcohol use or smoking 1 day before the test
- Rule out upper and lower respiratory viral infections.
- No vigorous exercise within 1 hour before the procedure
- Do not perform spirometry or peak flow for 1 hour before the test is scheduled.
- Continue to take all the medicines as usual.

Steps in Performing FeNO (Fig. 22)

1. Explain regarding procedure.
2. Seat in comfortable position or stand upright.
3. Avoid nose clips as nasal NO accumulated will leak into nasopharynx affecting the value.
4. Take a deep inhalation to reach TLC and exhale immediately at a constant flow rate of 50 mL/s for a sufficient duration.
5. The indicator on the machine shows the rate in which the flow is to be maintained.
   FeNO levels are shown on screen and interpreted.

Interpretation of FeNO Values

A rising FeNO >20% change and >20 ppb in children and >20% change and >25 ppb in adults is considered significant, suggesting increasing airway inflammation. A decrease in FeNO >20% for values above 50 ppb and >10 ppb for values <50 ppb may also be considered as a clinically relevant reduction **(Tables 4 to 6)**.

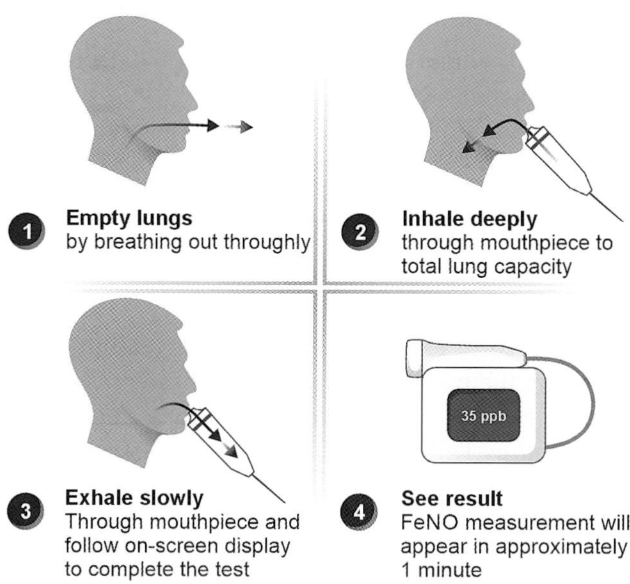

Fig. 22: Technique of performing FeNO.

TABLE 4: FeNO levels and assessment of airway inflammation as per the new ATS guidelines.

FeNO (ppb)	*Low*	*Intermediate*	*High*
Adults	<25	25–50	>50
Children	<20	20–35	>35
Type 2 inflammation	Unlikely	Possible	Likely

TABLE 5: Approach to diagnosis depending on FeNO values.

	FeNO <25 ppb (<20 ppb in children)	*FeNO 25–50 ppb (20–35 ppb in children)*	*FeNO >50 ppb (>35 ppb in children)*
Diagnosis			
Symptoms present during past 6+ weeks	• Eosinophilic airway inflamma-tion unlikely • Alternative diagnoses • Unlikely to benefit from ICS	Be cautious Evaluate clinical context Monitor change in FeNO over time	Eosinophilic airway inflammation presentLikely to benefit from ICS

(ICS: inhaled corticosteroid)

Factors Other than Asthma that Raise FeNO

- Male sex
- *Increasing age:* Effect is greater in people over age 60 or 64 years, but data conflict in adults and are more consistent in children

TABLE 6: Approach to disease monitoring depending on FeNO values.

	FeNO <25 ppb (<20 ppb in children)	*FeNO 25–50 ppb (20–35 ppb in children)*	*FeNO >50 ppb (>35 ppb in children)*
Monitoring (in Patients with Diagnosed Asthma)			
Symptoms present	Possible alternative diagnosis Unlikely to benefit from increase in ICS	Persistent allergen exposure Inadequate ICS dose Poor adherence Steroid resistance	Persistent allergen exposure Poor adherence or inhaler technique Inadequate ICS dose Risk for exacerbation Steroid resistance
Symptoms absent	Adequate ICS dose Good adherence ICS taper	Adequate ICS dosing Good adherence Monitor change in FeNO	ICS withdrawal or dose reduction may result in relapse Poor adherence or inhaler technique

(ICS: inhaled corticosteroid)

- *Increased height:* Because of increases in the airway mucosal surface area.
- Chronic rhinosinusitis, nasal polyposis, and AR. Perennial sensitization leads to higher FeNO than seasonal allergens.
- *Atopy:* Acute exposure to allergens can increase FeNO by up to 50%.
- Rhinovirus infections can increase FeNO by 50–150%.
- Nitrate-containing foods such as beetroot, spinach, etc., can increase FeNO levels by 20–60%.
- Air pollution (particulate matter and ozone), possibly because of oxidative potential

Factors Other than Asthma that Decrease FeNO

- Cigarette smoking decreases FeNO by 40–60%
- Physical exercise
- FeNO generally is sensitive to inhaled steroids and therefore will be low in most patients who are adherent to treatment
- Alcohol ingestion—avoid before testing.
- Spirometry may cause a marginal decrease.

- *Certain drugs:* Leukotriene receptor antagonists, prostaglandins—inhaled prostaglandin E2 and iloprost downregulate inducible NO synthase expression
- Respiratory syncytial virus (RSV) and influenza reduce FeNO, and bacterial infections of the respiratory tract do not affect FeNO.

Clinical Applications of FeNO

Diagnosis

- *Supports asthma diagnosis:* While not solely diagnostic, elevated FeNO levels support an asthma diagnosis, in eosinophilic inflammation and FeNO levels can help to differentiate allergic asthma from other types.
- *Evaluating rhinitis:* FeNO levels can be significantly higher in atopic AR compared to nonatopic rhinitis.
- *Predicting asthma in AR:* Studies have shown that higher baseline FeNO levels in individuals with persistent AR can be predictive of future asthma development indicating asymptomatic bronchial hyperresponsiveness.

Monitoring and Management

- *Assessing response to corticosteroids:* FeNO levels tend to decrease with effective corticosteroid treatment, making FeNO a valuable tool to monitor treatment response and adjust medication dosages. FeNO can also aid in assessing adherence to treatment.
- *Asthma control:* Elevated FeNO levels are associated with poor asthma control and increased risk of exacerbations. Monitoring FeNO helps track disease activity and may guide changes in therapy.
- *Targeted biologic therapies:* FeNO can help identify patients who are more likely to respond to certain biologic treatments for severe asthma, particularly dupilumab, omalizumab, and tezepelumab.

Limitations of FeNO

- FeNO alone cannot diagnose asthma or other conditions; it must be interpreted alongside clinical history, symptoms, and other diagnostic tests.
- Many factors can influence FeNO levels including exercise, which require careful patient preparation and consideration of potential confounders.
- Equipment can be expensive and not routinely available in all centers.

Key Learning Points

- FeNO is a simple noninvasive method to detect airway inflammation.
- FeNO has a supportive role in diagnosing asthma.
- FeNO can be used for monitoring asthma treatment and phenotyping children with severe asthma.
- Role of FeNO in other diseases is still unclear.

IMPULSE OSCILLOMETRY

Oscillometry is a newer less-invasive technique for measuring the mechanical properties of the respiratory system. Forced oscillation technique (FOT) was introduced by Dubois et al. more than 60 years, and it can be performed in very young children and elderly and is a more sensitive indicator of small airways, which are primarily involved in the pathophysiology of asthma. This technique characterizes respiratory mechanics during tidal breathing with no forced maneuver and hence is more suitable for children than spirometry. Oscillometry assesses lung function by measuring respiratory impedance, providing insights into airway resistance and reactance.

Principle of Oscillometry (Fig. 23)

Ohm's law states that Resistance = Pressure/flow. In a similar way, airway resistance can be identified by the relationship between pressure and flow.

- Oscillometry equipment generates pressure oscillations that are applied to the mouth.
- The impulses generated by the loudspeaker travel superimposed on normal tidal breathing through the large and small airways, with higher frequencies reflecting back from the large airways and lower frequencies traveling deeper into the lung before returning **(Fig. 24)**.
- A pressure and flow transducer measures inspiratory and expiratory flow and pressure.

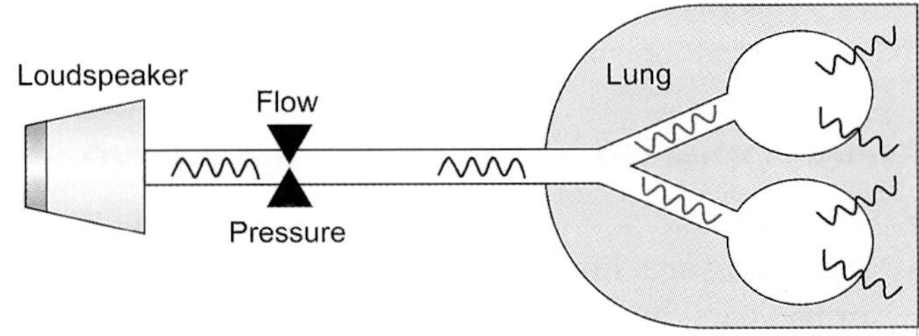

Fig. 23: Principle of impulse oscillometry.

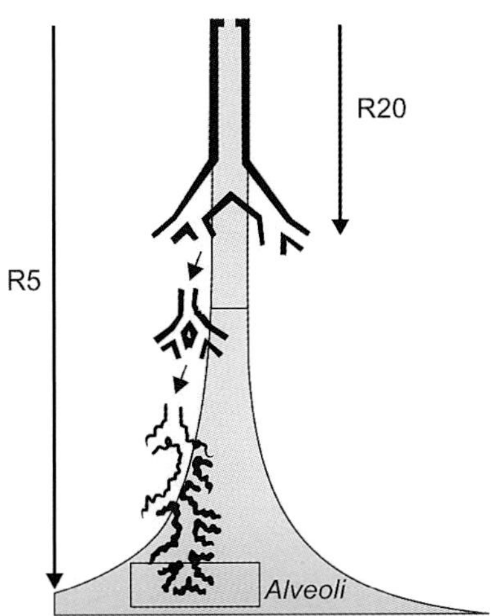

Fig. 24: Penetration of different frequency waves.

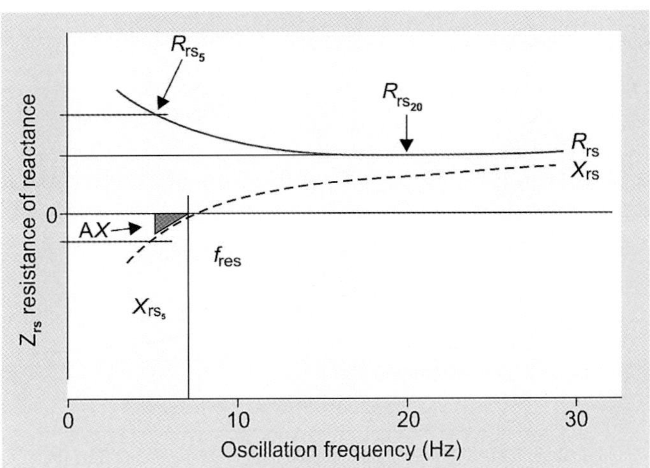

Fig. 25: Impedance spectrum: Impedance = Resistance + Reactance.

- The resultant signals of pressure and flow are separated from the breathing pattern by signal filtering.
- Respiratory impedance is the sum of all the forces (resistance and reactance) opposing the pressure impulses (oscillations) and is calculated from the ratio of pressure to flow at each frequency.

The FOT has two approaches:

1 Classic (FOT)—with the excitation wave being the sum of several sinusoidal waves
2. IOS—using pressure pulses

Physiology and Performance of Oscillometry

Oscillometry measures the mechanical impedance of the respiratory system, representing the resistive and reactive forces that must be overcome to drive an oscillating flow signal into the respiratory system **(Fig. 25)**.

The forces arise in the respiratory system from:

- The resistance of the airways and tissues (Rrs)
- The elastance (stiffness) of the lung parenchyma and chest wall in response to changes in volume (encompassed in reactance, Xrs)
- The inertance of accelerating gas in the airways (Irs)

Terminologies in Oscillometry

- *Impedance (Xrs):* The total force needed to propagate a pressure wave through the lungs which includes resistance and reactance
- *Resistance (R):* Energy required to propagate a pressure wave through the airways which is determined when a pressure wave is unopposed by airway recoil and is in phase with airflow
- *Reactance (X):* Energy generated by the recoil of the lungs after distention by a pressure wave out of phase with airflow. Reactance includes elastance and inertance.
- *Resonance frequency:* The frequency at which the lung tissue moves from passive distention to active stretch in response to the force of the pressure wave signal, graphically when reactance is zero.
- *Area of reactance (AX):* Area under the curve between the reactance values for 5 Hz and the resonance frequency
- *Coefficient of variability (CV):* Statistical determinant of the trial-to-trial variability serving as an index of reproducibility and coherence is an estimate of the quality of impedance measurements which provides an index of discrepancy between input and measured signals

Coherence

Coherence between flow and pressure at each frequency should be used to determine whether a measurement contained too many artifacts and thus should be discarded. Coherence values range between 0 and 1 but values <0.90 or 0.95 are discarded.

Resistance

Resistance is due to frictional losses in gases as they flow along airways, lung tissues, and chest wall, as they are stretched and deformed and almost 80% of the resistance is composed of central airways and only 20% of distal airways (<2 mm) **(Fig. 26)**.

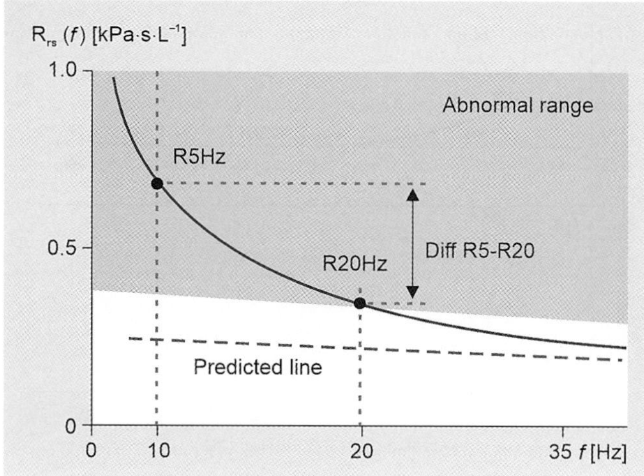

Fig. 26: Resistance spectrum.

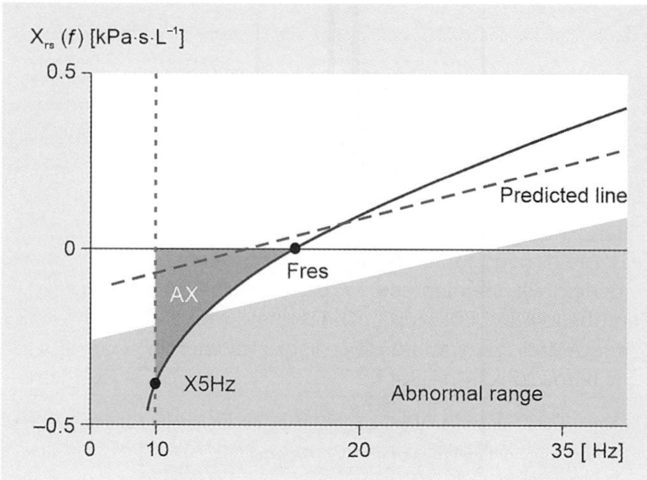

Fig. 27: Reactance spectrum.

R5: Represents the total resistance of the airways as low-frequency signals (5 Hz) penetrate the periphery of the lung

R20: Represents resistance of the proximal airways as high-frequency signals (20 Hz) reach only the proximal airways

R5 - R20: Resistance of the distal airways is calculated by the difference between R5 and R20.

The R5 value increases more in disease of distal airways and R20 will be more elevated in the proximal airway defects. Resistance reflects opposition to changes in flow, and it is in phase with flow and increased resistance will decrease flow for a given pressure input. It will not cause a time delay or phase lag in flow change, in relation to pressure change.

Reactance (Xrs)

Reactance is comprised of both inertance and elastance. It represents pressures changes that are out of phase with flow but in phase with volume changes and has also been called the "out of phase" component or the "imaginary" component. Respiratory system elastance (Ers), which is 1/compliance, is a measure of the stiffness of the entire system including chest wall, lungs, and airway and at commonly used oscillometry frequencies, it includes compressibility of gas in the airways and alveoli. As volume changes, the resultant elastic forces cause pressure changes to lag behind flow changes and hence elastance causes reactance to be negative. More negative reactance therefore indicates greater elastance or stiffness.

Reactance also includes inertance, the inertia of the air column. The capacitance component of the reactance presents a negative signal and the inertia component presents a positive signal. At higher frequencies, the air column inertia in the proximal airways dominates and total reactance is positive **(Fig. 27)**.

Resonant Frequency or Fres

When inertance and elastance are equal, the elastic contribution exactly equals the inertive contribution; hence, being in opposite directions, they cancel each other and reactance becomes zero. This point is termed resonant frequency (Fres) and its corresponding frequency typically occurs in healthy adults at about 8–12 Hz and increases with decreasing age, where Fres can be >30 Hz in young children.

Hence, when Xrs = 0 and Zrs = Rrs. At frequencies above Fres, Xrs is positive in value because it is dominated by the apparent inertia of the gas and tissues. Fres may be elevated in both restrictive and obstructive disorders **(Fig. 28)**.

Area Under the Reactance Curve (AX)

Area of reactance includes the area under the reactance curve from the lowest frequency to the Fres. It is the area between the *x*-axis below zero and reactance curve in the graph. It reflects the elastic properties of the lung **(Fig. 28)**.

Impulse Oscillometry Indications in Pediatrics

- Diagnosis of obstructive lung disease
- Suspected upper airway obstruction

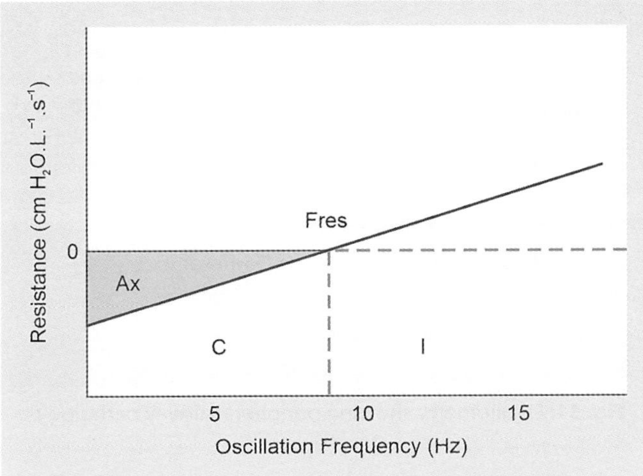

Fig. 28: Area under the curve and resonant frequency.

- To study the respiratory mechanics
- For screening purpose in healthy children

Prerequisites

- Get detailed history and clinical examination and decide on the indication.
- Avoid bronchodilators short-acting beta-agonist (SABA) for 4 hours and long-acting beta-agonist (LABA) for 24 hours.

Technique

- Explain the procedure to the child and bystanders and make them comfortable.
- Describe the nature of the sensations generated by the pressure oscillations that they will sense a "gentle vibration" or "fluttering" in their mouth and chest and it is better to have a practice run prior to data acquisition.
- Before the oscillation starts, ensure that breathing is normal and stable.
- The subject should have a sitting posture at a comfortable height with back straight with slight "chin-up" position with legs uncrossed. Swallowing should be avoided.
- A firm seal on the mouthpiece to avoid leaks; even small gaps in mouthpiece create remarkable pressure drops and hence a nose clip should be put
- Tongue should be kept relaxed below the mouthpiece to not block the orifice. Cheeks should be supported with the palm and fingers and the floor of the mouth should be held with the thumb positioned below the chin, to avoid upper airway shunt.

A suggested minimum acquisition time that would be suitable for children >12 years and adults is 30 seconds and for children aged <12 years is 16 seconds which would allow recording of at least three artifact-free breaths. It is recommended to use at least three replicates, which are deemed acceptable after application of specified quality criteria:

- Visual inspection
- Within-session coefficient of variability (CoV) (CoV ≤ 10% in adults and ≤ 15% in children)
- Automated signal processing

Identification of Artifacts

- There are no pauses in volume signal accompanied by zero flow, sudden changes, or spikes in resistance and pressure, which may represent swallowing, breath-holds, glottic closures, and mouth leaks.
- Leaks manifest as sudden large decreases in impedance |Zrs|, although the changes in flow–time and volume–time traces may be subtle at times.
- Swallowing or transient airway occlusion manifest as large values of impedance at zero flow.
- Artifact removal can be based on statistical filtering of impedance values from individual windows or on the basis of complete breaths.

Interpretation of Oscillometry

Oscillometry is a simple test to perform but its interpretation remains a challenge.

- *Normal lung function:* Respiratory resistance R5Hz and lung reactance X5Hz are in the normal range. The resistance spectrum Rrs shows a linear, frequency-independent response. The pattern of the reactance spectrum Xrs is normal which continually decreases toward lower frequencies **(Fig. 29)**.
- *Central obstruction:* Respiratory resistance R5Hz is elevated compared to its reference and abnormal, whereas X5Hz still lies in the normal range. The resistance spectrum Rrs shows no frequency dependence and runs parallel to the predicted line in the abnormal range. The reactance spectrum Xrs remains normal. Proximal obstruction leads to frequency-independent elevations in resistance and should have little to no effect on reactance, because the capacity of the lung to recoil and the signal to return to the sensor is relatively unaffected **(Fig. 30)**.

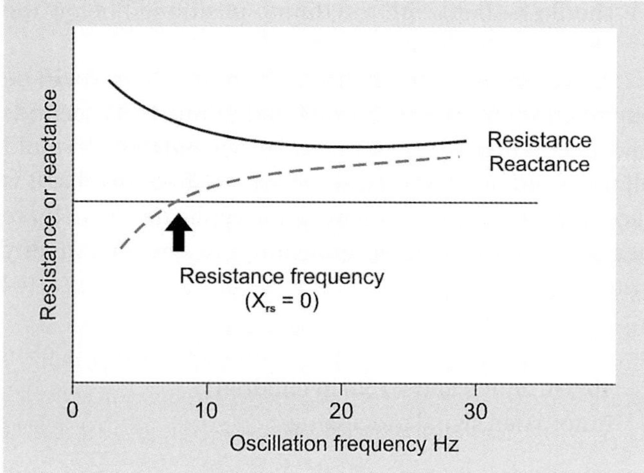

Fig. 29: Oscillometry showing normal lung function.

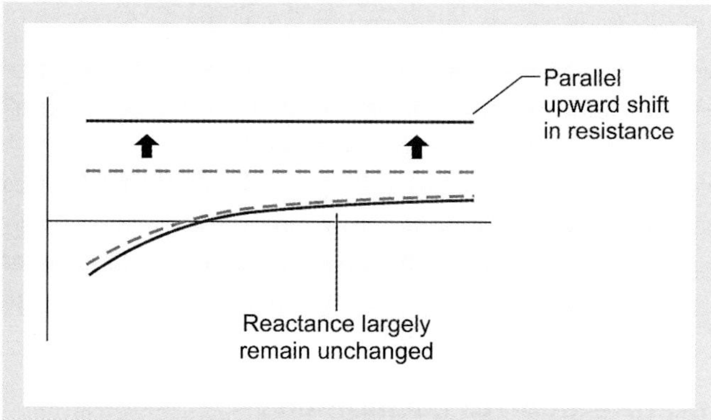

Fig. 30: Oscillometry showing central obstruction.

- *Peripheral obstruction:* Both R5Hz and X5Hz are abnormal. The resistance spectrum Rrs has a marked frequency dependency and it continually rises as oscillation frequency decreases. The reactance spectrum Xrs simultaneously shifts into the lower negative range.

Distal obstructive diseases, such as asthma and chronic bronchitis, result in a frequency-dependent increase in resistance (high R5–R20) because the pressure signal wave propagating out to the lung periphery (R5) encounters greater resistance than the more proximal higher-frequency (R20) impulse.

Distal obstruction also results in a decrease in reactance because the signal returning from the lung periphery to the sensor also has to navigate these same narrowed airways **(Fig. 31)**.

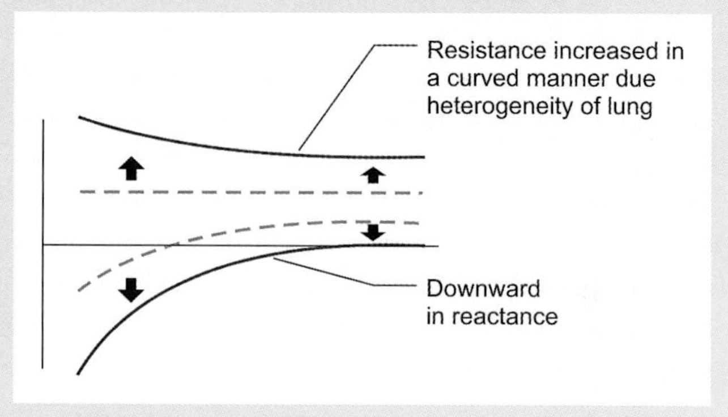

Fig. 31: Oscillometry showing peripheral airway pathology.

- *Restriction:* Restrictive lung diseases will result in a decrease in reactance, because the elastic recoil, and therefore the ability of the lung parenchyma to reflect the signal back, will be decreased. Restrictive processes will not affect resistance because the airway diameter is unchanged. Oscillometry is a sensitive tool for the diagnosis of restrictive airway disease. The clinical application of oscillometry in restrictive lung disease is less established in comparison to obstructive disease. Restrictive lung diseases like ILD and obstructive lung diseases are clinically distinct, but their corresponding Zrs spectra demonstrate similar patterns of abnormalities, perhaps due to the higher airway resistance found at lower lung volume in ILD and hence are difficult to differentiate through oscillometry.

Bronchodilator response testing: Recent technical standard cutoffs indicating a significant BDR using oscillometric indices reported in healthy adults and children are:

- 40% decrease in Rrs at 5 Hz
- 50% increase in Xrs at 5 Hz
- 80% decrease in AX relative to baseline

Different machines have different cutoffs for the parameters, and hence the definition of BDR varies according to the machine and the availability of the scientific data pertaining to that particular machine, especially in an Indian setting.

Interpreting Z-Scores in IOS

- *Normal range:* *z*-scores within a certain range (e.g., between –1.64 and 1.64) are typically considered normal.
- *Abnormal findings:* Values outside this normal range are considered abnormal.

TABLE 7: Impedance spectrum in obstructive and restrictive airway disease.

	R5	*R20*	*X5*	*Fres*	*R5–R20*
Distal obstruction	↑↑↑	Normal or ↑	More negative	↑	R5 >R20
Proximal obstruction	↑↑	↑↑	Normal	Normal	R5 = R20
Restriction	Normal	Normal	More negative	↑↑	Normal

TABLE 8: IOS parameters in various diseases.

Disease	*IOS Parameters*
Asthma	↑ R5, normal R20, X5 more negative, ↑ Fres
Cystic fibrosis	↑ R5, R20, Fres, and AX; X5 more negative
Infection by rhinovirus	↓ X5
Postinfectious bronchiolitis obliterans	↑ R5 and X5 more negative
Gastroesophageal reflux disease	↑ R5 and R5–R20
COPD	↑ Fres, R5, and R5–R20; X5 more negative

(COPD: chronic obstructive pulmonary disease; IOS: impulse oscillometry)

- A *z*-score greater than +1.64 for parameters like R5 (airway resistance at low frequency) is often flagged as potentially abnormal.
- A *z*-score less than −1.64 for parameters like X5 (reactance at low frequency) can indicate abnormality.

Role of Oscillometry in Childhood Asthma (Tables 7 and 8)

It can be used in the diagnosis of asthma along with bronchodilator reversibility response and also to monitor the treatment response and level of control, as oscillometry parameters are more sensitive than spirometry. Increase in airway resistance occurs in asthma; especially in peripheral airways, there will be an increase in R5, normal R20, more negative X5, and increase in Fres. Reactance area (AX) can be used to assess the response to asthma treatment. Oscillometry is better than spirometry for assessing the BDR in children which is an important predictor of asthma. The main parameter to evaluate the BDR is R5.

Comparison with Spirometry (Fig. 32)

- *Patient cooperation and effort:* Spirometry requires forceful expiratory maneuvers following maximal inhalation which is challenging in young children and elderly. Impulse oscillometry measures lung function during normal tidal breathing.
- *Airway assessment:* Spirometry assesses large airway function primarily and overall lung capacity by measuring airflow and volume over time, and parameters like FEV_1 and FVC are the key indicators. Oscillometry provides detailed information on airway resistance (R) and reactance (X) at various frequencies, allowing for the assessment of both central and peripheral airways. Lower frequencies penetrate deeper into the lungs, revealing abnormalities in the small, peripheral airways that might be missed by spirometry.
- *Early detection and monitoring:* Spirometry can be normal in early-stage disease, but oscillometry can detect subtle changes in small airway function even when spirometry results are normal. It may be more sensitive in detecting early stages of diseases like COPD and identifying peripheral airway obstruction in asthma.

Limitations of Oscillometry

- Detection of restrictive diseases is possible only in higher degree of the disease and differentiation between distal obstruction and restriction is only possible with additional investigations like spirometry or body plethysmography.
- Not freely available due to the cost factor
- The limitation of this representation of the respiratory system is that it is assumed to behave in a linear manner, whereas there is likely nonlinear behavior even in healthy lungs (primarily in the proximal and upper airways) and even more so in diseased lungs. Also, ventilation is heterogeneous in healthy lungs and much more so in disease, which also affects this relationship.

CONCLUSION

Functional assessments and advanced diagnostic technologies add substantial value to pediatric allergy practice by objectively evaluating airway structure,

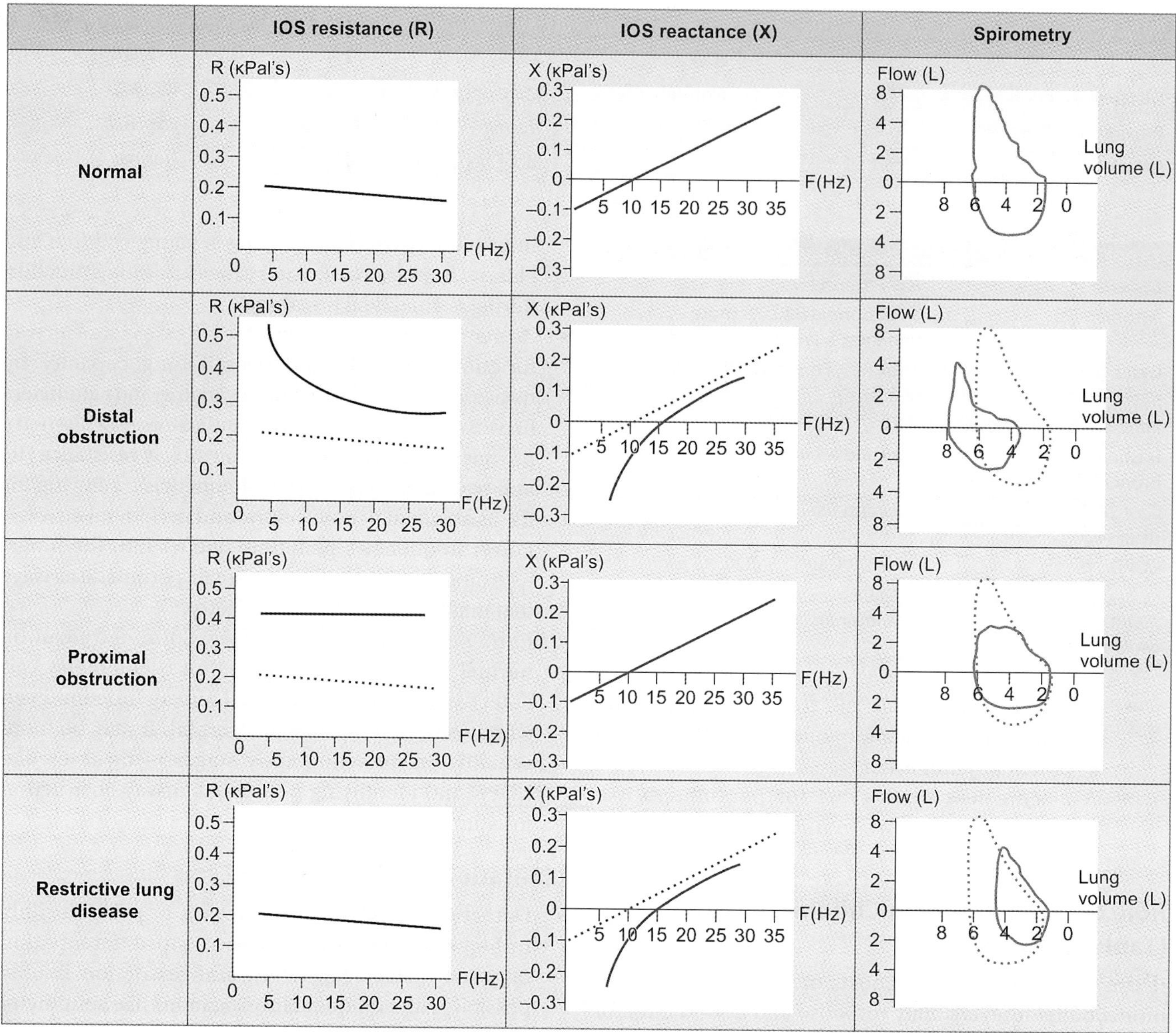

Fig. 32: Comparison between spirometry and oscillometry parameters in various diseases.

function, and inflammation. Tools such as DNE, rhinometry, rhinomanometry, spirometry, impulse oscillometry, and FeNO measurement enhance diagnostic precision, guide phenotyping, and allow monitoring of therapeutic response. While some modalities remain research-oriented or require specialized expertise, their integration—when clinically indicated—enriches understanding of disease severity and airway dynamics, particularly in asthma and AR. These technologies, used alongside meticulous history and examination, support a comprehensive approach to personalized, evidence-based pediatric allergy care.

KEY POINTS

- Impulse oscillometry is an effort-independent test based on the FOT which measures pulmonary function in children in whom a reliable spirometry is difficult to obtain.
- Oscillometry is not a replacement for spirometry, but should be used as a complement as of now; however, it

may later replace spirometry, especially in the pediatric age group.

- Interpretation of the oscillometry parameters is challenging, and more studies are needed to decide on the standard cutoffs.
- It has a significant role in asthma diagnosis and monitoring and assessment of the treatment response in children.

SUGGESTED READING

Nasal Procedures

1. Bang JH, Kim SJ, Lee YC, Lee KH. Representative Nasal Endoscopic Findings Suggestive of Allergic Rhinitis and Their Influencing Factors. J Rhinol. 2025;32(2):84-90.
2. Gotlib T, Samoliński B, Szczesnowicz-Dabrowska P. [Acoustic rhinometry—examination technique and discussion of the recommendation of the Committee for Standardisation of Acoustic Rhinometry, European Rhinologic Association]. Pol Merkur Lekarski. 2003;14(79):79-81.
3. Ko J, Kang M, un YJ. Deep learning-based allergic rhinitis diagnosis using nasal endoscopy images. Sci Rep. 2025;15:24341.
4. Melo AC, de Oliveira de Camargo Gomes A, Santos Cavalcanti A, da Silva HJ. Acoustic rhinometry in mouth breathing patients: a systematic review. Braz J Otorhinolaryngol. 2015;81:212-8.
5. Uzzaman A, Metcalfe DD, Komarow HD. Acoustic rhinometry in the practice of allergy. Ann Allergy Asthma Immunol. 2006;97(6):745-51; quiz 751-2, 799.
6. Vogt K, Bachmann-Harildstad G, Lintermann A, Nechyporenko A, Peters F, Wernecke KD. The new agreement of the international RIGA consensus conference on nasal airway function tests. Rhinology. 2018;56(2):133-43.

Spirometry

1. Altalag A, Road J, Wilcox P (Eds). Pulmonary Function Tests in Clinical Practice. New York: Springer; 2019.
2. Beydon N, Davis SD, Lombardi E, Allen JL, Arets HGM, Aurora P, et al. An official American Thoracic Society/European Respiratory Society statement: pulmonary function testing in preschool children. Am J Respir Crit Care Med. 2007;175(12):1304-45.
3. Chhabra SK, Kumar R, Mittal V. Prediction Equations for Spirometry for Children from Northern India. Indian Pediatr. 2016;53:781-5.
4. Davis SD, Eber E, Koumbourlis AC. Diagnostic Tests in Pediatric Pulmonology. New York: Springer; 2015.
5. Global Initiative for Asthma (GINA). (2025). Global Strategy for Asthma Management and Prevention. [online] Available from https://ginasthma.org/wp-content/uploads/2025/05/GINA-2025_tracked-for-archive-WMSA.pdf [Last accessed December, 2025].
6. Graham BL, Steenbruggen I, Miller MR, Barjaktarevic IZ, Cooper BG, Hall GL, et al. Standardization of Spirometry 2019 Update: An Official American Thoracic Society and European Respiratory Society Technical Statement. Am J Respir Crit Care Med. 2019; 200(8). https://doi.org/10.1164/rccm.201908-1590ST.
7. Miller MR, Hankinson J, Brusasco V, Burgos F, Casaburi R, Coates A, et al. Standardisation of spirometry. Eur Respir J. 2005;26(2):319-38.
8. National Asthma Council Australia. Spirometry quick reference guide. Melbourne: National Asthma Council Australia; 2020.
9. Queensland Health. Spirometry (Paediatric) Respiratory Science: Document Number QH-GDL-393:2013.
10. Stanojevic S, Kaminsky DA, Miller MR, Thompson B, Aliverti A, Barjaktarevic I, et al. ERS/ATS technical standard on interpretive strategies for routine lung function tests. Eur Respir J. 2022;60:2101499.

Peak Expiratory Flow Rate

1. Ahmed M, Gavhane J, Goel S. Age Specific Peak Expiratory Flow Nomogram in Children. Indian J Pediatr. 2017;84(4):271-5.
2. Al-Amin Mrindha M, Ruhul Amin A, Luthful Kabir ARM. Peak Expiratory Flow Rate (PEFR)-A Simple Ventilatory Lung Function Test. J Shaheed Suhrawardy Med Coll. 2011;3(2):44-7.
3. Davis SD, Eber E, Koumbourlis AK (Eds). Diagnostic Tests in Pediatric Pulmonology: Applications and Interpretation. New York: Springer; 2015.
4. Dr Jason Long, University of Glasgow. Peak Expiratory Flow Rate: Monograph. [online] Available from https://www.gla.ac.uk/media/Media_678202_smxx.pdf [Last accessed December, 2025].
5. Global Initiative for Asthma (GINA). 2025 GINA Strategy Report Global Strategy for Asthma Management and Prevention. [online] Available from https://ginasthma.org/2025-gina-strategy-report/ [Last accessed December, 2025].
6. Miller MR, Hankinson J, Brusasco V, Burgos F, Casaburi R, Coates A, et al. ATS/ERS Task Force. Standardisation of spirometry. Eur Respir J. 2005;26(2):319-38.
7. Srisingh K, Phuaksaman C. The reference values of peak expiratory flow rate in Thailand children. J Thorac Dis. 2021;13(1):31-8.
8. Taussig LM, Landau LI (Eds) Pediatric Respiratory Medicine, 2nd edition. Philadelphia: Elsevier; 2008.

FeNO

1. Dweik RA, Boggs PB, Erzurum SC, Irvin CG, Leigh MW, Lundberg JO. Interpretation of exhaled nitric oxide levels (FeNO) for clinical applications. Am J Respir Crit Care Med. 2011;184:602-15.

2. Hoggins R, Velpula M, Woodward S, Tighe MP. How to use the fractional exhaled nitric oxide test. Arch Dis Child Educ Pract Ed. 2022;107(2):133-40.
3. Ragnoli B, Radaeli A, Pochetti P, Kette S, Morjaria J, Malerba M. Fractional nitric oxide measurement in exhaled air (FeNO): perspectives in the management of respiratory diseases. Ther Adv Chronic Dis. 2023;14:20406223231190480.
4. Sen P, Khatri SB, Tejwani V. Measuring exhaled nitric oxide when diagnosing and managing asthma. Cleveland Clin J Med. 2023;90(6):363-70.

Oscillometry

1. Bickel S, Popler J, Lesnick B, Eid N. Impulse oscillometry: interpretation and practical applications. Chest. 2014;146(3):841-7.
2. Brashier B, Salvi S. Measuring lung function using sound waves: role of the forced oscillation technique and impulse oscillometry system. Breathe (Sheff). 2015;11(1):57-65.
3. Calverley PMA, Farré R. Oscillometry: old physiology with a bright future. Eur Respir J. 2020;56:2001815.
4. de Oliveira Jorge PP, de Lima JHP, Chong E Silva DC, Medeiros D, Solé D, Wandalsen GF. Impulse oscillometry in the assessment of children's lung function. Allergol Immunopathol (Madr). 2019;47(3):295-302.
5. Gupta N, Sachdev A, Gupta D, Gupta S. Oscillometry – The future of estimating pulmonary functions. Karnataka Paediatr J. 2020;35(2):79-87.
6. Kaminsky DA, Simpson SJ, Berger KI, Calverley P, de Melo PL, Dandurand R, et al. Clinical significance and applications of oscillometry. Eur Respir Rev. 2022;31:210208.
7. King GG, Bates J, Berger KI, Calverley P, de Melo PL, Dellacà RL, et al. Technical standards for respiratory oscillometry. Eur Respir J. 2020;55:1900753.
8. Shirai T, Kurosawa H. Clinical Application of the Forced Oscillation Technique. Intern Med. 2016;55(6):559-66.
9. Smith H, Reinhold P, Goldman MD. Forced oscillation technique and impulse oscillometry. Eur Respir Monogr. 2005;31:72-105.

3 SECTION

Respiratory, Ocular, and Food Allergies

***Section Editors:** Vikram Patra, Mitesh Kakkad*

10 CHAPTER

Allergic Rhinitis

Mitesh Kakkad

INTRODUCTION

Rhinitis is an inflammation of the nasal epithelium. It can be allergic, nonallergic, or infectious.

DEFINITION

Allergic rhinitis (AR) is an immunoglobulin E (IgE)-mediated, type-1 hypersensitivity response of the nasal mucosal membranes, resulting from allergen exposure in a sensitized individual.

PATHOPHYSIOLOGY

In a sensitized person, when an allergen is exposed, it is taken up by an antigen-presenting cell to T-lymphocytes. Depending on genetic predisposition, an antigen through major histocompatibility complex (MHC) class II induces TH2 response.

TH2 lymphocytes produce IL-4, IL-5, IL-13, and other cytokines.

IL-4 directs the lymphocytes to produce IgE-specific antibodies. These specific IgE antibodies will get attached to high-affinity receptors (FcRI) in mast cells or basophils. On re-exposure of these allergens, they will cross-link with this, causing release of preformed histamine mediators and also newly synthesized mediators such as prostaglandins, leukotrienes, and cytokines. Further, after 4–6 hours, cytokines and chemokines are generated, which are recruited from T-lymphocytes, eosinophils, and basophils and other inflammatory cells.

Pathophysiology of Symptoms (Fig. 1)

Sneezing and pruritus are mediated because of activation of sensory nerves. Rhinorrhea results from excessive activation of the nasal glandular apparatus producing

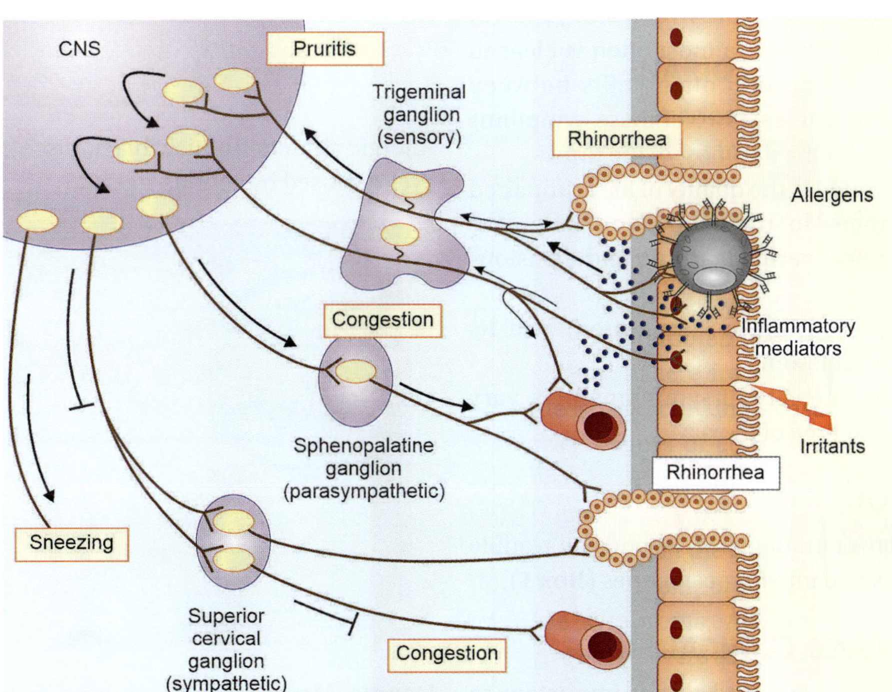

Fig. 1: Pathophysiology of symptoms.

TABLE 1: Differences between seasonal and perennial allergic rhinitis (AR).

Seasonal AR	***Perennial AR***
Intermittent (cyclical exacerbation)	Increase of symptoms in the night and early morning. *Persistent* (year-round symptoms)
Outdoor allergens • Tree pollen (spring) • Grasses (early summer) • Weeds (late summer)	*Indoor allergens* • House dust mites • Animal dander • Molds • Cockroaches • Pets

mucus. The nasal mucosa has a plethora of nasal glands, mucous and serous glands, and goblet cells. Nasal congestion occurs as a result of engorgement of the venous sinusoids of the nasal mucosa.

Factors that increase the risk of development of AR:
- Female gender
- Particulate air pollution
- Maternal smoking.

CLINICAL FEATURES

Classic symptoms of AR include sneezing, itching, rhinorrhea (anterior or posterior), and nasal congestion.

Sneezing is marked by explosive paroxysms of 5–10 sneezes or more. Rhinorrhea most often is clear to white in color. Nasal congestion often shifts between two nostrils. To diagnose, at least two of these symptoms should be present for 1 hour a day most of the time.

Because of the symptoms, the quality of life is impaired in the form of changes in the mood and cognitive disturbance; it may affect verbal learning and decision-making speed.

AR is underdiagnosed and under-treated, and its symptoms are more troublesome.

The duration and intensity of symptoms may vary according to season and time of the day.

CLASSIFICATION

According to symptoms duration and depends on trouble symptoms, AR is classified into four categories **(Box 1)**.

EXAMINATION AND CLINICAL SIGNS

Examination of nose, ear, eye, and skin is important to assess a patient of AR.

BOX 1: Classification of allergic rhinitis.

1. *Intermittent* • <4 days/week or • <4 weeks	3. *Persistent* • >4 days/week or • > 4 weeks
2. *Mild* • Normal sleep • No impairment of daily activities • No troublesome symptoms in untreated patients	4. *Moderate–Severe* • Abnormal sleep • Impairment of daily activities • Troublesom symptoms

Oropharyngeal examination reveals cobblestone appearance and postnasal drip.

Examination reveals signs as follows:

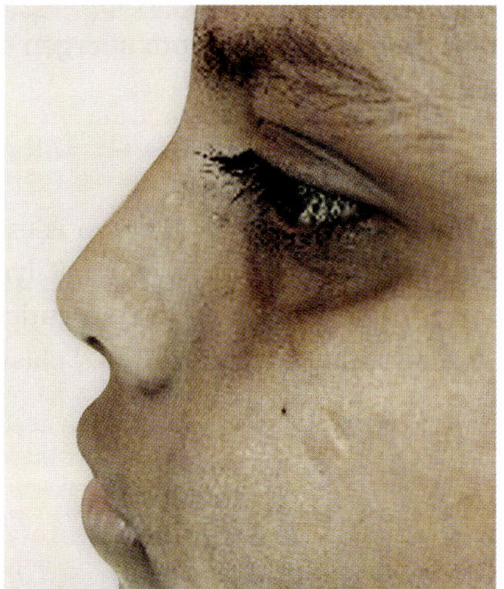

Allergic shiners—bluish-black discoloration under lower eyelid caused by venous stasis.

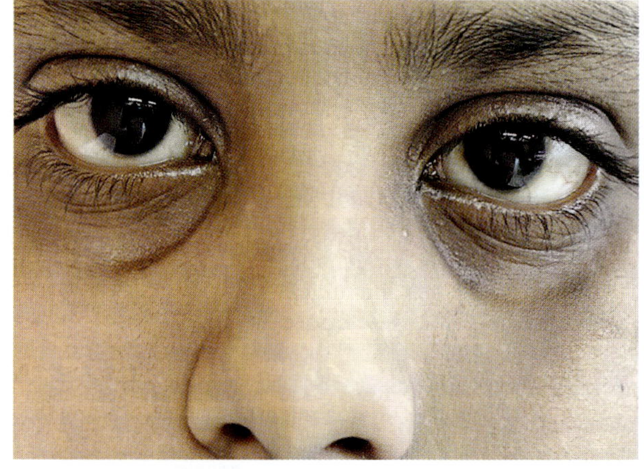

Dennie-Morgan folds—creases in lower eyelid due to Mueller's muscle spasm.

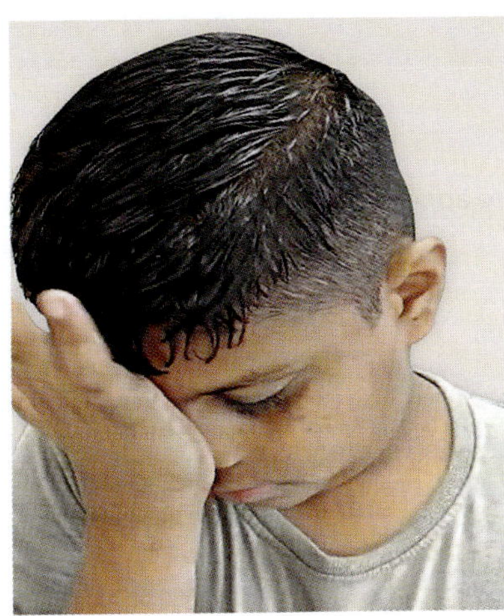

Allergy salute—due to itching and congestion, continuous rubbing of the nose upward with hands.

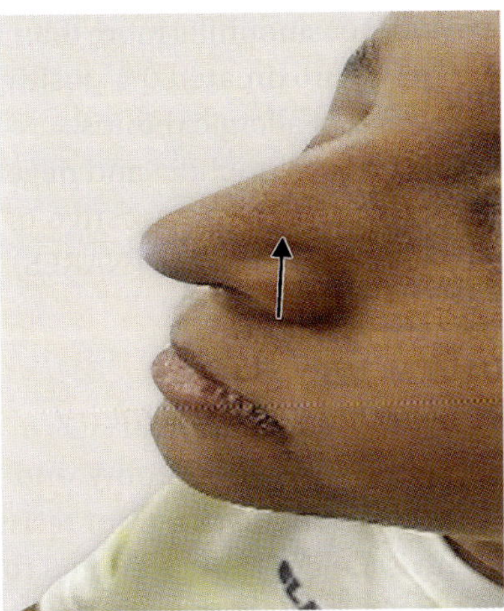

Transverse nasal crease—over the lower portion of the nose caused by repetitive pushing of the nose upward in response to nasal itching or discharge.

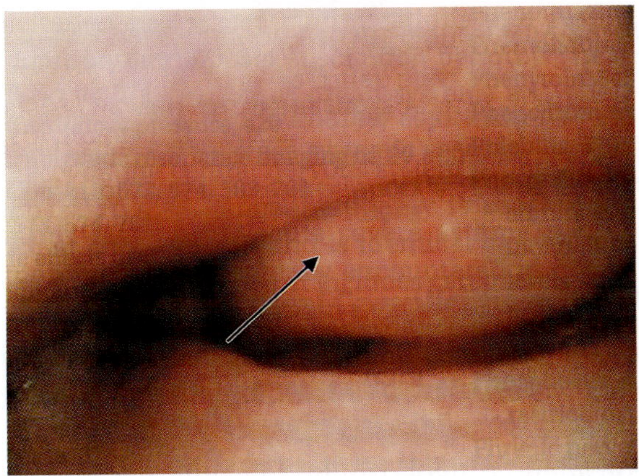

Hypertrophied inferior turbinate—pale bogy mucosa with clear secretions.

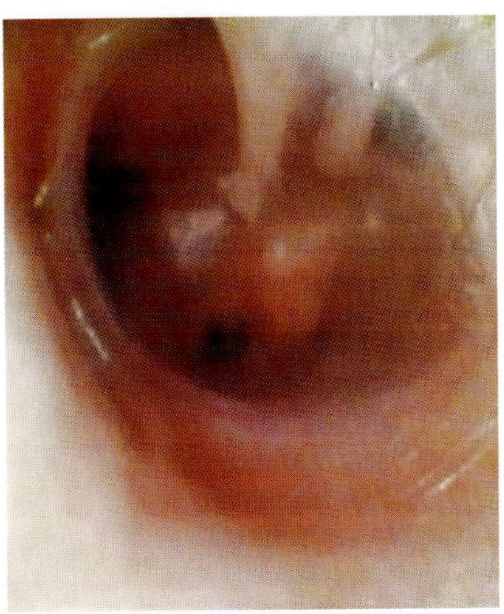

Serous otitis media with effusion (OME)

COMORBIDITIES

Asthma	AR	Allergic conjunctivitis
Atopic dermatitis		• Rhinosinusitis • Adenoid hypertrophy
Food allergy		• Hearing impairment OME • Gastroesophageal reflux (GER) • Laryngitis

- *Asthma:* 30% of the patients with AR have asthma and more than 80% of patients with asthma have AR. It is important to treat AR for better asthma control.
- *Rhinosinusitis:* Nasal allergy mostly likely precipitates acute sinusitis by causing sinus ostial edema resulting in impairment of sinus drainage and bacterial proliferation.
- *Adenoid hypertrophy:* Nasopharyngeal lymphoid tissue causes nasopharyngeal obstruction which leads to snoring, mouth breathing, hypopnea, and apnea.
- *Otitis media with effusion (OME):* This is associated with AR due to eustachian tube dysfunction, which induces negative pressure in the middle ear and leads to accumulation of fluid.

DIFFERENTIAL DIAGNOSIS

Differential diagnosis of AR is given in **Table 2**.

Mechanical Factors:

- Deviated nasal septum—unilateral nasal blockage and congestion
- Choanal atresia
- Foreign body—unilateral foul-smelling discharge

TABLE 2: Differential diagnosis of AR.

Characteristics	*Allergic Rhinitis*	*Sinusitis*	*Common cold*
Duration of cold	>10 days	>10 days	7–10 days
Onset of symptoms	Begin immediately after exposure to allergen	Take few days to appear after infection	Take few days to appear after infection
Treatment	Antihistamines	Antibiotics	Symptomatic
Constitutional symptoms	Usually no constitutional symptoms	Headache	Usually, severe malaise, headache
Nasal discharge	Usually clear	Clear mucus/thick yellowish	Thin mucus
Fever	No	Sometimes	Low-grade
Tooth pain/retro-orbital pain	No	Yes	No
Eyes	Itchy and watery	No	Sometimes watery

- Ciliary dyskinesia—thick viscid mucopurulent discharge with recurrent otitis media, sinusitis
- Cystic fibrosis—nasal polyps with recurrent pneumonia, failure to thrive, chronic diarrhea
- Tumors
- Granulomas

INVESTIGATIONS

Testing for Allergen Sensitization

Total IgE and blood eosinophils—increased value suggestive of Th2—mediated inflammation. They have a limited role in the diagnosis.

Skin Prick Test (In Vivo Test)

Skin prick test (SPT) is the gold standard test for allergen sensitization. It is cheap, rapid, and detects bound IgE.

Specific IgE is detected by FEIA-ImmunonoCap (Fluoro-Immuno-Enzymatic Assay on ImmunoCAP; in vitro). It can be done when SPT is not possible. It is expensive, takes 24–48 hours for result, and detects free IgE.

Singleplex ImmunoCAP

This test is done to identify true allergen or cross-reactive component. It helps in guiding immunotherapy for true major allergens.

Nasal Provocation test

Nasal challenge/provocation test is the use of allergens to elicit responses within the nose. It is relatively safe and gold standard for nasal allergy. It also helps to diagnose local allergic rhinitis (LAR).

Nasal Cytology

The presence of nasal eosinophilia more than 10 cells/high power field has an approximate 80% positive predictive value for the diagnosis of allergic rhinitis.

Patients with nasal eosinophilia and negative reaction on SPT/specific IgE are likely suggestive of nonallergic rhinitis with eosinophilia syndrome (NARES).

Tests for Nasal Patency

Measurement of Acoustic Rhinometry

This examines nasal airway anatomy and serves as a valuable aid in assessing nasal airflow or resistance.

The provocative challenge has a limited role in clinical practice.

Nasal peak flow—measured as either inspiratory or expiratory flow rates. It is simple, quick, inexpensive, effort dependent.

Active Rhinomanometry

It is effort independent and measures airway resistance. Anterior or posterior rhinomanometry can be done. Anterior rhinomanometry is more practical and easy to do in clinical practice.

Testing for Inflammation and Pathology

CT of paranasal sinuses detects mucoperiosteal thickening seen in AR and NARES. It is considered in chronic rhinosinusitis.

For adenoid hypertrophy—flexible nasopharyngoscopy for diagnosis and grading of adenoid hypertrophy.

X-ray lateral neck—for adenoid hypertrophy.

DIAGNOSIS—STEPWISE APPROACH

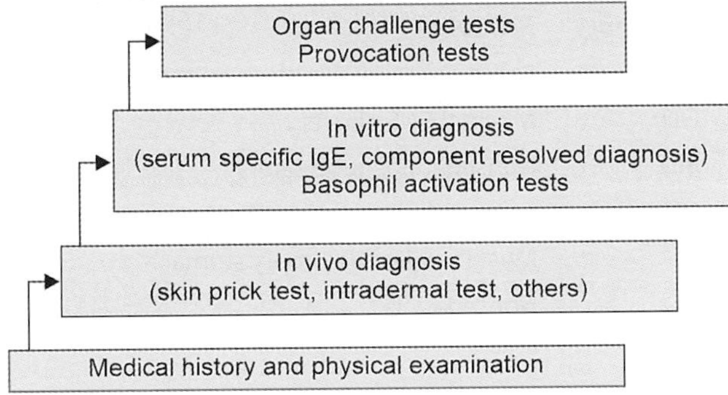

TREATMENT

- Parent education
- Counseling of the patient on severity of disease, environmental-control measures, and need of long-term treatment are the most important aspects of management.
- Allergen- and irritant-avoidance measures
- Parents should be educated about details on avoidance of allergens and irritants.
- Treatment according to Allergic Rhinitis and its Impact on Asthma (ARIA; **Fig. 2**)

Oral Antihistamines

Oral antihistamines are rapidly absorbed after oral administration and provide relief within 1–2 hours.

Some have anti-inflammatory effect. They reduce symptoms of sneezing, itching, and rhinorrhea. They are less effective for nasal congestion.

- *First generation*
  - Highly lipophilic, crosses blood–brain barrier
  - *Drugs:* Diphenhydramine, chlorpheniramine maleate
  - *Side effects:* Sedation, affect cognition, dry mouth
- *Second generation* ***(Table 3)***
  - Less lipophilic, less side effects
  - *Drugs:* Cetirizine, Levocetirizine, Loratadine, Desloratadine, Fexofenadine, Bilastine
  - *Side effects:* Less sedation so preferred over first generation

Intranasal Antihistamine

Drugs: Azelastine, Olopatadine hydrochloride

- Onset of action within 15 minutes
- Administered twice daily
- *Side effects:* Altered and bitter taste.
- Because of the bitter taste reformulated with sucrose for better compliance.
- Intranasal antihistamines are used usually with combination of intranasal corticosteroids for better efficacy.

Decongestants

They reduce nasal congestion but have no effect on other symptoms of rhinitis.

They act by alfa adrenergic stimulation which causes vascular constriction and leads to reduction of nasal blood supply to the sinusoids.

Oral decongestants:

- Phenylephrine, pseudoephedrine hydrochloride, phenylpropanolamine
- Less effective than nasal decongestants

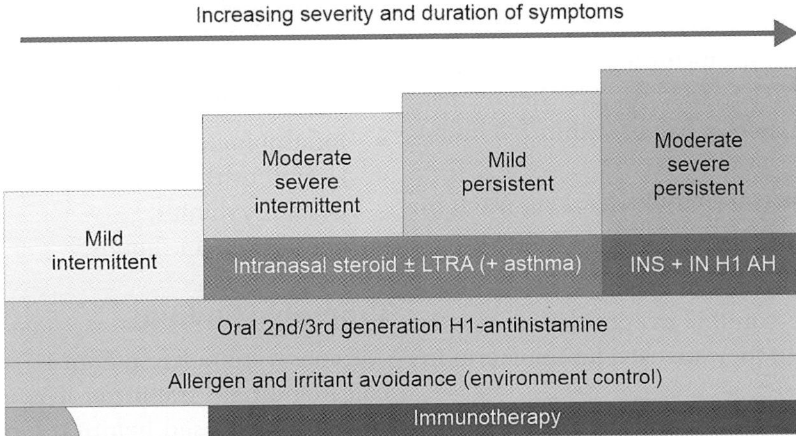

Fig. 2: Treatment of allergic rhinitis according to allergic rhinitis and its impact on asthma (ARIA) guidelines.

TABLE 3: Second-generation oral H1 antihistamines.

Molecule	Age group	Pediatric dose	Frequency	Remarks
Cetirizine	>6 months	2.5–5 mg (<6 years); 10 mg (>6 years)	OD	Rapid onset (30 minutes), mild sedation
Levocetirizine	>6 months	2.5–5 mg	OD	Minimal CNS effects
Fexofenadine	>6 months	30–60 mg	BID	Nonsedating, good safety
Loratadine	>2 years	5–10 mg	OD	Long half-life
Bilastine	≥6 years	10 mg (6–12 years); 20 mg (>12 years)	OD	Must be taken on empty stomach
Desloratadine	>6 months	2.5–5 mg	OD	Nonsedating

TABLE 4: Preparations of intranasal steroids (INS).

Drug	Dose	Age group	Comments
Fluticasone propionate	*4–12 years:* 1 spray/nostril (50 µg) od *>12 years:* 2 spray/nostril od.	>4 years	Bioavailability <1%
Fluticasone Furoate	27.5 µg/nostril od 55 µg/nostril od	2–12 years >12 years	Bioavailability <1%
Mometasone furoate	*2–12 years:* 1 spray/nostril (50 µg) od *>12 years:* 2 sprays/nostril od	>2 years	Bioavailability <1%

- Side effects are irritability, insomnia, aggravated hypertension, and arrhythmia.

Nasal decongestants:
- Nasal decongestants include imidazole derivatives such as xylometazoline or oxymetazoline.
- They have more rapid onset of action and are stronger than oral drugs. They are used only for 3–5 days
- They do not have systemic side effects. Longer use can lead to rhinitis medicamentosa.

Intranasal Steroids

Mechanism of action: Inhibition of mediator release during both early and late phase reactions

Inhibition of influx of basophils, neutrophils, eosinophils, reduction of Th2 cytokines and chemokines in nasal secretions. Their action begins within 7–8 hours of dosing.

Preparations of intranasal steroids (INS) are given in **Table 4**.

Side effects: Local nasal irritation, epistaxis, rarely nasal septal perforations, and candida overgrowth. Systemic side effects are very rare if they are used for long term in high dose.

Growth monitoring every 6 monthly if used for longer duration

Technique should be 45° toward turbinate away from the nasal septum.

Leukotriene Inhibitors

- *Zileuton:* Inhibitors of 5-lipooxygenease pathway
- *Montelukast and Zafirlukast:* Leukotriene receptor antagonists.
- Not used alone as a preferred drug for allergic rhinitis
- Less effective than INS and antihistamine
- *Side effects:* Agitation, hyperactivity, suicidal tendency
- In adolescence [Food and Drug Administration (FDA) issued black box warning]
- *Saline irrigation:* Prior to steroid, mucociliary clearance and removal of irritants

Anticholinergic

- Ipratropium bromide
- Useful for rhinorrhea, watery nasal discharge in AR, gustatory rhinitis,
- and vasomotor rhinitis.

Cromolyn Sodium

Intranasal cromolyn sodium 4% solution is used as A mast cell membrane stabilizer. It is mainly effective against sneezing and used before the onset of action. Dosage frequency is 4–6 times a day.

TABLE 5: Effect of drugs on various symptoms of allergic rhinitis.

Drug class	*Sneezing*	*Itching*	*Rhinorrhea*	*Congestion*	*Ocular symptoms*
Intranasal steroids	+++	++	+++	++	+
Intranasal antihistamines	++	++	++	+	++
Oral H1 antihistamines	+	+	+	+/–	+/–
LTRA	+	+	+	+	+/–

(LTRA: leukotriene receptor antagonists)

Role of Disease-modifying Therapy

Allergen Immunotherapy

It decreases the number of mast cells, basophils, eosinophils, and TH2 cells. Production of IgG/IgG4 antibodies inhibit IgE activation. It also decreases TH2 immune response and increases Treg cells. The minimum duration required is 3 years. It improves the symptom score as well as medication score in AR. Currently, sublingual immunotherapy and subcutaneous immunotherapy are practiced in India.

Role of Surgery in Allergic Rhinitis

- Septoplasty—for deviated nasal septum
- Adenoidectomy—for adenoidal hypertrophy
- Video endoscopic sinus surgery—associated with chronic sinusitis, where maximum
- Medical treatment fails

Management of Allergic Rhinitis According to Control

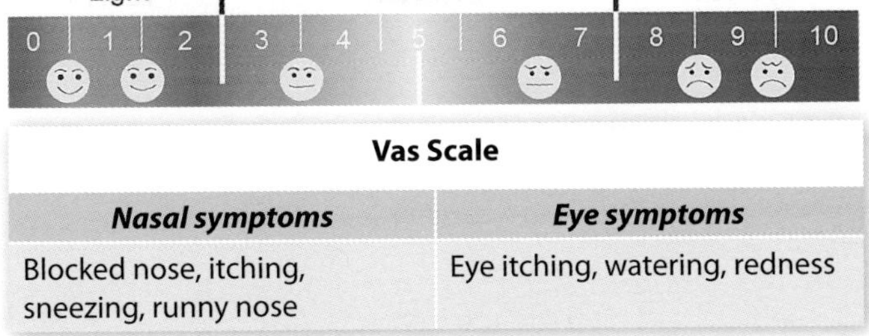

Vas Scale	
Nasal symptoms	***Eye symptoms***
Blocked nose, itching, sneezing, runny nose	Eye itching, watering, redness

LOCAL ALLERGIC RHINITIS

In patients with a negative SPT and absence of specific IgE antibody in peripheral blood, LAR is an underdiagnosed/misdiagnosed disease.

The diagnosis of LAR is based on a clinical history, a positive response to nasal allergen provocation test, and/or the detection of nasal IgE.

CAUSES OF NONALLERGIC RHINITIS

- Infective
- Acute rhinosinusitis
- Chronic rhinosinusitis
- Viral, bacterial
- *Noninfective:*
  - *Vasomotor:* Weather changes, smoke, strong smell. Mainly congestion and secretions
  - *Drug induced:* Nasal decongestant, cocaine
  - *Structural:* Deviated nasal septum (DNS)
  - *Immunopathological:* Primary ciliary dyskinesia (PCD), Primary immunodeficiency (PID)
  - *NARES:* Symptoms same as AR. Plenty of nasal eosinophils. SPT, specific IgE normal.

KEY POINTS

- Allergic rhinitis burden is increasing.
- Sneezing, itching, rhinorrhea, and nasal congestion are the main symptoms.
- SPT is the gold standard test for aeroallergen sensitization.
- Mainly a clinical diagnosis
- Identification of sanitization by allergen is important.
- Intranasal steroid is the main pharmacological treatment of moderate to severe persistent AR.
- Allergen avoidance and allergen immunotherapy are nonpharmacological treatment options.

CONCLUSION

Allergic rhinitis is a common, chronic, IgE-mediated inflammatory disorder of the nasal mucosa that significantly affects quality of life and is frequently associated with comorbid conditions such as asthma, sinusitis, otitis media with effusion, and allergic conjunctivitis. A thorough understanding of its pathophysiology, clinical presentation, and differential diagnosis is essential for accurate recognition and effective management. Diagnosis is largely clinical, supported by appropriate allergen sensitization testing when required. Management should follow a stepwise, individualized approach emphasizing patient and parent education, allergen avoidance, and pharmacotherapy, with intranasal corticosteroids forming the cornerstone of treatment for moderate to severe disease. Allergen immunotherapy offers a disease-modifying option in selected patients, while surgical intervention is reserved for associated structural abnormalities or complications refractory to medical therapy. Early diagnosis, optimal treatment, and regular follow-up are crucial to achieving good symptom control, preventing complications, and improving long-term outcomes in patients with allergic rhinitis.

SUGGESTED READING

1. Berger WE, Meltzer EO. Intranasal spray medications for maintenance therapy of allergic rhinitis. Am J Rhinol Allergy. 2015;29(4):273-82.
2. Bernstein IL, Li JT, Bernstein DI, Hamilton R, Spector SL, Tan R, et al. Allergy diagnostic testing: an updated practice parameter. Ann Allergy Asthma Immunol. 2008;100(3 Suppl 3):S1-148.
3. Bousquet, et al. Oral antihistamines in allergic rhinitis. Clin Exp Allergy; 2005.
4. Bousquet J, Khaltaev N, Cruz AA, Denburg J, Fokkens WJ, Togias A, et al. Allergic Rhinitis and its Impact on Asthma (ARIA) 2008 update (in collaboration with the World Health Organization, GA(2)LEN and AllerGen). Allergy. 2008;63(Suppl 86):8-160.
5. Bousquet J, Lockey R, Malling HJ. Allergen immunotherapy: therapeutic vaccines for allergic diseases. A WHO position paper. Allergy. 1998;53:4-42.
6. Brożek JL, Bousquet J, Agache I, Agarwal A, Bachert C, Bosnic-Anticevich S, et al. Allergic Rhinitis and Its Impact on Asthma (ARIA) guidelines-2016 revision. J Allergy Clin Immunol. 2017;140(4):950-8.
7. Hellings PW. Uncontrolled allergic rhinitis and chronic rhinosinusitis: where do we stand today? Allergy. 2013;68:1-7.
8. Hellings PW, Fokkens WJ, Akdis C, Bachert C, Cingi C, de Loos DD, et al. Uncontrolled allergic rhinitis and chronic rhinosinusitis: where do we stand today? Allergy. 2013;68:1-7.
9. Jonathan Corren, Fuad M. Baroody, Alkis Togias.
10. Major Nagaraju. Treatment of allergic rhinitis. In: Manual of Pediatric Allergy. New Delhi: Jaypee Brothers Medical Publishers; 2020. pp. 104-11.
11. Scaddling SK. Corticosteroids in the treatment of pediatric allergic rhinitis J Allergy Clin Immunol. 2001;108(1 Suppl):S59-64.
12. Seidman M, Gurgel RK, Lin SY, Schwartz SR, Baroody FM, Bonner JR, et al. Clinical Practice Guideline. Allergic Rhinitis. Otolarynogol Head Neck Surg. 2015;152:S1-43.
13. Sohrab S, et al. Allergo J 2013;22(2):128-34.
14. Wise SK, Lin SY, Toskala E, Orlandi RR, Akdis CA, Alt JA. International Consensus Statement on Allergy and Rhinology: Allergic Rhinitis. Int Forum Allergy Rhinol. 2018;8(2):108-352.

11 CHAPTER

Asthma and Allergy

Dhanesh Volvoikar

INTRODUCTION

Asthma is a heterogeneous disease characterized by chronic airway inflammation, with variable respiratory symptoms (wheezing, shortness of breath, chest tightness, and/or cough) and variable expiratory airflow limitation. These symptoms and airflow limitation can fluctuate over time and in intensity. Allergic asthma can be considered as asthma associated with sensitization to aeroallergens. Identification of allergic sensitization (in vivo and/or in vitro) and association between aeroallergen exposure and asthma symptoms are required to consider that one is having allergic asthma.

EPIDEMIOLOGY/INCIDENCE

The incidence of asthma varies between 1 and 29% of population in different countries. According to the Global Burden of Disease report, asthma accounts for roughly 4.2 lakhs death every year. The estimated prevalence in India is estimated at 7.9%, but regional variation ranges from 2 to 23%. The prevalence was higher among boys and in urban areas.

Asthma can begin at any age, onset is most common during early childhood, and 80% of cases begin before the age of 6 years.

PHENOTYPES AND ENDOTYPES OF ASTHMA

Asthma has been proposed as an umbrella term under which different phenotypes and endotypes frequently overlap, with allergic asthma holding a key position. Phenotypes refers to observable characteristics or traits, while endotype refers to specific biological mechanisms that contribute to those traits. In simple terms, phenotype is what you see (like symptoms) and endotype is what is happening (the underlying biological process).

Phenotypes

There are several clinical phenotypes of asthma. The common ones include the following:

- *Allergic asthma:* The most easily recognized phenotype, often commencing in childhood, and is associated with past or family history of allergic diseases such as eczema, allergic rhinitis, or food or drug allergy. Sputum examination often reveals eosinophilic airway inflammation, and the patients usually respond to inhaled corticosteroid (ICS) treatment.
- *Nonallergic asthma:* Not associated with allergy, often experiencing a minor short-term response to ICS. The cellular profile of the sputum of these patients can be neutrophilic and eosinophilic or contain few inflammatory cells.
- *Cough-variant asthma and cough-predominant asthma:* Cough may be the only symptom of asthma, and evidence of airflow limitation may be absent except during bronchial provocation testing. ICS-containing treatment is effective, but some of them can later develop wheezing and bronchodilator responsiveness.
- *Adult onset (late-onset asthma):* Usually nonallergic, often requires high doses of ICS or is relatively refractory to ICS
- *Asthma with persistent airflow limitation:* Patients with longstanding asthma can develop airflow limitation that is persistent or incompletely responsive ("reversible") to treatment due to airway wall remodeling **(Figs. 1A to C)**.
- *Asthma with obesity:* Obese patients with asthma may have a different pattern of airway inflammation with little eosinophilic inflammation.
- *Occupational asthma:* Usually found in adults due to agent exposed at workplace.

Endotype

Asthma is stratified into two main endotypes: T2 (Th 2) and non-T2 (non-Th2).

80% of childhood asthma and 50% of adult asthma have an allergic or Th2 (T2) endotype.

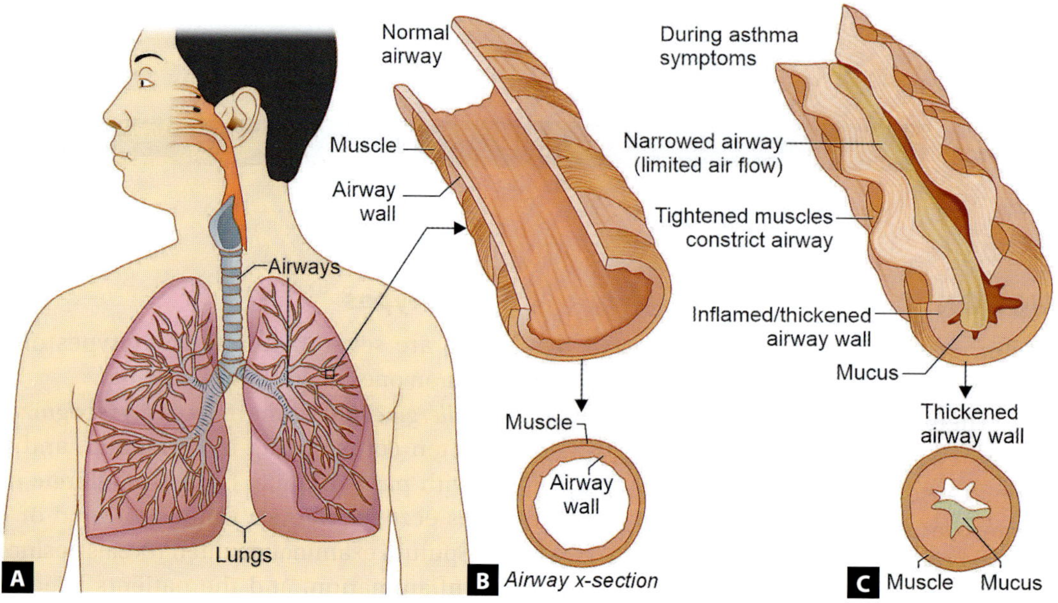

Figs. 1A to C: Factors limiting airflow.
Source: Adapted from Expert Panel Report 3: Guidelines for the Diagnosis and Management of Asthma. Bethesda: National Heart, Lung, and Blood Institute (US); 2007.

Th2 Endotype

This is one of the extensive and possibly the best-defined asthma endotypes. It is characterized by a type 2 immune response that involves Th2 cells, B cells, basophils, eosinophils, mast cells, major cytokines secreted from immune cells [interleukin (IL)-4, IL-5, IL-9, and IL-13], and others secreted from epithelial cells [IL-25, IL-31, IL-33, and thymic stromal lymphopoietin (TSLP)]. This is the endotype underlying allergic asthma and is strongly linked to atopy, IgE production, and eosinophilic inflammation. This is one of the most important endotypes in childhood, as is closely associated with the early-onset asthma phenotype that usually onsets during childhood and early adolescence. This endotype is certainly prevalent in adulthood, seeing that about 50% of mild asthmatics have an endotype that is associated with eosinophilia, mast cell activation, development of allergen-specific IgE, and Th2 cytokine production. Subset of T2-high phenotype could also be nonallergic where innate immunity is mediated with nonspecific mechanisms, as pollutants, parasites, and pathogens can trigger airway hyperresponsiveness and eosinophilia through alarmin-mediated ILC2 activation. Clinically, nonallergic eosinophilic patients have late-onset asthma and often develop chronic rhinosinusitis with nasal polyps (CRSwNP) **(Fig. 2)**.

Non-Th2 Endotype

Approximately half of adult asthmatic patients have non-T2 or Th2-low endotype. From the clinical perspective, these patients show less airway obstruction and hyperreactivity than Th2-high asthmatics. It is important to note that these are generally nonatopic patients, and there is little to no evidence of allergy in childhood or beyond. Two major mechanisms leading to non-type 2 asthma have been hypothesized: (1) Activation of the IL-17-dependent pathway and (2) innate immune response dysregulation bringing about neutrophil inflammation. It is generally characterized by neutrophilic (sputum neutrophils >40–60%) or paucigranulocytic (i.e., normal sputum levels of both eosinophils and neutrophils) inflammation, and a lack of response to corticosteroid therapy. T2-low asthma has been linked to the activation of Th1 and/or Th17 cells, and recent studies have found that the imbalance of Th17/Treg cells may play an important role in steroid-resistant, severe, and neutrophilic asthma.

ATOPIC MARCH AND NATURAL HISTORY

Allergic march can be labeled as the natural progression of start of allergic diseases. Often, the allergic disease initially manifests as eczema, occurring during infancy or early childhood. Alongside this, food allergies also develop in the early stages of life. Such early allergic diseases are

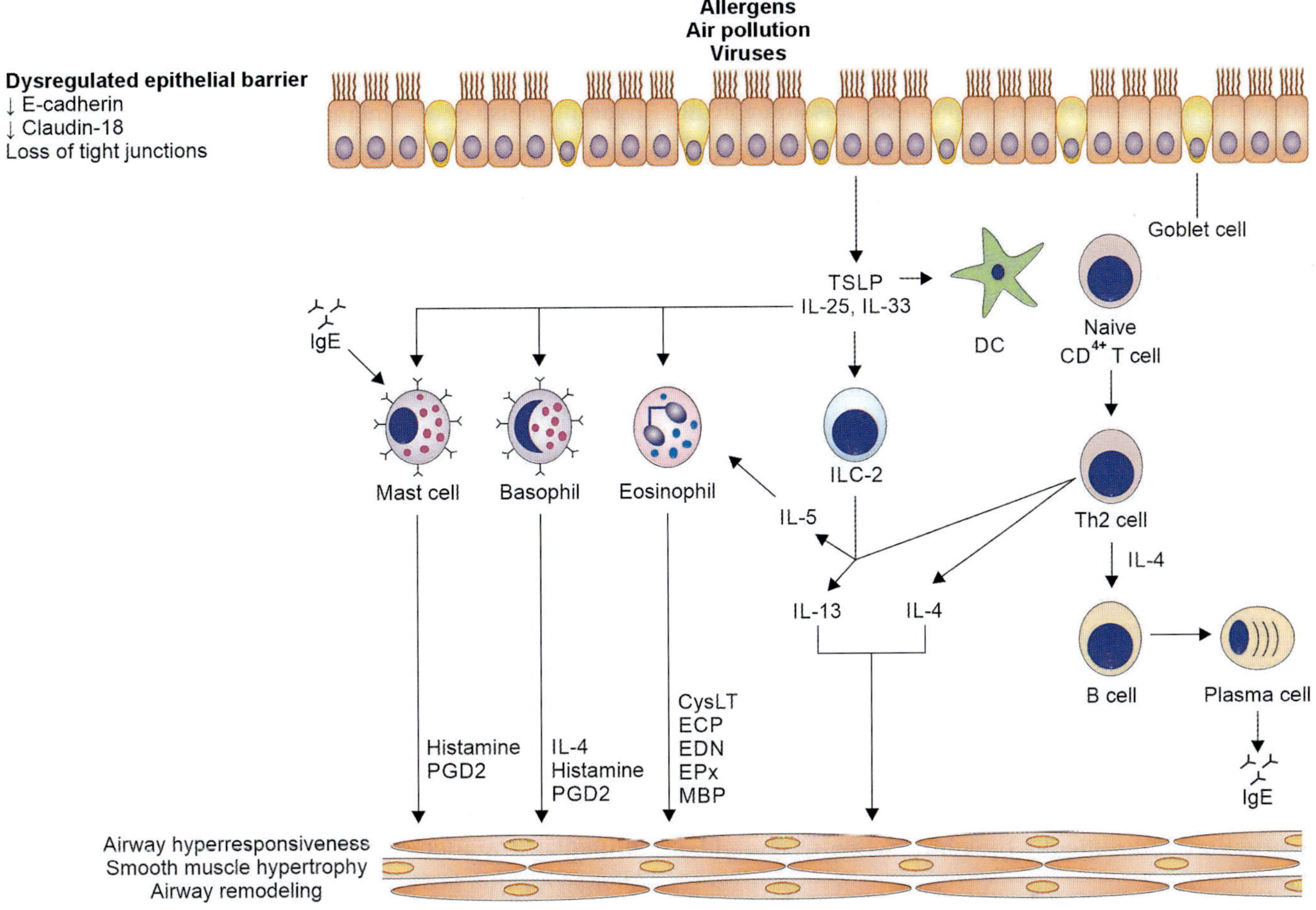

Fig. 2: T2-high inflammatory pathways in asthma. A dysregulated epithelial barrier enables translocation of allergens, air pollution, and viruses, leading to release of alarmins such as TSLP, IL-25, and IL-33. TSLP primes dendritic cells to induce the differentiation of naïve T cells into Th2 cells. Th2 cells activate B cells via IL-4 to differentiate into plasma cells that generate IgE required for mast cell responses to allergens. The alarmins IL-25 and IL-33 can activate group 2 innate lymphoid cells (ILC2s), mast cells, eosinophils, and basophils. Activated ILC2s, like Th2 cells, produce IL-5 and IL-13. IL-5 promotes eosinophil differentiation and survival. IL-13, IL-4, and inflammatory mediators from mast cells, basophils, and eosinophils have effects on airway hyperresponsiveness, smooth muscle hypertrophy, and airway remodeling. (CysLT: cysteinyl leukotrienes; ECP: eosinophil cationic protein; EDN: eosinophil-derived neurotoxin; EPx: eosinophil peroxidase; MBP: major basic protein; PGD2: prostaglandin D2)

generally followed by asthma and hay fever (allergic rhinitis). It is this natural progression of these diseases from eczema to food allergies to asthma to allergic rhinitis that constitutes the allergic march, also known as the atopic march. This trend is not seen strictly in all children, and some variations are observed. Some children outgrow their allergies, while others develop asthma and allergies for the first time later in adulthood. Both allergies and asthma are a result of a dysfunction of the immune system.

Rise of Atopic Diseases

There has been a noticeable increase in atopic diseases in the last couple of decades. Researchers have theorized that this increase may be attributed to dietary, genetic, epigenetic, environmental, and lifestyle factors—in utero and during childhood.

Patients who have a particular mutation in the filaggrin gene have been found to be more susceptible to atopic dermatitis. This gene is of vital function in the epidermis of the skin. Though atopic diseases have a genetic component and are more prevalent in individuals presenting a family history of allergic disease, the examined rapid increases in allergic diseases cannot be attributed to changes in genes alone. Atopic diseases are complicated and potentially caused by a range of factors rather than a singular cause. For instance, dietary changes in the past decades were thought to have altered the type of microbes in the gut, making one more vulnerable to allergies.

Another concept that strives to explain the increase in atopic disease is the hygiene hypothesis. It is an evolving theory that states an abnormally clean environment that limits childhood exposure to triggers and infections, which causes a "naive" immune system and increases the incidence of asthma and allergies. This theory suggests that the implementation of modern lifestyles limits one's exposure to the natural substances in the environment, and excessive cleanliness habits prevent one's body from acclimatizing to the environment while still in the womb, as an infant, or in childhood. Regular exposure to the outdoor environment and recurrent contact with animals and pets—as was common in previous generations—is believed to have protected people from allergies and asthma, by increasing exposure to various microbes and substances in the natural environment, and desensitizing the body to common environmental allergens.

PATHOPHYSIOLOGY

Allergic asthma pathophysiology involves a complex interplay of immune responses, airway inflammation, and bronchial hyperresponsiveness, resulting in airway obstruction and difficulty breathing when triggered by allergens.

Children with atopic predisposition identify certain allergens, like house dust mite (HDM), pollens, pet dander, etc., as harmful substances, triggering an immune response by producing allergen-specific antibodies which get attached to mast cells. When exposed to the same antigen, it can cause an antigen–antibody reaction and break mast cell, which releases a variety of inflammatory mediators like histamines, leukotrienes, prostaglandins, etc. These mediators cause the smooth muscles of the airway to contract, leading to bronchoconstriction. It also stimulates mucus production, which further obstructs the airway. The initial release of mediators attracts other inflammatory cells like eosinophils and neutrophils to the airways. *Late-phase response and chronic inflammation*: If not treated, a late-phase response can occur hours after the initial reaction. During this phase, inflammatory cells such as eosinophils, basophils, neutrophils, and helper and memory T-cells migrate to the lungs, prolonging and intensifying inflammation and bronchoconstriction, which further obstructs airflow. The sustained presence of these cells, particularly eosinophils, leads to the continued release of inflammatory cytokines, further perpetuating the inflammatory response. These cells contribute to prolonged airway inflammation, leading to airway hyperresponsiveness (increased sensitivity to triggers). In some cases, continuous airway inflammation can lead to permanent structural changes in the airways, collectively termed airway remodeling by way of irreversible thickening in their walls with increased mucous production which can make the airways permanently narrowed. These changes may include thickening of the airway walls, hyperplasia (increased number of cells) and hypertrophy (increased size) of airway smooth muscle, and subepithelial fibrosis (scarring and stiffening of the airway wall). This remodeling can lead to a more fixed and less reversible airflow obstruction, making asthma harder to manage. Another key feature in asthma is airway hyperresponsiveness, where airways constrict excessively in response to various stimuli, not just allergens.

WHAT IS ALLERGIC ASTHMA?

Allergic asthma which is the most common phenotype of asthma is defined as asthma associated with sensitization to aeroallergens, which leads to asthma symptoms and airway inflammation. A T2 inflammatory pathway influences the mechanisms of allergic asthma **(Fig. 3)**. Allergic asthma is the most common asthma phenotype. The onset of allergic asthma is most often in childhood and is usually accompanied by other comorbidities including atopic dermatitis and allergic rhinitis. It is often persistent although there is a wide variation in disease severity. It is a TH2-driven process. Biomarkers have been identified to distinguish patients with allergic asthma, particularly serum IgE levels, tests to indicate sensitization to aeroallergens such as specific IgE or skin prick test positivity, blood and sputum eosinophil levels, fraction of exhaled nitric oxide, and periostin. Treatments for allergic asthma include environmental-control measures, allergen immunotherapy, and glucocorticoids. Biologics, targeting the TH2 pathway, have been shown to be effective in the treatment of allergic asthma.

CLINICAL FEATURES

Asthma is usually characterized by chronic airway inflammation and variable symptoms including cough, chest tightness, shortness of breath and wheezing, along with variable expiratory airflow limitation, which can become persistent due to airway remodeling.

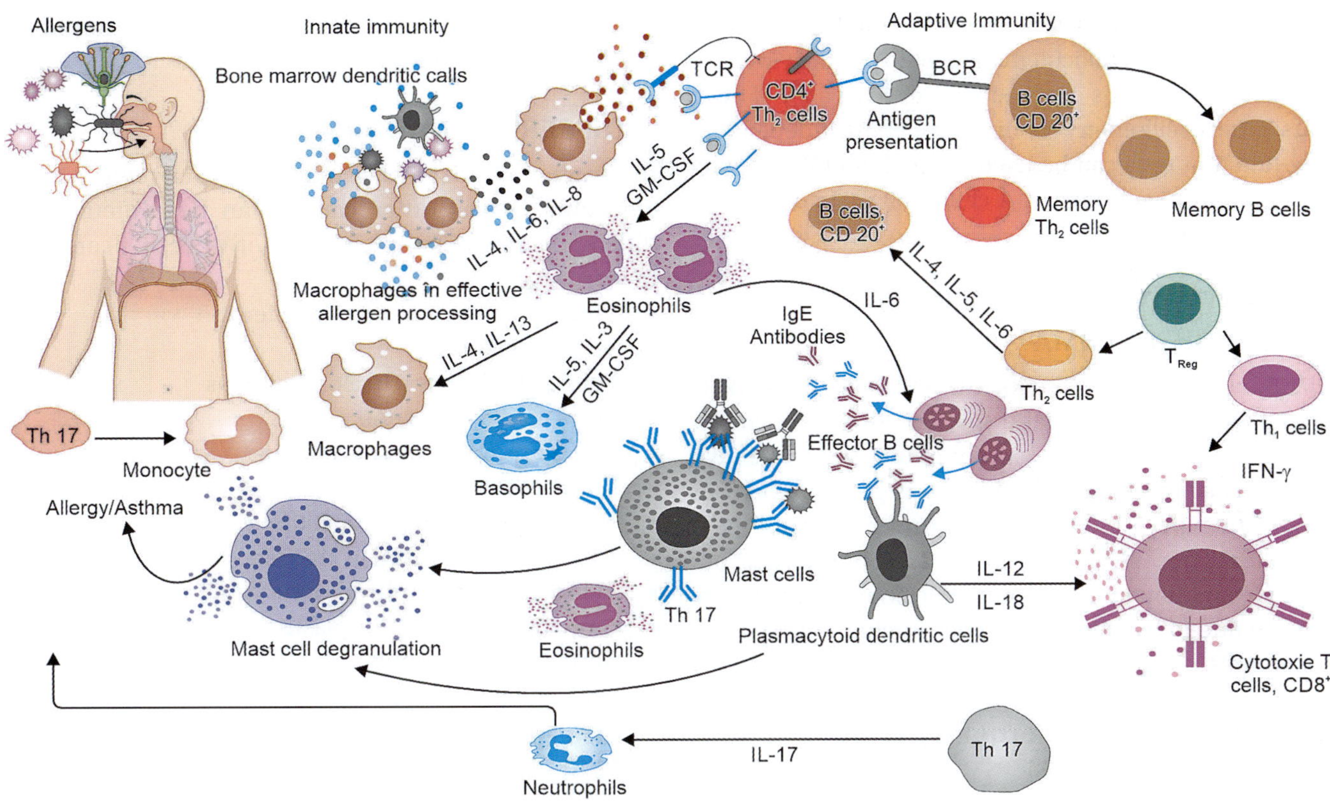

Fig. 3: Immune mechanism in allergic asthma.

DIAGNOSIS

Asthma diagnosis is based on characteristic symptom patterns and evidence of variable expiratory airflow limitation. This should be authenticated by bronchodilator reversibility tests or other assessments via pulmonary function test (PFT) before starting ICS-containing treatment.

SPIROMETRY

An increase of forced expiratory volume in 1 second (FEV1) of 12% or more from baseline after administration of a short-acting bronchodilator indicates significant reversibility. The ongoing SABA (short-acting beta-agonist) inhaler has to be withdrawn for 4 hours and formoterol or salmeterol for 24 hours.

Another spirometry parameter FEV1/FVC will also be decreased in asthma.

The above finding after 4 weeks of ICS treatment will also confirm variable airflow.

In a resource-poor setup, a peak flow meter can be used. Peak expiratory flow rate (PEFR) will be increased >15% in children or 20% in adults after the SABA inhaler when measured after 10–15 minutes.

In case spirometry or PEF is not available fractional exhaled nitric oxide (FeNO) >50 ppb in children above 11 years or >35 in children, or increased eosinophils can help in the diagnosis of type II asthma (other causes cannot be fully ruled out in this criteria).

Diagnosing asthma in children aged 5 years or younger can be difficult. A clinician may need to anticipate the pattern of symptoms indicative of asthma alongside family history and physical examination findings.

As per Global Initiative for Asthma (GINA) guidelines, the following symptoms are found to be consistent with asthma in young children:

- Recurrent persistent cough which gets worse at night
- Cough that worsens after exposure to triggers such as laughing, crying, exercise, or tobacco smoke
- Decreased level of activity compared to other children
- In case of positive family history of allergic or atopic disease
- Improvement in symptoms after 2–3 months' trial of ICS or worsening after stopping a trial of controller medication

Although spirometry is recommended in children above 5 years, it is a difficult maneuver to perform even for children up to 7 years or sometimes even in a child of 10 years. Lung oscillometry (noninvasive effort-independent lung function test) can be used in smaller children who cannot perform spirometry. A child of 3 years of age can perform this test.

INVESTIGATIONS SPECIFIC TO ALLERGIC ASTHMA

Allergic asthma often presents with TH2-high biomarkers including elevated blood and sputum eosinophil counts and FeNO, as well as periostin in adults. More than 3% sputum eosinophils are considered as gold standard as important type 2 biomarker. Sputum eosinophils are considered the "gold standard" type 2 biomarker, but there is limitation in using sputum eosinophils in clinical practice due to technical difficulties in obtaining sputum eosinophils.

Skin Prick Test and Allergen-specific Immunoglobulin E

Allergen sensitization can be confirmed using skin prick test (SPT) or allergen-specific immunoglobulin E (SsIgE) which is positive in majority of children with asthma, aged 3 years or older. Selective allergy testing can help to prevent strategies for children exposed to HDM, mold, furry animals, cockroaches, pollens, etc. It can be a useful guide for initiating allergen immunotherapy also.

Measuring fractional exhaled nitric oxide: This is produced by cells in the airways, including eosinophils, during airway inflammation and it can be assessed. FeNO >50 ppb in adults and 35 ppb in children is associated with eosinophilic inflammation and response to the same. These levels can be elevated in cases of allergic rhinitis, atopy, eosinophilic bronchitis, and atopic dermatitis and reduced in smokers or during bronchoconstriction. Viral exposure also can result in either reduced or increased levels of FeNO.

Serum periostin: Periostin is a matricellular protein that is upregulated by T2 cytokines, IL-4, and IL-13 in bronchial epithelial cells. Measurement of the same in the serum of asthmatic patients makes it a useful biomarker in assessing T2 inflammation and remodeling. But in pediatric population, its use as a biomarker is yet to be explored due to bone growth and baseline periostin levels always being on the higher side in children. As of now, it is not freely available in India.

DIFFERENTIAL DIAGNOSIS

In smaller children distinguishing between asthma wheezing versus other causes can be difficult. The differential diagnosis in children for wheezing can be as follows:

- Viral upper respiratory tract infection
- Viral bronchiolitis
- Foreign body in trachea or bronchus
- Vocal cord dysfunction
- Vascular rings or laryngeal webs
- Gastroesophageal reflux
- Protracted bacterial bronchitis
- Laryngotracheomalacia, tracheal stenosis
- Enlarged lymph node or tumor
- Bronchopulmonary dysplasia
- Kartagener syndrome
- Congenital heart disease
- Pertussis
- Cystic fibrosis.

MANAGEMENT

There are multiple treatment considerations for allergic asthma, including environmental-control measures, immunotherapy, glucocorticoids, and biologics. Always give importance and treat allergic conditions as whole. Allergic asthma is invariably associated with allergic rhinitis and its comorbidities, atopic dermatitis, allergic conjunctivitis, and sometimes even food allergy. Adress all the issues and not just treat the patient's lung condition as comprehensive management is required when dealing with allergic conditions. Health education on a one-to-one basis with parents is the necessity in any chronic diseases, and it is the backbone of effective allergy asthma management.

Health Education and Counseling

Important components of management are: (1) Provide simple explanation of asthma and its symptoms, (2) explain treatment modalities and advantages of using inhaler therapy, (3) demonstrate the use of inhaler technique with return demonstration by parents at follow-up, (4) reinforce the importance of compliance to medication, (5) provide written asthma action plan, (6) discuss the common triggers of asthma and measures to avoid and control them, (7) address parent concern and some of the common myths about the use of inhalers and steroids, and (8) explain and inform all other means of therapies and prognosis.

Bronchodilaters and Inhaled Corticosteroids

While the use of ICSs constitutes the gold standard in maintenance treatment of asthma and biologic agents, there are many other treatment options also available for asthma management. Long-acting beta-2 agonists (LABAs) approved for use with asthma include formoterol, salmeterol, and vilanterol, and the combination of ICSs and LABAs is proposed for therapy in adults and adolescents in step 3 of the GINA report. In response to single maintenance and reliever in which a single inhaler is used as a controller and reliever medication, GINA recommends the use of as-needed low doses of ICS/formoterol as the preferred reliever medication for all levels of asthma severity in adults and adolescents. Leukotriene receptor antagonists (LTRAs) can be used in patients with mild asthma as an alternative to ICSs, but its neuropsychiatric adverse effects should be informed to parents/caregivers. LAMAs can be considered as an add-on therapy, using a separate inhaler for patients aged >6 years, or in a triple combination in patients aged >18 years if asthma remains uncontrolled despite medium- or high-dose ICS/LABA treatment. Theophylline and cromoglycate are controllers that are rarely used nowadays due to their increased side effects and inferior efficacy profiles compared to ICSs. The use of SABA is no longer considered the best choice in the form of single inhalers for patients with mild asthma and they are no longer the preferred reliever option for all other patients except in under-5 wheezing. The short-acting muscarinic antagonist ipratropium can be used in a hospital setting along with SABA in asthma flare-ups to improve exacerbation. Specific management of asthma in different age-groups as per GINA 2025 for children younger than 5 years has been presented in **Table 1**, in children between ages of 6 and 11 years in **Table 2**, and in children >12 years in **Table 3**.

Environmental Control

Environmental control consists of identifying and reducing exposure to asthma triggers at home, school or workplace, or outdoor environment. Irritants like tobacco smoke, smell of deodorants/perfumes, powders, cold air, or cold drinks if found to stimulate asthma symptoms need to be avoided.

Environmental control can significantly affect allergic asthma management. A systematic review assessing the effect of multiple component environmental interventions concluded that an overall improvement in productivity and quality of life was observed in children and adolescents with asthma, but the results regarding the adult population

TABLE 1: Long-term management of asthma in children 5 years and younger.

Options	*Step I*	*Step II*	*Step III*	*Step IV*
Preferred controller choice	Insufficient evidence for daily controller	Daily low-dose ICS	Double "low-dose" ICS	Continue controller and refer to a specialist
Other controller options (limited indications or less evidence for efficacy or safety)	Consider intermittent short course of ICS at the onset of viral illness	Daily LTRA or intermittent short courses of ICS at the onset of respiratory illness	Consider specialist referral	
Reliever: As needed short-acting β2 agonist				
Consider this step for children with	Infrequent acute (e.g., viral induced) wheezing episodes and no or minimal interval asthma symptoms	Asthma symptoms not well controlled (SABA requires >2 times a week on an average) or one or more severe exacerbations in the past 1 year	Asthma diagnosis not well controlled on low-dose ICS	Asthma not well controlled on double ICS
			Before stepping up, check out for alternative diagnosis and inhaler skills and review adherence and exposures	

(ICS: inhaled corticosteroids; SABA: short-acting beta-agonist)

TABLE 2: Long-term management of asthma in children aged 6–11 years.

Age	Options	Step I	Step II	Step III	Step IV	Step V
		Symptoms <twice a month	Symptoms >twice a month	Symptoms most days or waking with asthma once a week or more	Symptoms most days or waking with asthma once a week or more and low lung function	Short-course OCS may also be needed for patients presenting with severely uncontrolled asthma
	Preferred controller	Low-dose ICS taken whenever SABA taken	Daily low-dose ICS	Low-dose ICS-LABA or medium-dose ICS or very low dose ICS Formoterol MART	Medium-dose ICS-LABA or low-dose ICS formoterol MART or refer for expert advice	Refer for phenotypic assessment +/− higher dose ICS-LABA or add-on therapy, e.g., LAMA, anti-IgE, anti-IL4Ra, anti-IL5
	Alternative controller		Daily LTRA or low-dose ICS taken whenever SABA taken	Low-dose ICS + LTRA	Add Tiotropium or add LTRA	Only as last resort consider add-on low-dose OCS, but consider side effects
	Reliever: As needed SABA or ICS-Formoterol reliever for MART in steps 3 and 4.					

(ICS: inhaled corticosteroids; LABA: long-acting beta-2 agonist; LAMA: long-acting muscarinic antagonist; LTRA: leukotriene receptor antagonist; OCS: oral corticosteroids; MART: maintenance and reliever therapy; SABA: short-acting beta-agonist)

were inconclusive. The use of mite-impermeable covers in mite-sensitized children led to a reduction of asthma exacerbation, but no effect was observed from the use of oral corticosteroids. It can be used in sensitized patients. In India, dust mite is known to be associated with 60–80% cases of allergic asthma. Specific recommendation can be given on environmental control based on other clinically relevant allergens like molds, pet dander, or pollens.

ALLERGEN IMMUNOTHERAPY

Allergen immunotherapy (AIT) has a century-long history of use for allergic diseases, and it aspires to be the only etiologically based therapy for allergic asthma and allergic rhinitis and works by inducing immunologic tolerance. It may be considered for adults and children with asthma who have clinically significant sensitization to aeroallergens, including in those with allergic rhinitis. AIT has a disease-modifying effect, demonstrated by prevention of new allergen sensitizations and the ability to halt disease progression. Hence, it is recommended for patients with allergic rhinitis and allergic asthma according to multiple guidelines and should be used early in atopic march. AIT should be commenced once asthma is well controlled and it should never be started in severe uncontrolled asthma. Subcutaneous immunotherapy (SCIT) or sublingual immunotherapy (SLIT) are two routes of administrations available. According to the European Academy of Allergy and Clinical Immunology (EAACI) guidelines for the use of HDM immunotherapy as an add-on treatment for HDM-driven allergic asthma in children and adolescents, HDM SCIT is recommended in both children and adults with allergic asthma to reduce symptoms and medication needs. HDM SLIT tablets and drops are recommended for adults and children, respectively. GINA recommends the use of HDM SLIT in adults and adolescents with allergic rhinitis and HDM sensitization as an add-on treatment when asthma symptoms persist despite treatment with a low/medium dose of ICS-containing medication given that FEV1 is predicted to be above 70%.

Biologic Agents

In patients with severe uncontrolled asthma characterized by T2 inflammation, targeted therapies using biologic agents are available as add-on treatments to reduce the disease burden. Five monoclonal antibodies are currently licensed for children >6 years of age by both the Food and Drug Administration (FDA) and the European Medicines Agency (EMA) as add-on treatments for severe uncontrolled asthma: Benralizumab, dupilumab, mepolizumab, omalizumab, and reslizumab. Recently, tezepelumab, an anti-TSLP biologic, has been granted approval by the FDA for use in the treatment of severe asthma in adults and adolescents aged 12 years and older. Many more agents are under development with the aim to further optimize treatment for asthma patients.

TABLE 3: Long-term management of asthma in children 12 years and older.

Age	*Options*	*Step I*	*Step II*	*Step III*	*Step IV*	*Step V*
12 years onward		Symptoms less than 3–5 days/ week, with normal or mildly reduced lung function	Symptoms less than 3–5 days/ week, with normal or slightly reduced lung function	Symptoms most days or waking at night once a week or more or low lung function	Daily symptoms or waking at night once a week or more, and low lung function or recent exacerbation	Short-course OCS may also be needed for patients presenting during an exacerbation
	Controller and preferred reliever	As needed, low-dose ICS-formoterol	As needed, low-dose ICS-formoterol	Low-dose maintenance ICS-formoterol	Medium-dose maintenance ICS-formoterol	Add-on LAMA. Refer for phenotypic assessment. Consider a trial of high-dose maintenance ICS formoterol. Consider anti-IgE, anti-IL5/5R, anti IL4Ra, anti-TSLP
	Reliever: As needed low-dose ICS-formoterol					
		Less frequent asthma symptoms, e.g., 1–2 days/ week or less	*Symptoms:* Twice a month or more but less than 4–5 days a week	*Symptoms:* Most days or waking at night once a week or more or low lung function	Daily symptoms or waking at night once a week or more, and low lung function or recent exacerbation	Short-course OCS may also be needed for patients presenting during an exacerbation
	Controller and alternative reliever	Low-dose ICS taken whenever SABA is taken	Low-dose maintenance ICS	Low-dose maintenance ICS-LABA	Medium-dose maintenance ICS-LABA	Add-on LAMA. Refer for phenotypic assessment. Consider trial of high-dose maintenance ICS-LABA. Consider anti-IgE, anti-IL5/5R, anti-IL4Ra, anti-TSLP
	As needed ICS-SABA, or as needed SABA as Reliever					

(ICS: inhaled corticosteroids; LABA: long-acting beta-2 agonist; LAMA: long-acting muscarinic antagonist; OCS: oral corticosteroids; SABA: short-acting beta-agonist; TSLP: thymic stromal lymphopoietin)
Note: If LTRA is prescribed, advise parents/caregiver about the risk of neuropsychiatric adverse effects.

PROGNOSIS

59% of persistent wheezing go in remission by 6 years of age. Allergic asthma often commences in childhood, representing a large variation in disease severity, which can occasionally be persistent and continue into adulthood. 30–70% of children with asthma undergo substantial improvement or become symptom-free by early adulthood. However, nearly 75% of those with asthma and wheezing during adolescence continue to experience symptoms into adulthood. Persistent asthma is associated with factors such as atopy, low lung function, and increased airway hyperresponsiveness, with sensitization and exposure to indoor allergens posing a three-fold higher risk.

CONCLUSION

Globally, about 30–35% of children suffer from allergic disorders, and the prevalence of these illnesses has been rising in recent years. Of all the allergic disorders, asthma has a substantial financial impact on both patients and the healthcare system. Allergic asthma is a common phenotype within the diverse spectrum of this chronic disease and a T2-high inflammation profile. Several biomarkers exist to diagnose allergic asthma and many more are under investigation with the aim of proving their value in predicting and monitoring the course of the disease and response to treatment. With allergen immunotherapy being the only etiological therapy for allergic diseases, and asthma that works by promoting immunologic tolerance, other tailor-made interventions have risen. Biologics as add-on treatments for severe asthma patients are at the forefront but these still need to be investigated, not only for their impact on controlling the inflammation of asthma but also for their disease-modifying outcome.

KEY PONITS

- *Allergic asthma is the most common asthma phenotype,* typically beginning in childhood, associated with atopy, IgE sensitization to aeroallergens, eosinophilic inflammation, and a *Type 2 (Th2/T2-high) endotype.*
- *Asthma is a heterogeneous disease* with overlapping *phenotypes and endotypes;* while ~80% of childhood asthma is T2-high, nearly *50% of adult asthma is non–T2,* often neutrophilic, steroid-resistant, and non-atopic.
- *Atopic (allergic) march* describes the natural progression from eczema and food allergy in infancy to asthma and allergic rhinitis later in childhood, highlighting shared immune mechanisms and opportunities for early intervention.
- *Diagnosis of allergic asthma* relies on characteristic symptoms with *demonstration of variable airflow limitation,* supported by biomarkers such as eosinophils, *FeNO, IgE sensitization* (SPT/specific IgE), and lung function testing (spirometry or oscillometry in young children).
- *Management is comprehensive and personalized,* combining inhaled corticosteroids as the cornerstone, environmental control, treatment of comorbid *allergies, allergen immunotherapy as the only disease-modifying therapy, and biologics targeting T2 pathways* for severe uncontrolled asthma.

SUGGESTED READING

1. Agache I, Lau S, Akdis CA, Smolinska S, Bonini M, Cavkaytar O, et al. EAACI Guidelines on Allergen Immunotherapy: House dust mite-driven allergic asthma. Allergy 2019;74: 855-73.
2. Brożek JL, Bousquet J, Agache I, Agarwal A, Bachert C, Bosnic-Anticevich S, et al. Allergic Rhinitis and its Impact on Asthma (ARIA) guidelines-2016 revision. J Allergy Clin Immunol. 2017;140:950-8.
3. Crocker DD, Kinyota S, Dumitru GG, et al. Effectiveness of home-based, multi-trigger, multicomponent interventions with an environmental focus for reducing asthma morbidity: A community guide systematic review. Am J Prev Med. 2011;41 (Suppl. S1):S5-32.
4. Global Initiative for Asthma (GINA) 2025. [online] Available from https://ginasthma.org/2025-gina-strategy-report/ [Last accessed December, 2025].
5. Gohal G, Moni SS, Ali Bakkari M, Eltaib Elmobark M. A Review on Asthma and Allergy: Current Understanding on Molecular Perspectives. J Clin Med. 2024;13:5775.
6. IAP Standard Treatment Guidelines 2022: Bronchial Asthma:177-185.
7. Jutel M, Agache I, Bonini S, Burks AW, Calderon M, Canonica W, et al. International consensus on allergy immunotherapy. J Allergy Clin Immunol. 2015;136: 556-8.
8. Kuruvilla ME, Eun-Hyung Lee F, Lee GB. Understanding Asthma Phenotypes, Endotypes, and Mechanisms of Disease. Clin Rev Allergy Immunol. 2019;56(2):219-3.
9. Murray CS, Foden P, Sumner H, Shepley E, Custovic A, Simpson A. Preventing Severe Asthma Exacerbations in Children: A Randomized Trial of Mite-Impermeable Bedcovers. Am J Respir Crit Care Med. 2017;196: 150-8.
10. Myers TR, Tomasio L. Asthma: 2015 and beyond. Respir Care. 2011;56(9):1389-407; discussion 1407-10.
11. Pajno GB, Barberio G, De Luca F, Morabito L, Parmiani S. Prevention of new sensitizations in asthmatic children monosensitized to house dust mite by specific immunotherapy. A six-year follow-up study. Clin Exp Allergy. 2001;31:1392-7.
12. Papapostolou N, Makris M. Allergic Asthma in the Era of Personalized Medicine. J Pers Med 2022;12:1162.
13. Pijnenburg MW, Fleming L. Advances in understanding and reducing the burden of severe asthma in children. Lancet Respir Med. 2020;8:1032-44.
14. Pitsios C, Demoly P, Bilò MB, Gerth van Wijk R, Pfaar O, Sturm GJ, et al. Clinical contraindications to allergen immunotherapy: An EAACI position paper. Allergy. 2015;70:897-909.
15. Schatz M, Rosenwasser L. The allergic asthma phenotype. J Allergy Clin Immunol. Pract. 2014;2:645-8.
16. Tosca MA, Licari A, Olcese R, Marseglia G, Sacco O, Ciprandi G. Immunotherapy and Asthma in Children. Front Pediatr. 2018;6:231.

12 CHAPTER

Eosinophilic Lung Diseases

Indu Khosla, Geetesh Baijal

INTRODUCTION

Eosinophilic lung diseases (ELD) are a group of heterogeneous parenchymal lung diseases with diffuse eosinophilic infiltration into alveolar spaces and the lung interstitium with an intact lung architecture. A high index of suspicion of ELD in pneumonias unresponsive to appropriate antibiotic treatment should be kept as standardized diagnostic criteria are lacking. Early recognition and treatment are known to have improved outcomes. Corticosteroids are the mainstay of management. Even with pulmonary impairment at presentation, early corticosteroid therapy has shown resolution with no pulmonary sequelae. There is still a felt need for other treatment modalities due to significant adverse effects of long-term corticosteroids. Newer therapies targeting eosinophils are under research which may have promising outcomes.

EPIDEMIOLOGY

Pediatric ELD has been under-reported as there is a lack of epidemiological data and most data originates from adult case cohort studies.

ETIOPATHOGENESIS

Eosinophils in the body are involved in both physiological and pathological processes. They regulate tissue and organ homeostasis and contribute to defense against infections and helminths. They also play a role in tumor immunity. They have pathological roles in inflammation and tissue damage which results in remodeling in chronic cases. Eosinophilic asthma, idiopathic chronic eosinophilic pneumonia (ICEP), eosinophilic granulomatosis with polyangiitis (EGPA), and hypereosinophilic syndrome (HES) pose a challenge to treatment and are associated with significant morbidity. Understanding the pathobiology of eosinophils in ELD may help improve treatment principles.

Cytokines like interleukin (IL)-3, IL-5 and granulocyte macrophage colony stimulating factor (GM-CSF) lead to differentiation of precursor cells in bone marrow to eosinophils which then get recruited in blood and tissues. Cytokines like IL-5, eotaxin, and C-C chemokine receptor 3 cause recruitment of eosinophils in lungs **(Flowchart 1)**. Hence, development of anti-IL-5 antibodies is a potential therapeutic option.

ROLE OF EOSINOPHILS IN INNATE IMMUNITY (FLOWCHART 2)

Cell membranes of eosinophils have receptors (toll-like receptors, receptors for cytokines, immunoglobulins, and complement) which interact with basophils, endothelial cells, macrophages, platelets, fibroblasts, and mast cells contributing to innate immunity. Activated eosinophils release proinflammatory mediators, cytokines, arachidonic acid derivatives, reactive oxygen species, complement proteins, chemokines, chemoattractants, metalloproteases, and toxic granules like cationic proteins. Eosinophilic cationic proteins (ECP) are proinflammatory and cause upregulation of chemoattraction and expression of adhesion molecules. They also regulate vascular permeability and cause smooth muscle contraction. ECP are also responsible for the cardiac damage in HES and in tropical eosinophilia by inducing local thrombosis leading

Flowchart 1: Eosinophils in innate and acquired immunity.

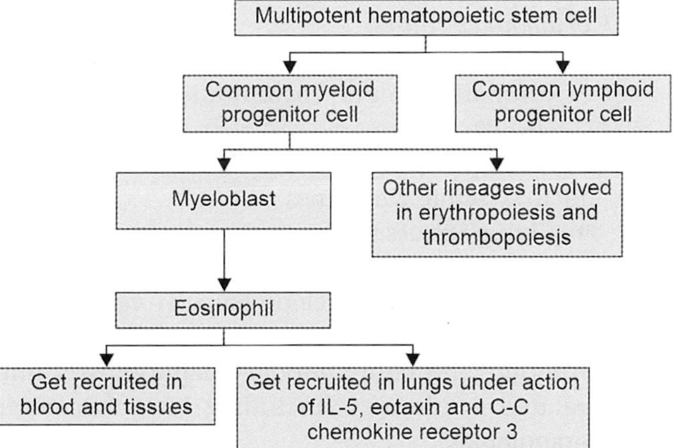

Flowchart 2: Development and recruitment of eosinophils in various organs and tissues.

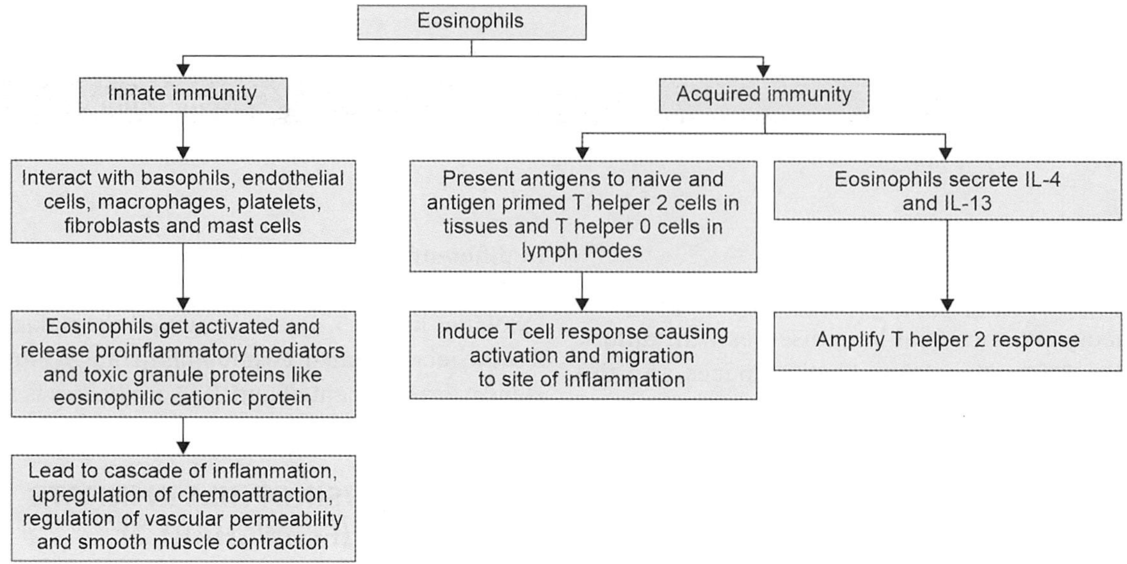

to necrosis and eventually fibrosis. Activated degranulated eosinophils are found in bronchoalveolar lavage (BAL) and lung of patients with eosinophilic pneumonias (EP).

ROLE OF EOSINOPHILS IN ADAPTIVE IMMUNITY

Eosinophils induce T-cell development, activation, and migration to sites of inflammation by presenting antigens to T helper 2 cells in tissues and T helper 0 cells in lymph nodes. Eosinophils secrete IL-4 and IL-13 which amplify T helper 2 response in lung. T helper 2 cell-derived cytokines like IL-4, IL-5, and IL-13 further enhance the recruitment and activation of eosinophils **(Flowchart 2)**.

CLASSIFICATION OF EOSINOPHILIC PNEUMONIA

- *EP of unknown causes:*
  - Solitary idiopathic EP
    - Idiopathic acute eosinophilic pneumonias (IAEP)
    - ICEP
  - EP in systemic syndromes
    - Churg–Strauss syndrome
    - Idiopathic hypereosinophilic syndromes (lymphocytic or myeloproliferative variant)
- *EP of known causes:*
  - Allergic bronchopulmonary aspergillosis and related syndromes (including bronchocentric granulomas)
  - EP of parasitic origin
  - EP of other infectious diseases
  - Drug-induced EP
- *Eosinophilic airway diseases:*
  - Idiopathic hypereosinophilic constrictive bronchitis
- *Other pulmonary syndromes with usually mild eosinophilia:*
  - Organizing pneumonia
  - Asthma
  - Idiopathic pulmonary fibrosis
  - Langerhans cell histiocytosis
  - Malignancy
  - Sarcoidosis
  - Rheumatological conditions

CLINICAL FEATURES

Dyspnea is commonly seen in patients with IAEP or ICEP and is associated with cough in almost 90% of patients. Acute EP can rapidly progress to respiratory failure requiring mechanical ventilation. In contrast, ICEP has an indolent presentation. Other symptoms include rhinitis and sinusitis.

History and examination:

- Drugs—antibiotics, nonsteroidal anti-inflammatory drugs (NSAIDs), antiepileptics, antileukotriene modifiers in EGPA
- New onset of smoking cigarettes or cocaine

- Environmental exposures to dust or inhaled chemicals
- Travel to areas endemic with parasites or coccidioidomycosis
- Poorly controlled asthma
- Allergic bronchopulmonary aspergillosis (ABPA) in patients with cystic fibrosis or asthma
- Extrapulmonary symptoms of vasculitis, neuropathy, heart failure, or neoplasm
- Rash in visceral larval migrans or ulcerations in EGPA

Investigations:

- *Blood eosinophil count:*
    - Degree of eosinophilia does not differentiate between ELD
    - Not elevated in IAEP
    - Occasionally normal in ICEP or after use of corticosteroids
- *Sputum eosinophil count:*
    - Gold standard for assessing eosinophilic airway inflammation
    - Limitations—sample processing within 2 hours of collection, requires experience, time consuming and expensive
- *Fractional excretion of nitric oxide (FeNO):*
    - Marker of eosinophilic airway inflammation
    - *High FeNO (>50 ppb):* Eosinophilic asthma
    - *Low FeNO (<25 ppb):* Noneosinophilic asthma
    - *Limitations:* Sensitivity 66% and specificity 76%, influenced by factors like age, cigarette smoking, use of inhaled corticosteroids, consumption of nitrate-rich food like green leafy vegetables, infections, and pollution
- *Radiography:*
    - Chest radiography:
        - Nonlobar infiltrates
        - Peripheral infiltrates—mirror image of pulmonary edema
        - Bilateral pleural effusion in IAEP
        - Central bronchiectasis in ABPA
    - *High-resolution CT (HRCT) chest:*
        - Middle and upper lobe infiltrates with ground-glass appearance
        - Mucus plugging, central bronchiectasis in ABPA
- *Total serum IgE:* Elevated in patients with ABPA with underlying cystic fibrosis or uncontrolled asthma
- Detection of parasites by serology or on stool examination
- *Perinuclear anti-neutrophil cytoplasmic antibodies (P-ANCA):* Positive in 40–70% cases of EGPA
- *BAL eosinophilia:*
    - ≥25% eosinophils diagnostic of IAEP
    - ≥40% eosinophils diagnostic of ICEP
    - Eosinophil percentages below these require lung biopsy
    - <25% eosinophils seen in connective tissue disorders, sarcoidosis, drug-induced eosinophilia, and interstitial pulmonary fibrosis.
- *Bone marrow biopsy:* In patients with blood eosinophil count ≥1,500/mm^3 to rule out hematological neoplasms with clonal eosinophilia or any other cause.

SYNDROMES IN EOSINOPHILIC PNEUMONIAS

Eosinophilic lung diseases is an umbrella term which encompasses a broad spectrum of diseases as given in the following text.

Loeffler Syndrome

Loeffler syndrome is now called transient pulmonary infiltrates with eosinophilia syndrome. It is caused by helminthic infections, *Ascaris lumbricoides* being the most common. On ingesting a fertilized egg from contaminated food, it transforms into larval form which penetrates the duodenum to enter the systemic circulation and reaches various organs like heart, liver, and lungs. The larvae break through the pulmonary capillaries and interstitial space to enter alveoli and ascend upward to the trachea, where they get expectorated or swallowed.

Helminths like *Toxocara canis* and *Toxocara cati*, *Strongyloides stercoralis*, *Baylisascaris procyonis*, and *Lagochilascaris minor* cause visceral larva migrans and may cause ELD.

Clinical features include recurrent cough and dyspnea. Larva can migrate to other organs and multiply in intestinal and biliary tract, producing symptoms like abdominal pain, vomiting, cholecystitis, pancreatitis, and rarely obstruction. Diagnosis is made by stool microscopy for egg detection. Radiology may reveal peripheral pulmonary infiltrates and blood may show eosinophilia. It is self-limiting and treatment is with antihelminthics and during a pulmonary phase aggravated inflammatory response may require corticosteroids.

Idiopathic Acute Eosinophilic Pneumonia

Idiopathic acute eosinophilic pneumonia mimics infectious pneumonia or acute respiratory distress syndrome due to its rapid onset and marked hypoxemia. Majority of patients present within 7 days of onset of symptoms with dyspnea, cough, fever, and chest pain. Examination findings include tachypnea, tachycardia, and crackles in lung fields. Many may require mechanical ventilation. It has been associated with onset, re-initiation, or change in smoking frequency or following massive secondary smoke exposure. Crack lung refers to diffuse alveolitis with pulmonary hemorrhage within 48 hours of cocaine inhalation.

Diagnostic Criteria

- Acute onset with febrile respiratory manifestations (≤1 month, and especially ≤7 days duration before medical examination)
- Bilateral diffuse infiltrates on imaging
- PaO_2 on room air ≤60 mm Hg or PaO_2/FiO_2 ≤300 mm Hg or oxygen saturation on room air < 90%
- Lung eosinophilia with ≥25% eosinophils at BAL differential cell count
- Absence of determined cause of acute EP. Recent onset of tobacco smoking or exposure to inhaled dusts may be present

Idiopathic Chronic Eosinophilic Pneumonia

Idiopathic chronic eosinophilic pneumonia is characterized by symptoms like cough, dyspnea, malaise, and weight loss which progress within few weeks to an infiltrative pulmonary disease. It is common in nontropical areas where the prevalence of parasitic infections is low. It has a predilection for females (F:M 2:1) and is more common in adults but has no genetic predisposition. Underlying asthma is found in 67%, and 50% have history of atopy in the form of drug allergy, nasal polyposis, urticaria, and/or eczema. Examination findings include tachypnea, crackles, and wheezing. Salient differentiating points are mentioned in **Table 1**.

Diagnostic Criteria

- Respiratory symptoms present for at least 2–4 weeks.
- Diffuse pulmonary alveolar consolidation with air bronchogram and/or ground-glass opacities at chest imaging with peripheral predominance
- Eosinophilia at bronchoalveolar lavage differential cell count ≥40% (or peripheral blood eosinophils ≥1,000/mm^3) **(Fig. 1)**
- Absence of other known causes of ELD

Allergic Bronchopulmonary Aspergillosis or Mycosis

Allergic bronchopulmonary aspergillosis or allergic bronchopulmonary mycosis (ABPM) is a type 2 hypersensitivity response to fungus in airways, the most common being *Aspergillus*. Other fungi associated include *Candida*, *Penicillium*, and *Curvularia*. ABPA should be suspected in patients with difficult-to-control or nonresponding asthma (1–2%) and progressive cystic fibrosis (7–15%) although ABPM can occur in the absence of any underlying lung condition. Development of fixed airway obstruction is indicative of ABPA in asthmatics.

Asano criteria for ABPM (presence of six or more are diagnostic):

- Current or previous history of asthma or asthmatic symptoms
- Peripheral blood eosinophilia (>500 cells/mm^3)
- Elevated levels of total serum IgE (>417 IU/mL)
- Immediate cutaneous hypersensitivity or specific IgE for filamentous fungi
- Presence of precipitins or specific IgG for filamentous fungi
- Filamentous fungi in sputum or bronchial lavage culture
- Fungal hyphae in mucus plugs of bronchi
- Central bronchiectasis on HRCT **(Figs. 5A and B)**
- Mucus plugs in central bronchi on HRCT/bronchoscopy, or in expectoration **(Fig. 5C)**
- High-attenuation mucus in bronchi on HRCT **(Fig. 5C)**

Antineutrophil Cytoplasmic Antibody Associated Vasculitis

These are multisystemic autoimmune diseases with involvement of small vessels which are rare in children. They are classified as either granulomatosis with polyangiitis (GPA), EGPA, or microscopic polyangiitis (MPA).

Eosinophilic granulomatosis with polyangiitis presents as difficult-to-control asthma, allergic rhinitis, and peripheral eosinophilia (>10% or >1,500 cells/mm^3). Evidence of vasculitis should be present in at least two

TABLE 1: Differentiating features between IAEP and ICEP.

	IAEP	*ICEP*
Onset	<1 month	>2–4 weeks
History of asthma	No	Yes
Smoking history	2/3rd of smokers, often recent initiation	10% of smokers
Respiratory failure	Usual	No
Peripheral blood eosinophilia	No	Yes (as high as 5,000/mm^3)
BAL eosinophilia	>25%	>40%
Spirometry	Restrictive pattern	Obstructive and restrictive patterns
Chest imaging	Bilateral patchy areas of ground-glass attenuation, mixed alveolar and interstitial opacities along Kerley lines, airspace consolidation, interlobular septal thickening, bilateral pleural effusion **(Fig. 2)**	Homogeneous peripheral airspace consolidation, characteristic X-ray finding of "radiographic negative of pulmonary edema or reverse bat wing appearance" **(Figs. 3 and 4)**
Treatment	Corticosteroids (methylprednisolone 1–2 mg/kg/day IV or orally)	Corticosteroids (oral prednisolone 0.5 mg/kg/day recommended for 2 weeks following which dose is reduced to half and given for additional 2 weeks if symptoms have abated. Remaining dose is tapered over 6 months, Alternatively IV methylprednisolone given with 10–30 mg/kg/dose for either 3 consecutive days per month or 1 day per week)
Relapse	No	Yes

(BAL: bronchoalveolar lavage; IAEP: idiopathic acute eosinophilic pneumonia; ICEP: idiopathic chronic eosinophilic pneumonia)

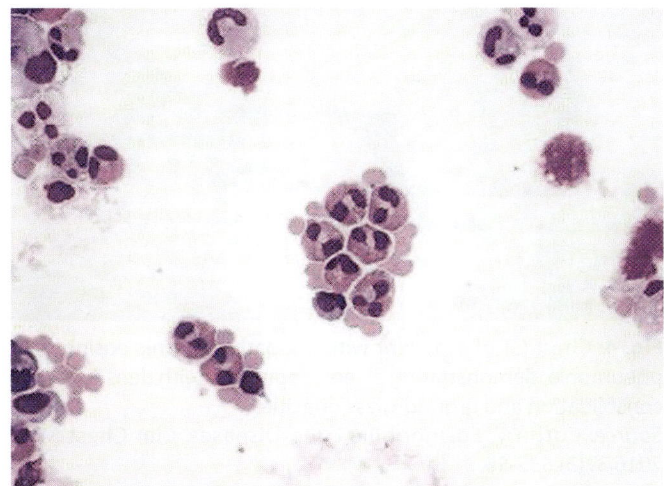

Fig. 1: Light microscopy of eosinophils in bronchoalveolar lavage fluid.
Source: Kleigman RM, St Geme III JW (Eds). Nelson Textbook of Pediatrics, 22nd edition. Philadelphia: Elsevier; 2024.

organs. Organs affected include skin, central nervous system, heart, sinuses, kidneys, and gastrointestinal tract. The progression of disease occurs in three phases:

1. Rhinitis and asthma
2. Tissue eosinophilia
3. Systemic vasculitis

European Respiratory Society Task Force EGPA Diagnostic Criteria

Asthma plus eosinophilia ($>1\times10^9$/L and/or >10% leukocytes) plus at least two of the following features **(Table 2)**:

- Biopsy showing histopathological evidence of eosinophilic vasculitis, or perivascular eosinophilic infiltration, or eosinophil-rich granulomatous inflammation
- Mono- or polyneuropathy (motor deficit or nerve conduction abnormality)
- Nonfixed pulmonary infiltrates
- Sinonasal abnormality
- Cardiomyopathy (established by echocardiography or magnetic resonance imaging)
- Glomerulonephritis
- Alveolar hemorrhage by BAL
- Palpable purpura
- ANCA-positive (MPO or proteinase 3)

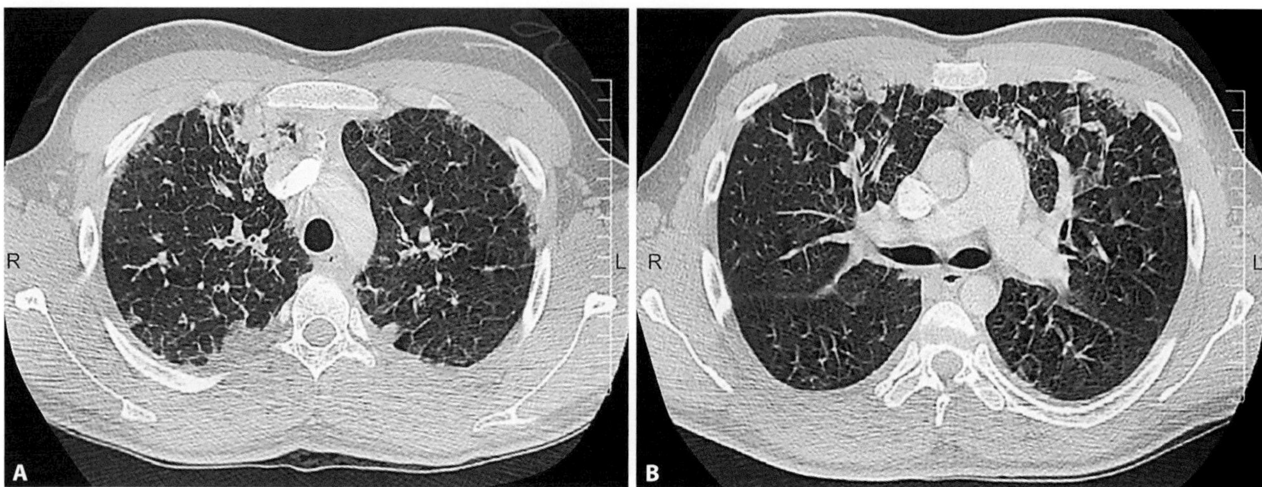

Figs. 2A and B: HRCT of an IAEP patient showing (A) bilateral subpleural consolidations and septal thickening in upper pulmonary lobes and (B) diffuse ground-glass opacities with septal thickening in lower pulmonary lobes. Presence of pleural effusion in the right lobe. (HRCT: high-resolution CT; IAEP: idiopathic acute eosinophilic pneumonia)

Source: Giovannini-Chami L, Blanc S, Hadchouel A, Baruchel A, Boukari R, Dubus JC, et al. Eosinophilic pneumonias in children: A review of the epidemiology, diagnosis, and treatment. Pediatr Pulmonol. 51(2):203-16.

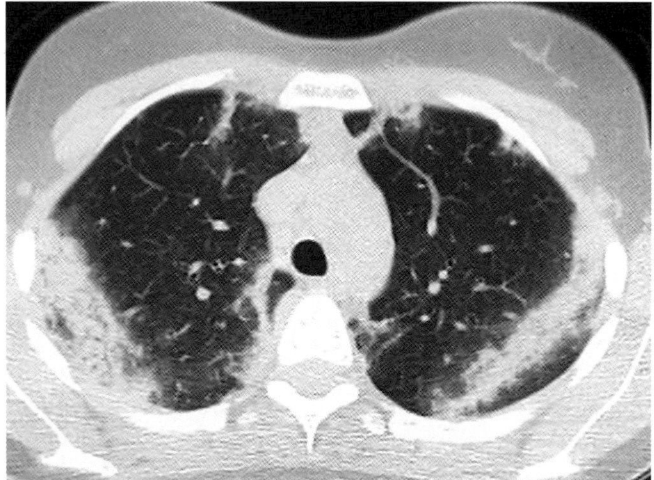

Fig. 3: Chest CT of a patient with idiopathic chronic eosinophilic pneumonia, demonstrating peripheral airspace consolidation predominating in upper lobes.

Source: Cottin V. Eosinophilic Lung Diseases. Clin Chest Med. 2016;37(3):535-56.

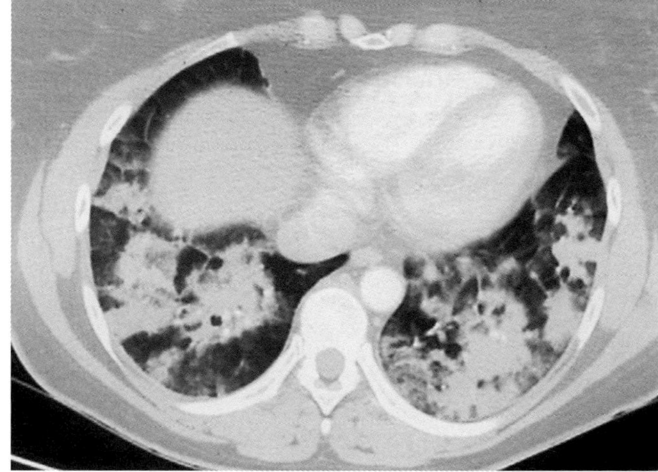

Fig. 4: Chest CT of a patient with idiopathic chronic eosinophilic pneumonia, demonstrating alveolar opacities, with dense airspace consolidation and ground-glass opacities.

Source: Cottin V. Eosinophilic Lung Diseases. Clin Chest Med. 2016;37(3):535-56.

Drug-induced Eosinophilic Pneumonia

Drug-induced EP can have a transient, acute, or chronic presentation. A causal relationship has not been established for many of these drugs listed below:

- *NSAIDs:*
  - Acetylsalicylic acid
  - Diclofenac
  - Fenbufen
  - Ibuprofen
  - Naproxen
  - Oxicam
  - Para-aminosalicylic acid
  - Phenylbutazone
  - Piroxicam
  - Sulindac

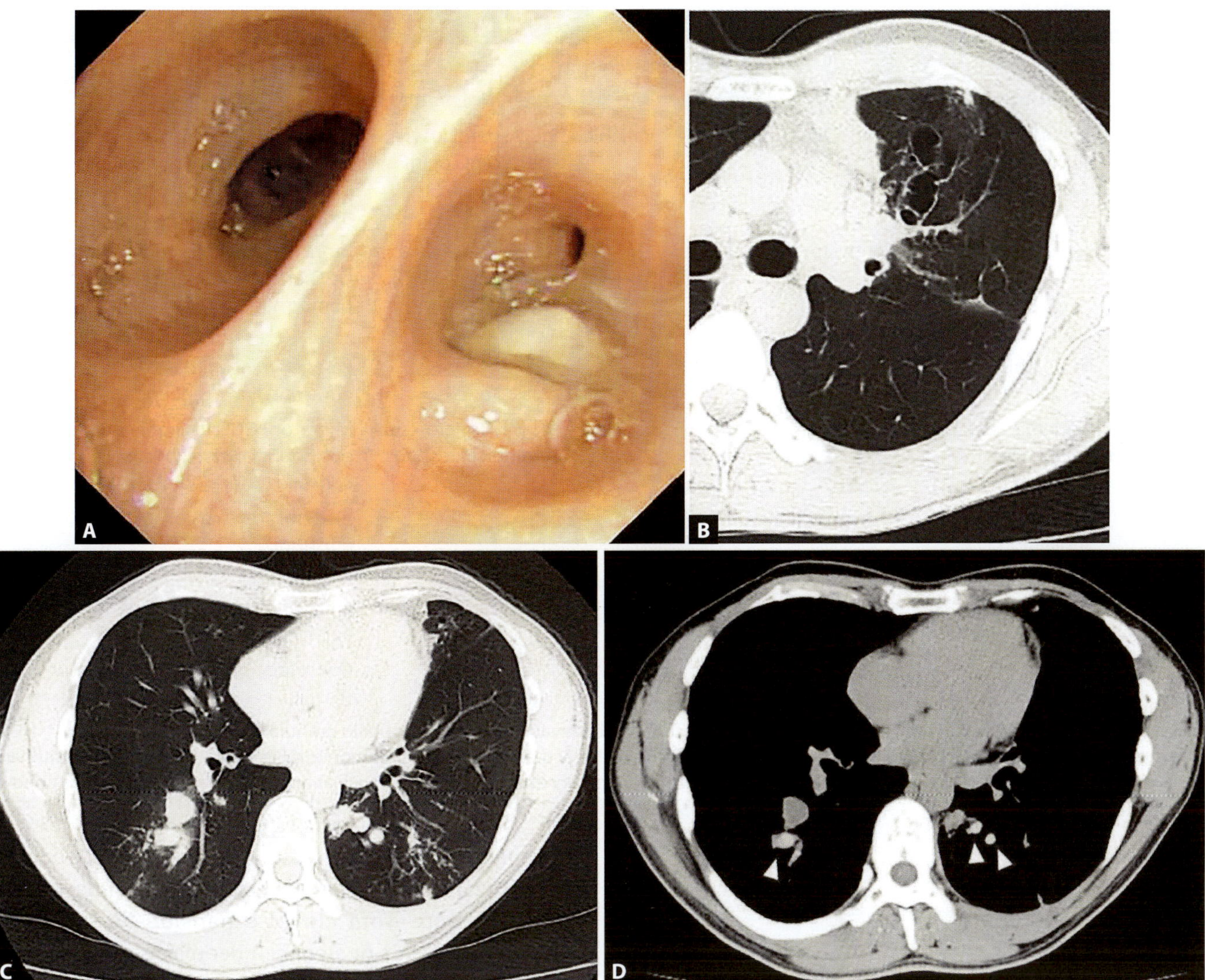

Figs. 5A to D: *Clinical findings of allergic bronchopulmonary mycosis (ABPM):* (A) Bronchoscopic findings of impacted mucus plug in right lower lobe bronchus; (B) central bronchiectasis in the left upper lobe; (C) mucus plugs in both lower lobes; and (D) high attenuation mucus.
Source: ERS Monograph: Eosinophilic Lung Diseases. p. 130.

TABLE 2: Types of EGPA.

	Vasculitic phenotype	***Eosinophilic tissular disease phenotype***
Frequency	40%	60%
ANCA	Present (mostly perinuclear ANCA with anti-MPO specificity)	Absent
Predominant manifestations	• Glomerular renal diseases • Peripheral neuropathy • Purpura • Biopsy-proven vasculitis	• Cardiac involvement (eosinophilic myocarditis) • Eosinophilic pneumonia • Fever

(ANCA: antineutrophil cytoplasmic antibody; EGPA: eosinophilic granulomatosis with polyangiitis; MPO: myeloperoxidase)

TABLE 3: Differential diagnosis of hypereosinophilic syndrome.

Disorder	*Association*	*Duration of symptoms*	*Eosinophilia*		*Other investigations*	*Chest imaging*
			Serum	*BAL*		
ABPA	H/o asthma, cystic fibrosis, or prior tuberculosis	Months to years	++	Variable	IgE, Aspergillus-specific IgG or IgE	Transient GGO, centrilobular nodules, upper lobe saccular bronchiectasis, mucoid impaction, high attenuation mucus (finger in glove)
EGPA	H/o asthma	Months to years	++	+	ANCA (usually P-ANCA anti-MPO), extrapulmonary manifestations	Bronchial wall thickening, migratory GGO or consolidation, diffuse alveolar hemorrhage
HES	Idiopathic, Male > Female	>1 month	+++	++		Parenchymal infiltrates, pleural effusions, lymphadenopathy
Parasitic infections	Endemic areas or recent travel	Variable	++	Variable	Stool for microscopy, serological testing	Migratory GGO in simple pulmonary eosinophilia, cystic or coin lesions, consolidation, pleural effusion
IAEP	Smoking, dust inhalation	<1 month	–	+		Bilateral airspace consolidation, pleural effusion
ICEP	H/o asthma, atopy or allergic rhinitis, females > males	>1 month	++	++	IgE, anemia, thrombocytosis	Peripheral GGO, typically upper lobe and nonmigratory, reverse bat wing appearance
Drugs	NSAIDs, antibiotics, anticonvulsants	Variable	+	+		Consolidation, pleural effusion

(ABPA: allergic bronchopulmonary aspergillosis; BAL: bronchoalveolar lavage; EGPA: eosinophilic granulomatosis with polyangiitis; HES: hypereosinophilic syndrome; GGO: ground-glass opacity; IAEP: idiopathic acute eosinophilic pneumonia; ICEP: idiopathic chronic eosinophilic pneumonia; MPO: myeloperoxidase; NSAIDs: nonsteroidal anti-inflammatory drugs; P-ANCA: perinuclear antineutrophil cytoplasmic antibody)

- *Antibiotics:*
  - Ethambutol
  - Minocycline
  - Penicillins
  - Pyrimethamine
  - Sulfonamides
  - Trimethoprim–sulfamethoxazole
- *Cardiovascular medications:*
  - Angiotensin-converting enzyme inhibitors
  - Amiodarone
  - Beta blockers
- *Anticonvulsants:*
  - Carbamazepine
  - Phenytoin
- *Miscellaneous:*
  - GM-CSF
  - L-tryptophan

Hypereosinophilic Syndromes

Hypereosinophilic syndrome is defined as persistent hypereosinophilia in the blood ($>1.5 \times 10^9$ cells/mm^3) on two separate occasions at least 1 month apart and evidence of end-organ injury. It can be classified as primary when eosinophils are from clonal expansion and includes myeloid neoplasms or stem cell neoplasms (eosinophilic leukemia), myelodysplastic syndromes, and systemic mastocytosis. HES is diagnosed by bone marrow analysis, molecular genetics, and cytogenetics.

Differential Diagnosis

Differential diagnosis of hypereosinophilic syndrome is given in **Table 3**.

Diagnostic Algorithm

Eosinophilic pneumonia can be subclassified into two groups: Primary EP with unknown causes and secondary EP related to a known cause **(Flowchart 3)**.

Stepwise approach:

1. Eliminate secondary causes by comprehensive history taking and serological assessment. Parasitological assessment is to be done, especially in developing and

Flowchart 3: Diagnostic algorithm for eosinophilic pneumonias.

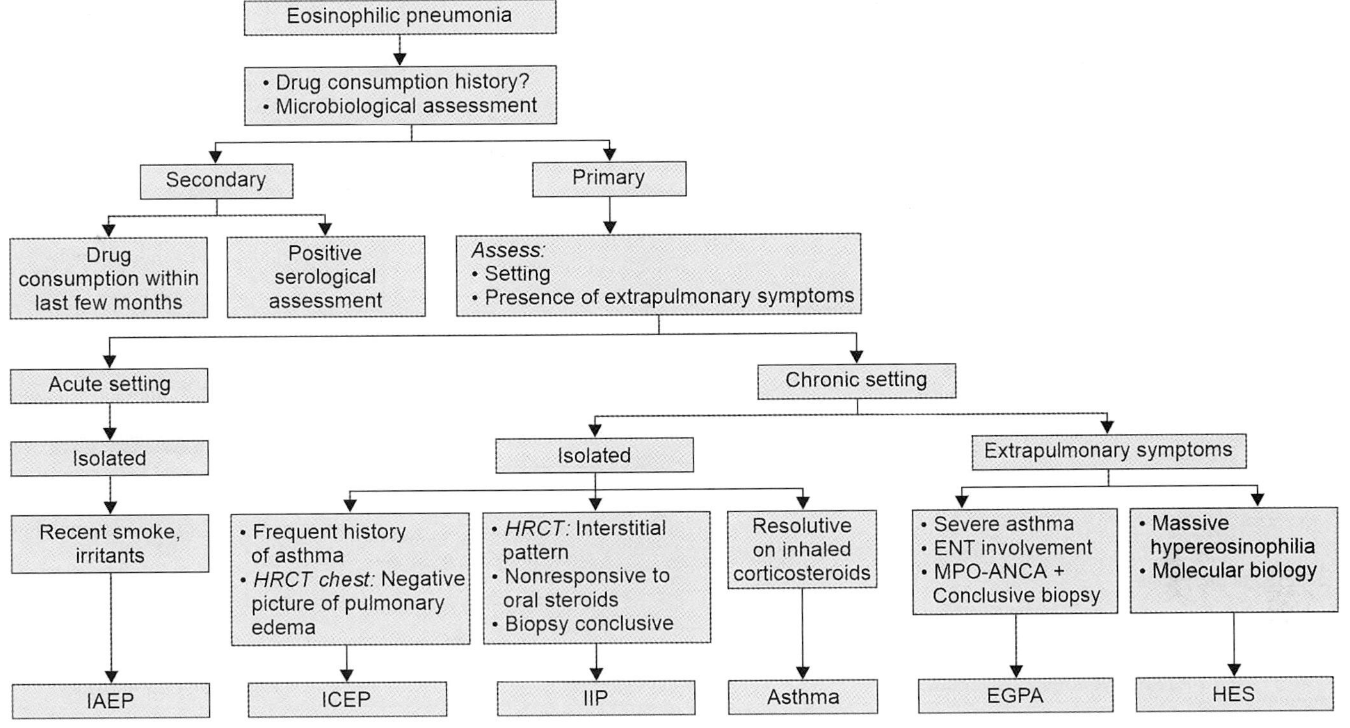

underdeveloped countries. Underlying conditions like asthma and cystic fibrosis predispose to EP secondary to Aspergillus (ABPA) and should be excluded. Look for history of drug consumption.

2. If no cause is found, then it is suggestive of primary EP. Look at the duration of symptoms—whether acute or chronic. IAEP is acute in onset with rapid progression to respiratory failure and associated with exposure to smoke, irritants, tobacco, and drugs like cocaine. Chronic symptoms can be seen with ICEP, asthma, idiopathic interstitial pneumonia, EGPA, and HES which can be differentiated based on clinical and radiological features.

RECENT ADVANCES

- *Eosinophil biomarkers:* Many biomarkers to assess eosinophilic inflammation of airways are under evaluation but most are still under research.
  - *ECP:*
    - Cytotoxic protein stored in eosinophil granules and released by activated eosinophils
    - Measured in serum and sputum
    - Indicative of asthma control
    - Levels have shown to decrease after initiation of benralizumab anti-IL-5 receptor (anti-IL-5R) antibody
    - In a systematic review by Koh et al., ECP correlated well with inflammation but not with airway hyperresponsiveness. It was found to be useful in assessing asthma severity, compliance with anti-inflammatory therapy, and guide to taper inhaled corticosteroids.
  - *Eosinophil peroxidase (EPX):*
    - Released by activated eosinophils and found in nasal and pharyngeal swabs
    - Autoantibodies against EPX have been found in sputum of patients with specific autoimmune endotype of severe asthma.
    - Nair et al. concluded EPX as a reliable marker of eosinophilic degranulation.
    - *3-Bromotyrosine:*
      - Urinary eosinophil-derived biomarker
      - Produced during inflammation by activated eosinophils and EPX during respiratory burst
      - In a study by Wang et al., it was observed that patients with severe asthma had significantly elevated urinary total conjugated bromotyrosine levels. It showed independent

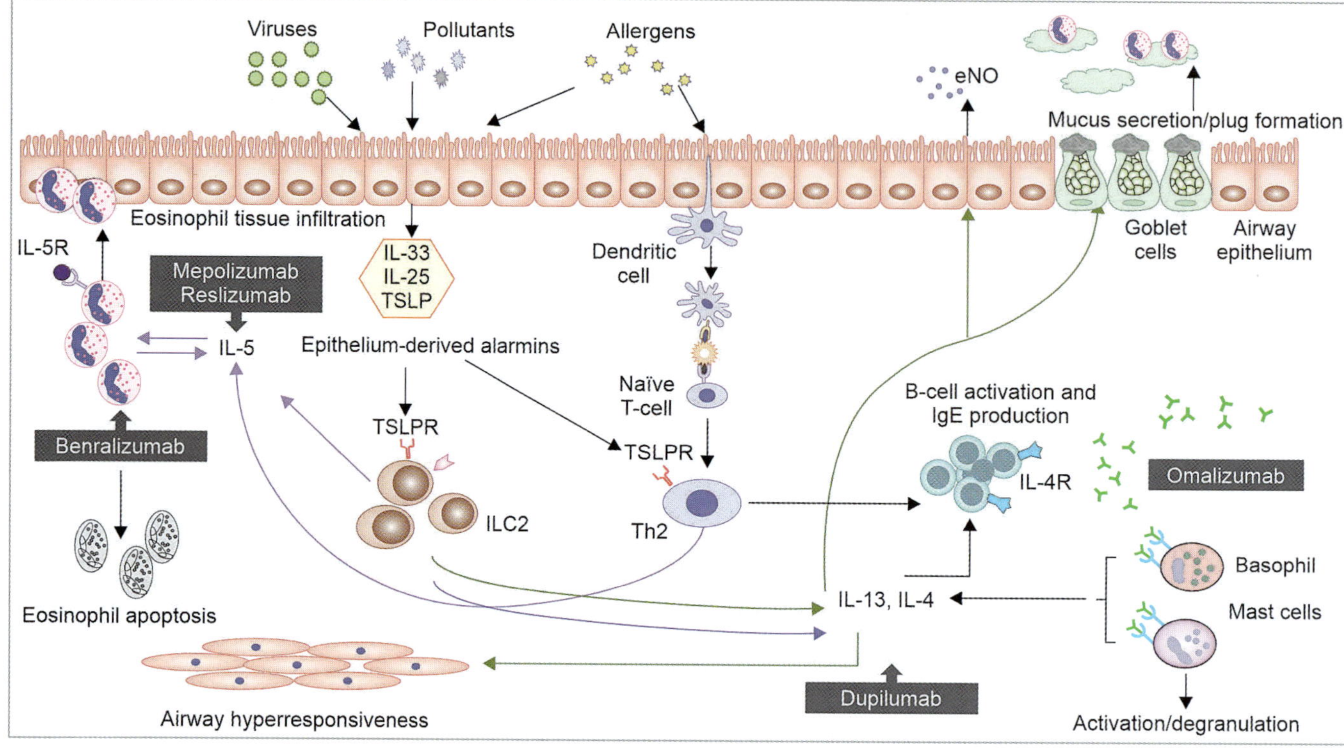

Fig. 6: Currently available biological therapies with their site of action.

association with asthma severity and showed correlation with the number of asthma exacerbations and also served as a predictor of exacerbation.

- *Eosinophil-derived neurotoxin (EDN):*
- Measured in serum and urine
- Elevated levels of eosinophils, EDN and ECP are associated with asthma exacerbations and bronchial hyperresponsiveness

- *Biologicals **(Fig. 6)**:* They are monoclonal antibodies which target pathways associated with eosinophil activation and inflammation.
  - *Omalizumab:*
    - Approved for children >6 years
    - Used in severe uncontrolled asthma
    - Role in ABPA as a corticosteroid-sparing agent
  - *Mepolizumab:*
    - Binds to IL-5 preventing its interaction with the receptor
    - Approved between 6 and 11 years for severe asthma
    - Approved for >12 years of age with HES and add-on treatment for patients with relapsing-remitting or refractory EGPA
    - Ortega et al. concluded that administration of mepolizumab significantly reduced asthma exacerbations with improved asthma control. However, more data and further research are required for its use.
  - *Reslizumab:*
    - Humanized IgG4 antibody which binds IL-5 and prevents receptor interaction
    - Approved in severe asthma in ≥18 years of age
  - *Benralizumab:*
    - It binds to α subunit of IL-5 receptor which is expressed on eosinophils and basophils and blocks IL-5 signaling and also leads to eosinophil and basophil apoptosis through antibody-dependent cell-mediated cytotoxicity.
    - Approved in children aged 6–11 years with severe asthma and for EGPA.
  - *Dupilumab:*
    - Acts against α subunit of IL-4 receptor, also has low affinity to IL-13 receptor
    - Approved in age group 6–11 years with severe asthma

CONCLUSION

Eosinophilic lung diseases in children represent a diverse group of conditions characterized by pulmonary eosinophilic infiltration with variable clinical presentation and severity. Early suspicion is essential, especially in pneumonias unresponsive to routine antibiotics or in children with asthma and pulmonary infiltrates. A combination of clinical evaluation, eosinophil markers, imaging, and bronchoalveolar lavage guides diagnosis. Corticosteroids remain the mainstay of therapy, with biologics emerging as promising options for severe or refractory cases. Timely diagnosis and targeted treatment usually result in excellent outcomes, underscoring the importance of clinician awareness.

KEY POINTS

- ELD with the exception of parasitic infection are rare in pediatric population and data is limited
- In developing countries, ELD secondary to parasitic infections should be kept as a differential in an acutely wheezing child having pulmonary infiltrates.
- ELD is a differential in pneumonia not responding to conventional antibiotics and ABPA should be considered in difficult-to-control asthma and cystic fibrosis.
- *The diagnosis can be made by:*
  - Peripheral blood eosinophilia and chest X-ray infiltrates.
  - Lung biopsy (gold standard)
  - Bronchoalveolar lavage demonstrating eosinophilia
- Presence of extrapulmonary symptoms and history of asthma-like symptoms suggest primary ELD.
- Corticosteroids are the mainstay of management.

SUGGESTED READING

1. Bjermer L, Alving K, Diamant Z, Magnussen H, Pavord I, Piacentini G, et al. Current evidence and future research needs for FeNO measurement in respiratory diseases. Respir Med. 2014;108(6):830-41.
2. Bush A, Deterding R, Li AM, Ratjen F, Sly PD, Zar HJ, et al. Kendig and Willmott's Disorders of the Respiratory Tract in Children. Philadelphia: Elsevier; 2024.
3. Cottin V. Eosinophilic Lung Diseases. Clin Chest Med. 2016;37(3):535-56.
4. Giovannini-Chami L, Blanc S, Hadchouel A, Baruchel A, Boukari R, Dubus JC, et al. Eosinophilic pneumonias in children: A review of the epidemiology, diagnosis, and treatment. Pediatric Pulmonol. 2016;51(2):203-16.
5. Jackson DJ. Eosinophilic Lung Diseases. Sheffield: European Respiratory Society; 2022. 1 p. (ERS Monograph Ser).
6. Kleigman RM, St Geme III JW (Eds). Nelson Textbook of Pediatrics, 22nd edition. Philadelphia: Elsevier; 2024.
7. Koh GCH, Shek LPC, Goh DYT, Van Bever H, Koh DSQ. Eosinophil cationic protein: Is it useful in asthma? A systematic review. Respir Med. 2007;101(4):696-705.
8. Nair P, Ochkur SI, Protheroe C, Radford K, Efthimiadis A, Lee NA, et al. Eosinophil peroxidase in sputum represents a unique biomarker of airway eosinophilia. Allergy. 2013;68(9):1177-84.
9. Ortega HG, Liu MC, Pavord ID, Brusselle GG, FitzGerald JM, Chetta A, et al. Mepolizumab Treatment in Patients with Severe Eosinophilic Asthma. N Engl J Med. 2014;371(13):1198-207.
10. Suzuki Y, Suda T. Eosinophilic pneumonia: A review of the previous literature, causes, diagnosis, and management. Allergol Int. 2019;68(4):413-9.
11. Wang Z, Xu W, Comhair SAA, Fu X, Shao Z, Bearden R, et al. Urinary total conjugated 3-bromotyrosine, asthma severity, and exacerbation risk. Am J Physiol-Lung Cell Mol Physiol. 2022;323(5):L548-57.

13 CHAPTER

Hypersensitivity Pneumonitis

Barnali Bhattacharya

INTRODUCTION

Hypersensitivity pneumonitis (HP) is a complex and a heterogenous interstitial lung disease (ILD). It happens due to an aberrant immunological response provoked by an overt or occult inhaled antigen in predisposed individuals. While it is more commonly diagnosed in adults due to occupational exposures, HP is increasingly recognized in children, often triggered by domestic antigens such as bird droppings, mold, or food particles.

EPIDEMIOLOGY

Globally, the incidence of HP in adults is estimated at 1–2 per 100,000 per year. Pediatric HP is significantly rare at approximately 4 per million. Pediatric HP accounts for 10–15% of chronic ILDs in children.

In India, there is limited pediatric data, but adult studies suggest that HP is the most common form of ILD.

ETIOPATHOGENESIS

The pathogenesis of HP in children is principally related to two factors: The type of allergen inhaled and the host immune response. In order to trigger the disease, the antigen should be able to enter the small airways; thus, its size must be within the respirable range (<5 mm).

Hypersensitivity pneumonitis develops from a repeated immune response to an inhaled antigen like fungal spores, thermophilic bacteria, avian proteins, or aspiration of lentil-based foods. In children, common domestic exposures are bird droppings (particularly pigeons), moldy homes, biomass fuel, and hobbies like flute playing.

Genetic predispositions [e.g., specific human leukocyte antigen (HLA) types] and host factors (age, nutrition, immune status) affect susceptibility. Not all exposed individuals develop HP, which indicates the critical role of individual immune reactivity induced by multiple allergens. However, an individual genetic predisposition is considered fundamental to develop HP. The interaction between environmental allergens and the immune system in genetically predisposed individuals generates an inflammatory state in alveoli, terminal bronchiole, and lung interstitial tissue. Both innate and adaptive immune responses contribute to the development of HP. Specifically, the aberrant immune response leads to an exaggerated inflammatory reaction in the lungs. The pathophysiological features of the interaction between allergens and the immune system are expressed differently in acute and chronic HP at times leading to lung fibrosis, which represents the last step of this illness.

CLINICAL FEATURES

The clinical presentation of HP in children can range from acute, reversible episodes to insidious chronic disease. Classically, clinicians have described three forms—acute, subacute, and chronic HP—based on the duration and intensity of exposure and the tempo of symptoms. However, there is overlap between these forms, and recent perspectives often group them into nonfibrotic (acute/subacute) versus fibrotic (chronic) phenotypes for simplicity. In pediatric patients, recognizing the pattern is important but often challenging.

Acute HP: It develops within hours of exposure. Symptoms include fever, cough, malaise, and dyspnea, resembling flu or atypical pneumonia. Rapid resolution occurs with antigen withdrawal.

Subacute HP: It has gradual onset with persistent dry cough, fatigue, weight loss, and exercise intolerance. Misdiagnoses as asthma or recurrent pneumonia are common.

Chronic HP: It presents with clubbing, progressive breathlessness, failure to thrive, and hypoxemia. Long-standing inflammation leads to fibrosis, restrictive lung disease, and potentially pulmonary hypertension.

Overall, pediatric HP should be suspected in any child with recurrent or persistent "pneumonia," chronic cough, or diffuse lung disease that does not fit common diagnoses. Often, these children receive multiple rounds of antibiotics, inhalers, or even antitubercular therapy without improvement. Careful history-taking may reveal exposure to birds, mold, farming environments, or (in infants) a history of forceful feeding/aspiration events. Recognizing the constellation of exposure, respiratory symptoms, and lack of response to standard therapy is critical. Early in the disease (acute/subacute), removing the child from the offending environment typically results in dramatic improvement, whereas continued exposure can drive the illness toward chronic fibrosis. The key is to consider HP in the differential diagnosis of pediatric respiratory cases—as studies note, despite a "characteristic clinical presentation", HP is frequently not initially recognized in children due to its infrequency.

Differential diagnosis of pediatric HP include various conditions **(Table 1)**:

- Recurrent pneumonia
- Asthma
- Tuberculosis (especially in endemic areas)
- Aspiration syndromes
- Connective tissue disease-associated ILD
- Sarcoidosis
- Primary immunodeficiency disorder

TABLE 1: Differential diagnosis of pediatric HP.

Condition	*Key distinguishing features*
Asthma	Episodic, reversible, strong atopy history
Recurrent pneumonia	Localized consolidation, response to antibiotics
Tuberculosis	Contact history, caseating granulomas
Aspiration syndromes	Feeding difficulty, recurrent lower lobe disease
Connective tissue disease—ILD	Autoantibodies, systemic features
Sarcoidosis	Non-caseating granulomas, extrapulmonary involvement
Primary immunodeficiency	Recurrent infections, low Ig levels

(HP: hypersensitivity pneumonitis; ILD: interstitial lung disease)

DIAGNOSIS

Diagnosing HP in children requires correlating clinical findings with exposure history, imaging, and specialized tests. No single test is definitive for HP; instead, a constellation of evidence leads to the diagnosis. Notably, there are no separate pediatric HP diagnostic criteria published by major societies—pediatricians generally adapt adult guidelines [such as the 2016 European EAACI (European Academy of Allergy & Clinical Immunology) position paper or the 2020 ATS/JRS/ALAT (American Thoracic Society/Japanese Respiratory Society/Latin American Thoracic Association) criteria] to children, with the understanding that some tests (like lung function or provocation tests) **(Table 2)** may be more difficult to perform in young patients. A multidisciplinary approach—involving pediatric pulmonologists, radiologists, and pathologists—is often the best strategy.

Criteria used in the diagnosis of hypersensitivity pneumonitis:

- *Identified exposure to offending antigen(s) by:*
  - Medical history of exposure to suspected antigen in the patient's living environment
  - Investigations of the environment confirm the presence of an inciting antigen
  - Identification of specific immune responses (immunoglobulin G serum precipitin antibodies against the identified antigen) are suggestive of the potential etiology but are insufficient in isolation to confirm a diagnosis.
- *Clinical, radiographic, or physiologic findings compatible with HP:*
  - *Clinical*
    - Respiratory and often constitutional signs and symptoms **(Table 3)**

TABLE 2: Clinical criteria.

Acute	Fever, chills, cough of 4–6 hours after exposure	Diffuse or patchy air-space consolidation	Neutrophils early on, then lymphocytes, giant cells and foamy macrophages
Subacute	Insidious onset of cough, dyspnea, and malaise	Centrilobular nodules or widespread nodular opacities and ground-glass attenuation	Noncaseating granulomas
Chronic	Progressive dyspnea, fatigue, anorexia, weight loss, chronic cough	Mid-lung zone fibrosis with or without honeycombing	Interstitial fibrosis, air space destruction

TABLE 3: Clinical spectrum of pediatric HP.

Type	Clinical features	Radiology	Pathology
Acute	Fever, cough, dyspnea hours after exposure	Patchy consolidation	Neutrophils → lymphocytes, foamy macrophages
Subacute	Chronic dry cough, fatigue, weight loss	Nodular opacities, ground glass	Non-caseating granulomas
Chronic	Progressive dyspnea, clubbing, FTT	Fibrosis, honeycombing	Interstitial fibrosis

(FTT: failure to thrive; HP: hypersensitivity pneumonitis)

- Crackles on auscultation of the chest
- Weight loss
- Cough
- Breathlessness
- Episodic fever
- Wheezing
- Fatigue

(*NOTE:* These findings are especially suggestive of HP when they appear or worsen several hours after antigen exposure)

- *Radiological:*
  - A reticular, nodular, or ground-glass opacity on chest radiograph or high-resolution CT
- *Physiological:*
  - *Abnormalities in the following pulmonary function tests (PFTs):*
  - Spirometry (restrictive, obstructive, or mixed patterns)
  - Lung volumes (low or high)
  - Reduced diffusion capacity by carbon monoxide
  - Altered gas exchange either at rest or with exercise (reduced partial pressure of arterial oxygen by blood gas or pulse oximeter testing)

- *Bronchoalveolar lavage with lymphocytosis:*
  - Usually with a low CD4:CD8 ratio (i.e., CD8 is higher than normal)
  - Lymphocyte stimulation by offending antigen results in proliferation and cytokine production
- *Abnormal response to inhalation challenge testing to the offending antigen:*
  - Re-exposure to the environment
  - Inhalation challenge to the suspected antigen (rarely done now because of the risk of exacerbating the disease)

    Histopathology showing compatible changes with HP by one of these findings:
    - Poorly formed, noncaseating granulomas (most often found closer to the respiratory epithelium where deposition of the offending antigen occurs)
    - Mononuclear cell infiltrate in the pulmonary interstitium

TREATMENT

Management of HP in children centers around two main principles: Eliminate the offending antigen exposure and control the lung inflammation. Pediatric management closely parallels adult treatment guidelines, but with attention to growth and minimizing treatment side effects.

Antigen avoidance: The single-most important factor is identifying and removal of the inciting antigen from the child's environment. This is the only definitive way to halt lung injury. In the acute form, removing the child from exposure can lead to full symptom resolution in days.

Corticosteroids: Systemic corticosteroids are the mainstay for moderate-to-severe HP or when there is significant lung impairment. Corticosteroids have potent anti-inflammatory effects that can speed up recovery and suppress the immune response. In children with acute HP who have more than mild symptoms (e.g., significant hypoxia, severe cough, or extensive infiltrates on imaging), a course of oral prednisone is typically started. A commonly used regimen is prednisone 0.5–1 mg/kg/day (for 4–8 weeks, followed by a gradual tapering over a couple of months). In the infant lentil-HP series, for instance, all children received oral steroids for up to 8 weeks and showed remarkable clinical and radiologic improvement. In the severe form of acute disease, methylprednisolone injections may be given. In subacute/chronic HP, longer courses (3–6 months taper) might be needed. The goal is to induce remission of symptoms and allow lung healing. Most children respond with improved cough, weight gain, and better oxygenation within weeks. Objective improvements in PFTs and imaging can be seen by 6–12 weeks of therapy in responders. Monitoring is required for steroid side effects (growth suppression, hyperglycemia, blood pressure, etc.)

Second-line immunosuppressives: If a child's HP progresses despite corticosteroids or if steroid side effects are prohibitive (e.g., if long-term treatment is needed in chronic HP), additional immunosuppressive agents are considered. There is no pediatric-specific trial data, so choices are extrapolated from adult ILD practices and case reports.

Bronchodilators: Some HP patients with wheezing or an obstructive component may get symptom relief from bronchodilator inhalers. They can ease breathing in those with coexisting airway hyperreactivity.

Antibiotics: They are usually not indicated unless there is a suspicion of secondary infection. However, sometimes children with HP get empiric azithromycin if *Mycoplasma* was in differential (prior to diagnosis). Macrolide antibiotics have anti-inflammatory properties and are used in some chronic lung diseases (like bronchiolitis obliterans); their role in HP is not established but could be considered in certain scenarios.

Nutrition and growth: Chronic lung disease increases caloric needs. Nutritional support (high-calorie diet, feeding assistance) may be required, especially if the child has growth failure. Inhaled diseases like HP can cause expenditure of more calories due to the work of breathing.

Physical therapy: Chest physiotherapy can help mobilize secretions if present, and pulmonary rehabilitation (light exercise training, breathing exercises) can be useful in older children to improve endurance once an acute illness is controlled.

Vaccinations: Ensure that the child is up to date on immunizations, especially influenza and pneumococcal vaccines, since respiratory infections could be particularly severe in a child with underlying HP. Preventing infections helps avoid additional lung injury.

Avoiding smoke and pollutants: Parents should be counseled to avoid smoking around the child and to minimize indoor air pollution. Smoke exposure can exacerbate HP and further damage lungs.

PROGNOSIS

Prognosis in pediatric HP is generally excellent with early recognition and antigen avoidance. Lung function typically improves or normalizes over months. Delayed diagnosis, continuous exposure, or fibrotic transformation worsens outcomes and may require long-term therapy or rarely lung transplantation.

CONCLUSION

Hypersensitivity pneumonitis in children, though uncommon, is an important cause of preventable ILD. Early identification relies on careful correlation of exposure history, compatible imaging, and supportive immunologic or bronchoalveolar lavage (BAL) findings. Antigen avoidance is the cornerstone of management, with corticosteroids reserved for moderate-to-severe or chronic disease. Timely intervention leads to full recovery in most pediatric cases, whereas delayed diagnosis may result in irreversible fibrosis. Increasing awareness among clinicians and improving environmental assessment practices are essential to reduce morbidity and improve outcomes.

KEY POINTS

- HP is an *immune-mediated ILD* caused by repeated exposure to inhaled organic antigens.
- In children, HP is most often linked to *domestic exposures* such as bird droppings, mold, or aspiration of lentil-based foods.
- Clinical forms are best grouped as *nonfibrotic (acute/subacute)* and *fibrotic (chronic)* phenotypes.
- *High-resolution CT (HRCT)* with centrilobular nodules and air-trapping, combined with *exposure history*, strongly supports diagnosis.
- *Early antigen removal is crucial*; corticosteroids are useful in moderate-to-severe cases, while prognosis is generally excellent if diagnosed early.

SUGGESTED READING

1. Alberti ML, Rincon-Alvarez E, Buendia-Roldan I, Selman M. Hypersensitivity Pneumonitis: Diagnostic and Therapeutic Challenges. Front Med (Lausanne). 2021;8: 718299.
2. Buchvald F, Petersen BL, Damgaard K, Deterding R, Langston C, Fan LL, et al. Frequency, treatment, and functional outcome in children with hypersensitivity pneumonitis. Pediatr Pulmonol. 2011;46(11):1098-107.

3. Griese M, Haug M, Hartl D, Teusch V, Glöckner-Pagel J, Brasch F; National EAA Study Group, et al. Hypersensitivity pneumonitis: lessons for diagnosis and treatment of a rare entity in children. Orphanet J Rare Dis. 2013;8:121.
4. Gupta N, Moitra S, Nagarajan S. Comprehensive Textbook of Allergy: Striking the Right Balance. New Delhi: Jaypee Brothers Medical Publishers; 2024.
5. Kliegman R, St. Geme III JW. Nelson Textbook of Pediatrics, 21st edition. Philadelphia, PA: Elsevier; 2020.
6. Kumar D, et al. Pediatr Respirol Crit Care Med. 2024;8(4): 82-6.
7. Sankar J, Pillai MS, Sankar MJ, Lodha R, Kabra SK. Clinical profile of interstitial lung disease in children. Indian Pediatr. 2013;50(2):127-33.
8. Wawszczak M, Bielecka T, Szczukocki M. Hypersensitivity pneumonitis in children. Ann Agric Environ Med. 2021;28(2):214-9.
9. Zhang F, Yang T, Liu Z, Jia X, Yang L, Wu L, Tang L. Clinical Features of Hypersensitivity Pneumonitis in Children: A Single Center Study. Front Pediatr. 2022;9:789183.

14 CHAPTER Food Allergy

Sowmya Nagarajan, Vikram Patra, Mosam Maroo

INTRODUCTION

Food allergy is a growing global health concern, with an increasing incidence and diverse clinical phenotypes across all age groups. It significantly affects quality of life, healthcare utilization, and economic burden. Food allergies encompass immune-mediated reactions—both IgE-mediated and non-IgE-mediated—as well as nonimmune adverse reactions more appropriately termed food intolerance. Each category requires distinct diagnostic and management approaches.

The condition also poses a unique challenge because of its potential to cause sudden, severe, and sometimes life-threatening reactions such as anaphylaxis, even in otherwise healthy individuals. In addition, food allergy impacts nutrition, social participation, and emotional well-being, particularly in children and their families. The spectrum of common food allergens differs across regions, emphasizing the importance of understanding local dietary habits and genetic influences in order to develop effective prevention and management strategies.

EPIDEMIOLOGY

The estimated global prevalence of food allergy ranges from 1 to 10% of the population, with higher rates reported in children (up to 8%) than in adults (around 2–3%). While the profile of common food allergens reported globally—such as peanut, tree nuts, shellfish, fish, milk, egg, wheat, and soy—is well established, emerging Indian studies suggest a differing spectrum, including chickpea, lentils, vegetables like brinjal, and shrimp; however, such region-specific data remain limited.

ETIOPATHOGENESIS

Food allergy can be classified as:

- True food allergy
- Adverse reactions to food/food allergy mimics

True Food Allergy

It means a food reaction arising from a typical immune response, reproducible on every exposure of the given food. IgE-mediated disease or "classical food allergy" requires both compatible symptoms and evidence of IgE sensitization, while non-IgE-mediated primarily affects the gut and causes subacute or chronic symptoms.

The "true" food allergy is divided as per the mechanism of symptoms through disability and repeatability as IgE mediated and non-IgE mediated. A third category can be seen as mixed IgE and non-IgE mediated food allergy **(Table 1)**.

- *IgE-mediated food allergy:* Immediate-onset symptoms (typically within 2 hours) with reproducibility and evidence of sensitization by skin prick test (SPT)/specific IgE or effector cell tests.
- *Non-IgE-mediated food allergy:* Delayed presentations, often gastrointestinal [e.g., food protein-induced enterocolitis syndrome (FPIES), food protein-induced proctocolitis, enteropathy], diagnosed clinically and with elimination challenge.

The European Academy of Allergy and Clinical Immunology (EAACI) defines *IgE-mediated food allergy* as:

- Typical signs and symptoms **(Table 2)**
- Evidence of IgE sensitization

TABLE 1: Types of food allergies.

Non-IgE-mediated food allergy	*Mixed IgE and non-IgE-mediated food allergy*
• Contact dermatitis • Food protein-induced enterocolitis syndrome (FPIES) • Food protein-induced allergic proctitis and proctocolitis • Food protein-induced enteropathy • Dermatitis herpetiformis • Heiner syndrome • Coeliac disease (may also be considered an auto-immune condition)	• Exacerbation of atopic eczema • Eosinophilic esophagitis • Eosinophilic gastritis/enteritis • Exacerbation of asthma

TABLE 2: Clinical features of IgE-mediated food allergy.

Organ or system	*Symptoms and signs*
Skin	• Urticaria • Angioedema • Pruritus • Flushing • Erythema in the predilection sites of eczema • Ear or palm itching
Gastrointestinal	• Oral/pharyngeal pruritus • Oral/pharyngeal swelling • Vomiting • Nausea • Abdominal cramps • Diarrhea • Abdominal pain
Ocular	• Conjunctival erythema • Pruritus • Lacrimation
Cardiovascular	• Pallor • Cold sweats • Heart palpitations • Presyncope/syncope • Tachycardia • Hypotension • Shock
Respiratory	• Rhinitis (rhinorrhea, sneezing, nasal obstruction, pruritus) • Hoarseness • Stridor/laryngeal oedema • Cough • Dyspnea • Chest tightness • Wheezing • Cyanosis
Neurological	• Anxiety • "Feeling of impending doom" • Change in behavior • Irritability • Apathy • Lethargy • Seizures • Syncope/Loss of consciousness

Nonimmune Adverse Reactions/ Food Allergy Mimics

Metabolic, pharmacologic, toxic, or idiosyncratic reactions (e.g., lactose intolerance, sulfite sensitivity), which do not involve immune mechanisms, are:

- Psychological
- Organic
- Toxic (Microbiological pharmacological)
- Nontoxic (a.k.a food intolerance)

TABLE 3: Enzyme deficiencies.

Deficiency/Intolerance	*Food item*
Lactase deficiency	Lactose (milk)
Fructose intolerance	Fructose, especially fruit juices
Sucrose intolerance	Sucrose and starch
Alcohol intolerance	Alcohol
Sulfite intolerance	Sulfite preservatives
G6PD deficiency	Fava (broad) beans
Pancreatic insufficiency	Fatty food
Galactosemia	Lactose and galactose (milk and legumes)
Phenylketonuria	Phenylalanine (high protein foods) and aspartame sweetener

(G6PD: glucose-6-phosphate dehydrogenase)

Psychological or behavioral reactions to food include food refusal, food fixation, abnormal parental feeding practices, onset after a specific trigger, and presence of anticipatory gagging.

Organic or anatomical problems such as pyloric stenosis, hiatus hernia, Hirschsprung's disease, or irritable bowel syndrome.

Toxic reactions from food may be inflicted by any ingredient in the particular food item. These include bacterial toxins, like *Salmonella* or *Staphylococcus*, that spoil food resulting in nausea and vomiting, and nitrates contained in green vegetables like spinach.

Food intolerance: The well-known example is lactose intolerance as given in **Table 3**. So, this category is all about enzyme deficiencies, presenting as symptoms of intolerance on the injection of respective food. Food intolerance is often labeled as "nonimmune-mediated food allergy".

Why are IgE-mediated food allergies important?
IgE-mediated food allergy can lead to severe, life-threatening reactions like anaphylaxis and requires strict allergen avoidance. A detailed clinical history is the most crucial step in diagnosis, guiding further evaluation and testing. Let us now see how to approach the diagnosis of food allergy.

DIAGNOSTIC TOOLS IN FOOD ALLERGY

- Clinical history
- Physical examination

- *Allergy testing:*
  - SPT
  - Blood-specific IgE testing
  - Component-resolved diagnostics (CRD)
  - Oral food challenge (OFC)—*gold standard*

Importance of a food allergy diary

A food allergy diary helps establish the following:
- Temporal relationship
- Reproducibility of symptoms
- Differentiation between IgE-mediated, non-IgE mediated, and intolerance
- Avoids unnecessary food restrictions
- Aids in safe dietary practices

What to record in a food diary?
- Name and quantity of suspected food
- Time of symptom onset after ingestion
- Detailed symptoms observed (by patient and witnesses)
- Reproducibility—did symptoms recur on repeated exposure?
- Symptom relief on food avoidance
- Location of the reaction (home, school, restaurant, etc.)
- *Co-factors:* Exercise, stress, sleep deprivation, alcohol
- Treatment given and response

Diagnostic Tests for Allergy

Skin Prick Testing and Serum-specific IgE Testing

These are primary diagnostic tools used to evaluate sensitization to suspected food allergens. However, these tests must be interpreted after a good clinical history for assessing the likelihood of true food allergy **(Flowchart 1)**.

When to use these tests:
- For suspected IgE-mediated food allergies
- For identifying cross-reactive allergens
- *Avoid in non-IgE-mediated conditions like:*
  - FPIES
  - EoE (eosinophilic esophagitis)

Skin prick test—In vivo testing
- A bioassay that detects allergen-specific IgE on cutaneous mast cells
- Not a measure of reaction severity—a person can react even with a negative test.
- An increasing wheal size means a higher risk, which does not always mean a severe reaction.

Flowchart 1: Diagnostic tools in FA.

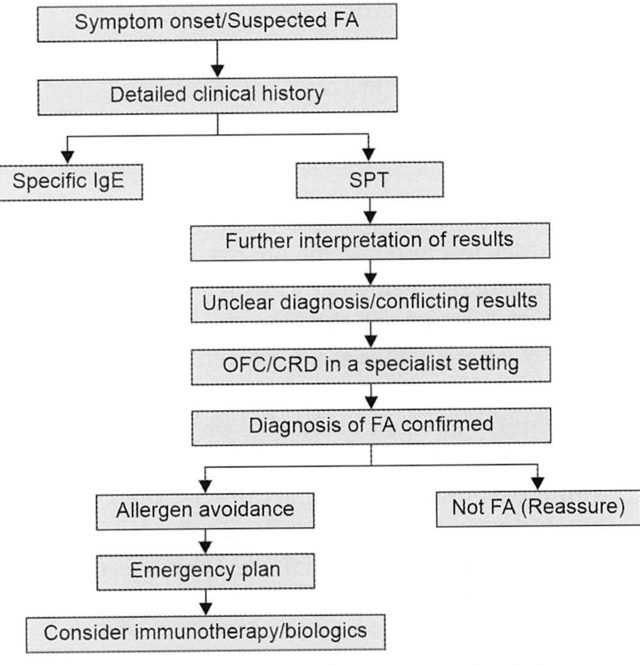

(CRD: component-resolved diagnostics; FA: food allergy; OFC: oral food challenge; SPT: skin prick test)

TABLE 4: Diagnostic accuracy.

Feature	***SPT and Specific IgE***
Sensitivity	High
Specificity	Low
Positive predictive value (PPV)	Low–moderate (↑ with high levels)
Negative predictive value (NPV)	High (with proper technique)

- High sensitivity, low specificity as seen in **Table 4**.
- Best used with strong clinical history to increase diagnostic accuracy
- SPT is to be avoided in chronic urticaria and atopic dermatitis as this may give false-positive results. In such cases, specific IgE testing is preferred (see the following text).

Serum specific IgE—In vitro test
- Blood test measuring circulating allergen-specific IgE antibodies
- *Types of methods in specific IgE testing include:*
  - *Fluorescence enzyme immunoassay (FEIA):* Preferred method
  - Chemiluminescence enzyme immunoassay
  - *Radio-allergosorbent assay technique (RAST):* Not to be used due to radiation exposure

- *Can be used when SPT is contraindicated, such as:*
  - Recent anaphylaxis
  - Current antihistamine use
  - Extensive eczema
  - Uncontrolled asthma
  - Cardiovascular disease
  - Pregnancy
  - Poor skin condition

Skin prick test and specific IgE have low-to-moderate positive predictive value (PPV) which can be improved with a very high wheal size/specific IgE level as seen in **Table 5**. These values are, however, not absolute and vary with age. A strong history is needed before advising the patient on allergen avoidance or allowing them to consume the suspected allergen.

Table 6 shows the comparison between SPT and specific IgE test. It is important to understand that the final decision on the choice of the test depends on a good clinical history by the allergist/clinician.

Prick-to-prick testing

- Used for labile allergens (e.g., fruits/vegetables) where commercial extracts are unavailable
- Less standardized but increases test relevance in certain foods (e.g., banana, apple, kiwi)

When to Escalate?

- *If clinical history is strong but SPT/specific IgE is negative or inconclusive, consider:*
  - CRD
  - Oral food challenge OFC—*gold standard*

TABLE 5: Predictive cutoff examples (not absolute!).

Food	SPT wheal ≥ (mm)	Specific IgE level ≥ (kUA/L)	Approximate PPV (~95%)
Egg	8	7	Yes
Peanut	8	14	Yes
Milk	8	15	Yes
Wheat	8	26	Yes
Soy	8	30	Yes

Component-resolved Diagnostics

Component-resolved diagnostics is an advanced in vitro test that detects IgE antibodies in blood to individual allergenic proteins (components) as opposed to sIgE test that detects IgE antibodies to whole food.

It provides greater precision than traditional specific IgE tests, which may react to nonallergenic parts of foods and lead to overdiagnosis.

Why use CRD?

- Differentiates between true allergy and cross-reactivity
- Predicts the severity and persistence of food allergies
- *Helps guide:*
  - OFC
  - Oral immunotherapy (OIT)
  - Safe food choices

Clinical benefits of CRD

- Differentiates *genuine allergy versus cross-reactivity*
- Guides *OFC and dietary decisions*
- Helps *stratify anaphylaxis risk*
- Supports *personalized treatment plans*
- Monitors *tolerance development* or *disease persistence*
- Especially helpful in *complex or polysensitized patients*

TABLE 6: Comparison of skin prick test (SPT) versus serum-specific IgE.

Parameter	SPT	Serum-specific IgE
Age consideration	May be less reactive in infants	Easier to perform in very young children
Influencing factors	Affected by antihistamines, skin condition	Affected by age, total IgE, laboratory standards
NPV (negative predictive value)	>95% (very high)	>90%
PPV (positive predictive value)	~50% (depends on cutoff and population)	~50% (improves with higher levels)
Sensitivity	>90% (high)	~70–90%
Specificity	~50–60% (moderate)	~50–60%
Speed of results	Immediate (15–20 minutes)	Delayed (laboratory-dependent; 1–2 days)
Utility	Best for ruling out allergy (high NPV)	Useful adjunct; consider component testing (component-resolved diagnostics)

Oral Food Challenge (Table 7)

- Gold standard for diagnosing food allergies
- Used when history and test results are inconclusive
- Always done in a controlled clinical setting with emergency precautions

Clinical applications

- Confirm or exclude a food allergy diagnosis
- Monitor for resolution of an existing food allergy
- Identify threshold dose that causes symptoms
- Aid in planning treatment or dietary expansion

Prechallenge considerations

- Nutritional importance of the food
- Patient and caregiver preferences and anxiety
- Previous reaction severity
- Parental understanding of procedure and risks

Advantages

- Reduces fear and dietary restrictions if negative
- Identifies safe exposure threshold
- May support tolerance induction
- Improves quality of life

TABLE 7: Types of food challenges.

Type	*Description*	*Bias level*
Open challenge	• Simple and quick • Both patient and doctor know the food	High
Single-blind placebo-controlled food challenge (SBPCFC)	Observer knows, patient does not	Moderate
Double-blind placebo-controlled food challenge (DBPCFC)	• Gold standard • Neither patient nor observer knows the food	None

Note: DBPCFC is mainly used in research settings due to complexity.

Disadvantages

- Risk of severe allergic reaction
- Time-consuming
- Requires trained staff and emergency setup

Table 8 summarizes all the diagnostic modalities and their applications. This is a quick reference chart for clinicians when they come across allergy patients. It is wise to counsel patients with complex allergies about the emergency action plan (EAP) and basic management **(Table 8)** before referring them to the allergy specialist.

MANAGEMENT

Allergen Avoidance

- Cornerstone of food allergy management
- Requires strict avoidance of identified allergens
- Read food labels and avoid cross-contamination
- Patients and caregivers must be vigilant in home, school, travel, and dining settings

Medications

- *For mild-to-moderate reactions:*
  - Oral antihistamines (e.g., cetirizine, loratadine)
    - Help manage symptoms like rash, itching, mild swelling
    - Not effective for preventing anaphylaxis
- *For severe reactions (anaphylaxis):*
  - Intramuscular (IM) adrenaline is the gold standard
    - Must be given into the anterolateral thigh
    - Immediate administration at the first sign of anaphylaxis

Emergency Preparedness

- *Education is critical:*
  - Recognize early signs of anaphylaxis (e.g., difficulty breathing, throat tightness, drop in BP)
  - Train in administration of IM adrenaline

TABLE 8: Allergy investigations at a glance.

Investigation	*Purpose*	*When to use*	*Notes*
Specific IgE	Detect IgE antibodies in blood	Suspected IgE-mediated FA	Easy to access but can overestimate FA
SPT	Detect immediate hypersensitivity	Done by trained personnel	Needs 5–7-day antihistamine washout
CRD	Detect reaction to specific allergen components	When specific IgE/SPT unclear/ multiple allergens	Use for peanut, milk, egg, etc.
OFC	Confirm diagnosis	When diagnosis uncertain or before reintroduction	Gold standard; hospital setup essential

(CRD: component-resolved diagnostics; FA: food allergy; OFC: oral food challenge; SPT: skin prick test)

- *Provide a personalized EAP:*
  - Patients and parents
  - Schools, daycare centers, and caregivers

Adrenaline Delivery in India

- Epinephrine autoinjectors are not yet authorized for routine use in India, and thus indigenous syringe adrenaline is prescribed to the patients.
- *Current recommendation:*
  - Use syringe + adrenaline ampoule
  - Prefilled, labeled kits with instructions
  - Kin of patients must be trained to administer adrenaline

Tables 9 and 10 shows the treatment modalities and and practical tips in the Indian scenario for food allergy management.

TABLE 9: Treatment options for food allergy.

Strategy	*When to use*	*Notes*
Avoidance	All confirmed cases	Label reading, school information essential
Emergency plan	All IgE-mediated cases	Include written plan, demonstration
Immunotherapy (OIT)	Select food allergens (peanut, milk)	Only under specialist care
Biologics (omalizumab)	Severe/multiple allergies	Specialist setting

(OIT: oral immunotherapy)

TABLE 10: Practical food allergy management tips in the Indian scenario.

Tip	*Details*
Allergen education	Provide visual aids, ingredient names in local languages
Label reading	Teach patients to identify allergen synonyms
Emergency kit	Include adrenaline ampoule, syringe, antihistamines, instructions
School coordination	Written action plan, trained staff, allergen-free meal policy
Family awareness	Educate extended family and domestic help
Periodic review	Reassess diagnosis, update management plans annually

ADVANCES IN DIAGNOSIS, MANAGEMENT, AND PREVENTION OF FOOD ALLERGY

Diagnostic Innovations

Basophil activation test (BAT):

- A functional assay using flow cytometry
- Measures activation markers (e.g., CD63, CD203c) on basophils after exposure to allergens
- Useful in ambiguous cases where specific IgE or SPT results are inconclusive

Emerging Therapies

- *OIT:*
  - Gradual introduction of increasing doses of the allergenic food under medical supervision
  - Aims to induce desensitization and potentially long-term tolerance
  - Requires careful patient selection and well-equipped allergy centers
- *Biologics (e.g., omalizumab):*
  - Anti-IgE monoclonal antibody
  - Can be used alone or along with OIT
  - Beneficial in patients with severe multifood allergies

New Anaphylaxis Rescue Options

Invasive Devices

The management of anaphylaxis in India has significantly improved with the growing availability and awareness of adrenaline (epinephrine) autoinjectors. While devices like EpiPen® and Jext® remain standard globally, they were not easily accessible in India until recently.

Newer indigenous devices, such as:

- Tirpal® auto-injector and
- Symjepi® (available via selected importers) are emerging as cost-effective alternatives.

In addition, prefilled adrenaline syringes and training kits are now being used in educational initiatives for schools, clinics, and caregivers. These options are making timely intramuscular adrenaline delivery more feasible, particularly in pediatric patients and high-risk groups.

However, standardized training protocols and prescription guidelines for adrenaline autoinjector use remain under development and vary across regions. Pediatricians are advised to remain updated with local regulatory approvals and patient accessibility.

Noninvasive Devices

A needle-free delivery device named Neffy®, which is a nasal adrenaline spray, has been recently approved by the US Food and Drug Administration (FDA) for anaphylaxis.

Prevention Strategies

Early Allergen Introduction

Early introduction of allergenic foods, especially peanuts, reduces the incidence of peanut allergy in high-risk infants.

- *LEAP randomized trial (2015):* Early peanut consumption from infancy substantially reduced peanut allergy by age 5 years in high-risk infants compared with avoidance.
- *LEAP-On and long-term follow-up to adolescence (LEAP-Trio):* Protection persisted after a year of avoidance and remained significant at age 12 years, with lower prevalence in the early-introduction group; findings align with the dual-allergen exposure hypothesis and support sustained population-level-prevention strategies.

Indian Dietary Practices

- The diverse and traditional Indian diet, with early exposure to a variety of spices and lentils, may contribute to a lower prevalence of food allergy in India.
- Continued breastfeeding and home-cooked meals may also be protective.

FOLLOW-UP AND NATURAL HISTORY

- Many childhood allergies to milk and egg resolve over time; peanut, tree nut, fish, and shellfish allergies are more likely to persist; periodic reassessment with history, testing, and OFC enables dietary liberalization when tolerance develops.
- Shared decision-making and psychosocial support are integral, given the anxiety and lifestyle burdens associated with food allergy.

CONCLUSION

Food allergies impose a significant burden on affected children and their families, with risks ranging from nutritional compromise to life-threatening anaphylaxis. Accurate diagnosis using history, testing, and oral food challenges is vital to avoid unnecessary avoidance and ensure safety. Management must be individualized, incorporating avoidance of confirmed allergens, nutritional support, emergency preparedness, and consideration of emerging therapies including immunotherapy. Education and family empowerment remain central to preventing reactions and improving quality of life.

KEY POINTS

- *Diagnosis requires a detailed history*, supported by tests like SPT, specific IgE, CRD, and OFC.
- *CRD helps differentiate between true allergy and cross-reactivity*, especially useful in cases like egg allergy and pollen-food syndrome.
- *OFC remains the gold standard* for diagnosing and monitoring food allergy but must be done in controlled settings due to the risk of severe reactions.
- *Management includes strict allergen avoidance, antihistamines for mild reactions, and intramuscular adrenaline for anaphylaxis.* Equip patients with action plans and ensure access and training for epinephrine.
- *Newer approaches* include BAT, OIT, and biologics. Patients should be reassessed regularly for tolerance development.
- *Prevention through early allergen introduction (4–6 months of age)* has been shown to reduce food allergy incidence, with Indian diets possibly playing a protective role.

CASE SCENARIOS

A set of case scenarios will help in better correlation of these diagnostic tools in allergy.

Scenario 1: Egg Allergy and Baked Egg Tolerance

A 3-year-old child develops hives within 5 minutes of consuming scrambled eggs but tolerates baked goods (e.g., muffins). There are no other systemic symptoms (like breathlessness, choking sensation, vomiting, diarrhea, dizziness, or loss of consciousness). These hives have occurred in the past and respond to antihistamines within 10 minutes.

When they visit the allergy specialist, it is deduced that there is a good temporal correlation and reproducibility of these symptoms. Also, these symptoms have not amounted to a severe allergic reaction or anaphylaxis. SPT to egg white is positive and the allergist counsels about the emergency action plan.

TABLE 11: CRD components.

Component	*Protein type*	*Clinical significance*
Gal d 1 (Ovomucoid)	Heat-stable	Persistent, higher-risk allergy
Gal d 2 (Ovalbumin)	Heat-labile	Often tolerates baked egg

(CRD: component-resolved diagnostics)

However, what is unclear here is the absence of symptoms on consuming baked egg. This is where we apply the CRD test **(Flowchart 1)**. A single plex CRD report has revealed the following:

CRD result **(Table 11)**:

- High IgE to Gal d 2
- Low/negative IgE to Gal d 1

On follow-up, the allergist counsels the parents that the patient is likely to tolerate baked egg in the form of muffins or cakes after a *negative OFC*. They are also informed that they should continue to give baked egg which will accelerate the tolerance development to the scrambled egg preparation (which is less cooked and has more egg protein exposure) in the future.

However, a large amount of baked egg may also lead to a severe reaction like the scrambled egg preparation wherein they should follow the emergency action plan.

Scenario 2: Pollen-Food Syndrome versus True Nut Allergy

A 10-year-old, with birch pollen allergy (presenting as allergic rhinitis), complains of mouth itching 5–10 minutes after eating apples and hazelnuts. The family is concerned and visits the allergist. After a thorough history taking and positive SPT to hazelnut and apple, the allergist informs them that these symptoms could be an oral allergy syndrome or less likely due to a true food allergy.

As shown in **Flowchart 1**, to confirm this diagnosis, a CRD panel is sent. The report is as follows:

CRD result **(Table 12)**:

- Positive to Cor a 1, Mal d 1, and Bet v 1
- Negative to Cor a 9 and Cor a 14

The allergist informs them that it is a pollen-food allergy syndrome (PFAS) due to the cross reactivity between hazelnut and birch pollen and apples and birch pollen. It is likely safe to eat hazelnuts and cooked apples as these will cause mild oral symptoms and not a systemic allergy.

TABLE 12: CRD components.

Hazelnut component	*Associated with*	*Risk*
Cor a 1 (PR-10)	Birch pollen cross-reactivity	Mild symptoms
Cor a 9/ Cor a 14	True hazelnut allergy	Severe reactions/ anaphylaxis
Mal d 1 (PR-10)	Birch pollen cross-reactivity	Mild symptoms
Bet v 1 (PR-10)	Birch pollen	Allergic rhinoconjunctivitis

(CRD: component-resolved diagnostics)

SUGGESTED READING

1. Anvari S, Miller J, Yeh CY, Davis CM. IgE-Mediated Food Allergy. Clin Rev Allergy and Immunol. 2019;57:244-60.
2. ASCIA guidelines for Anaphylaxis 2025.
3. Du Toit G, Huffaker MF, Radulovic S, Feeney M, Fisher HR, Byron M, et al. Follow-up to Adolescence after Early Peanut Introduction (LEAP-Trio). NEJM Evid. 2024;3(6): EVIDoa2300311.
4. Du Toit G, Roberts G, Sayre PH, Bahnson HT, Suzana Radulovic MPH, Santos AF, et al. Randomized trial of peanut consumption in infants at risk for peanut allergy (LEAP). N Engl J Med. 2015;372:803-13.
5. EAACI guidelines on the diagnosis of IgE-mediated food allergy. Allergy. 2023.
6. EAACI Guidelines on the Management of IgE-Mediated Food Allergy (Management summary with recommendations including omalizumab and OIT). EAACI Hub. 2024.
7. National Peanut Board. LEAP-Trio follow-up insights on early introduction and prevention. [online] Available from https://nationalpeanutboard.org/news/new-results-from-leap-trio-studies-unlock-additional-insights-on-allergy-prevention/ [Last accessed December, 2025].
8. ONU Pharmacy and Wellness Review. (2024). FDA Approves Neffy® – First Nasal Spray for Anaphylaxis. [online] Available from https://digitalcommons.onu.edu/cgi/viewcontent.cgi?article=1198&context=paw_review [Last accessed December, 2025].
9. ThermoFisher Scientific. EAACI Food Allergy and Anaphylaxis Guidelines (overview). [online] Available from https://www.thermofisher.com/diagnostic-education/dam/clinical/documents/EAACI-Food-Allergy-and-Anaphylaxis-Guidelines.pdf [Last accessed December, 2025].

15 CHAPTER

Allergic Conjunctivitis in Children

Sugaranjini Galiyugavaradhan, Shweta Agarwal

INTRODUCTION

Allergic conjunctivitis (AC) in children encompasses a spectrum of ocular hypersensitivity disorders which may coexist with other allergic diseases including asthma, rhinitis, and atopic dermatitis (AD). The World Health Organization (WHO) has recognized that individuals with allergies often experience a reduced quality of life, which in turn contributes to negative economic consequences. Similarly, the World Allergy Organization (WAO) has expressed concern over the growing global burden of allergic diseases, especially among children and in developing countries. Timely diagnosis and targeted management are essential. Notably, cases of AC unresponsive to initial therapy should be promptly referred by pediatricians and primary care providers to ophthalmologists to facilitate early intervention and prevent potentially sight-threatening complications.

EPIDEMIOLOGY

Allergic conjunctivitis affects up to 30% of children, either as an isolated condition or in association with allergic rhinitis. A cross-sectional study from a semiurban community in Chandigarh, India, reported a prevalence of 12.22% among children aged 5–15 years, with a higher occurrence in males. Seasonal allergic conjunctivitis (SAC) and perennial allergic conjunctivitis (PAC) are the most commonly encountered subtypes, while vernal keratoconjunctivitis (VKC) is the most severe and vision-threatening, particularly in the pediatric age-group. SAC and PAC affect both sexes and are estimated to occur in approximately 15–40% of the general population. SAC typically worsens from spring through fall and subsides during colder months, whereas PAC occurs year-round and tends to be milder in severity.

Vernal keratoconjunctivitis is most prevalent and severe in hot, dry climates such as the Mediterranean region, West Africa, and the Indian subcontinent. A recent population-based study in India found the prevalence of allergic eye disease (AED) and VKC to be 4.98% and 1.11%, respectively, with higher occurrence in rural areas. Prevalence rates of VKC range between 2 and 6% across various parts of Africa, whereas in Western Europe, the reported prevalence is <0.03%. An epidemiological survey across six European countries (Italy, France, the Netherlands, Norway, Finland, and Sweden) found VKC to be more prevalent in southern nations, particularly Italy, and least common in northern countries like Norway. These geographic and racial variations are likely influenced by a complex interplay of genetic susceptibility, environmental exposure, migration, and socioeconomic status.

Atopic dermatitis is a common chronic inflammatory skin condition affecting 15–20% of children, and approximately 25–40% of these individuals develop atopic keratoconjunctivitis (AKC) as an ocular manifestation.

Giant papillary conjunctivitis (GPC), commonly linked to soft contact lens wear, affects 1–5% of users—about ten times more than RGP lens users—likely due to greater allergen adherence. Though pediatric data are limited, risk is influenced by lens wear duration, daily use, and hygiene.

CLASSIFICATION

Ocular allergy (OA) encompasses a spectrum of conditions that can be classified based on clinical features and underlying immunopathogenesis into six major subtypes: SAC, PAC, VKC, AKC, GPC, and contact dermatoconjunctivitis (CDC). SAC and PAC represent the more common and milder forms and are predominantly mediated by immunoglobulin E (IgE)-dependent hypersensitivity mechanisms. In contrast, VKC, AKC, GPC, and CDC involve a more complex interplay of both IgE-mediated and non-IgE-mediated (cellular immune) pathways, often associated with chronic inflammation and tissue remodeling.

ETIOPATHOGENESIS

Seasonal and perennial allergic conjunctivitis are IgE-mediated type I hypersensitivity disorders triggered by airborne allergens. In sensitized individuals, allergen exposure leads to cross-linking of membrane-bound IgE on conjunctival mast cells, causing degranulation and release of histamine, leukotrienes, prostaglandins, and other inflammatory mediators. This initiates an immediate hypersensitivity reaction followed by a late-phase response, characterized by recruitment of eosinophils and other immune cells, sustaining conjunctival inflammation.

Vernal keratoconjunctivitis was traditionally considered a purely IgE-mediated type I hypersensitivity disorder. However, approximately 50% of VKC patients show no evidence of allergic sensitization, with negative skin prick tests and low or absent tear IgE levels, despite often elevated serum IgE. These findings indicate that VKC is not solely an IgE-driven condition. Recent insights have highlighted a significant non-IgE-mediated, T cell-driven response in VKC. Activated T helper 2 (Th2) lymphocytes in the conjunctiva release proinflammatory cytokines such as interleukin 4 (IL-4), IL-13, and tumor necrosis factor alpha (TNF-α), which promote corneal fibroblast activation and conjunctival remodeling through excessive extracellular matrix deposition. These cytokines also facilitate eosinophil recruitment and activation, leading to the release of matrix metalloproteinases that contribute to corneal epithelial degradation. Additionally, mucus hypersecretion—a hallmark of VKC—is associated with a marked increase in goblet cell density within giant papillae and is stimulated by Th2 cytokines and other allergic mediators. Neuroimmune and hormonal pathways also appear to influence disease expression. Elevated levels of nerve growth factor and increased expression of estrogen and progesterone receptors in conjunctival tissues have been observed. These findings may explain the male predominance of VKC and its tendency to resolve around puberty. Additionally, altered sphingolipid metabolism, particularly reduced tear levels of ceramide and sphingosine, has been linked to greater disease severity, likely through impaired barrier function and amplified inflammation.

Similarly, AKC is a chronic ocular surface inflammation in patients with AD, driven by IgE-mediated and delayed-type hypersensitivity. It involves cytokine release from mast cells, eosinophils, and T cells, with associated goblet cell loss, reduced corneal sensitivity, and elevated tear inflammatory markers.

Giant papillary conjunctivitis is primarily a mechanical irritation of the tarsal conjunctiva, most commonly associated with soft contact lens wear, likely due to greater allergen adherence on soft lens surfaces compared to rigid lenses.

CLINICAL PRESENTATION

Seasonal and Perennial Allergic Conjunctivitis

The most common forms of AC in children are SAC and PAC. These conditions are primarily distinguished by their duration and the nature of the allergens involved. SAC typically arises during the spring and summer months due to exposure to outdoor allergens like pollen from trees and grasses. It often coexists with allergic rhinitis and asthma. In contrast, PAC is triggered by indoor allergens such as dust mites, mold, pet dander, and tends to cause year-round symptoms with intermittent flare-ups. Some children may be polysensitized, experiencing ongoing PAC symptoms with seasonal exacerbations. Both conditions are usually bilateral and present with itching (the hallmark symptom), tearing, redness, conjunctival swelling (chemosis), and papillary hypertrophy **(Fig. 1A)**. Corneal involvement is very unusual and thus very rarely patient presents with visual complaints. Importantly, symptoms may fluctuate or be absent at the time of examination, so a detailed history—particularly regarding seasonal patterns, associated atopic conditions, and environmental exposures—is essential for accurate diagnosis.

Vernal Keratoconjunctivitis

Vernal keratoconjunctivitis is a chronic bilateral, recurrent allergic disorder which primarily affects boys with peak incidence between 7 and 13 years of age. It usually resolves by puberty; however, in the last few years an adult-onset VKC-like disease has also been reported. Adult-onset VKC presents with clinical features largely similar to the childhood form, albeit with subtle differences and generally a milder disease course. Other than the male predominance, there are no notable gender-based differences in clinical presentation or complications. VKC may be seasonal or perennial, with exacerbations during the spring and summer months—hence the term "vernal". It is more common and severe in tropical belts like Asia, Africa, and South America. VKC can be limbal, tarsal/palpebral, or mixed based on the part of conjunctiva primarily involved. Disease exacerbations are often

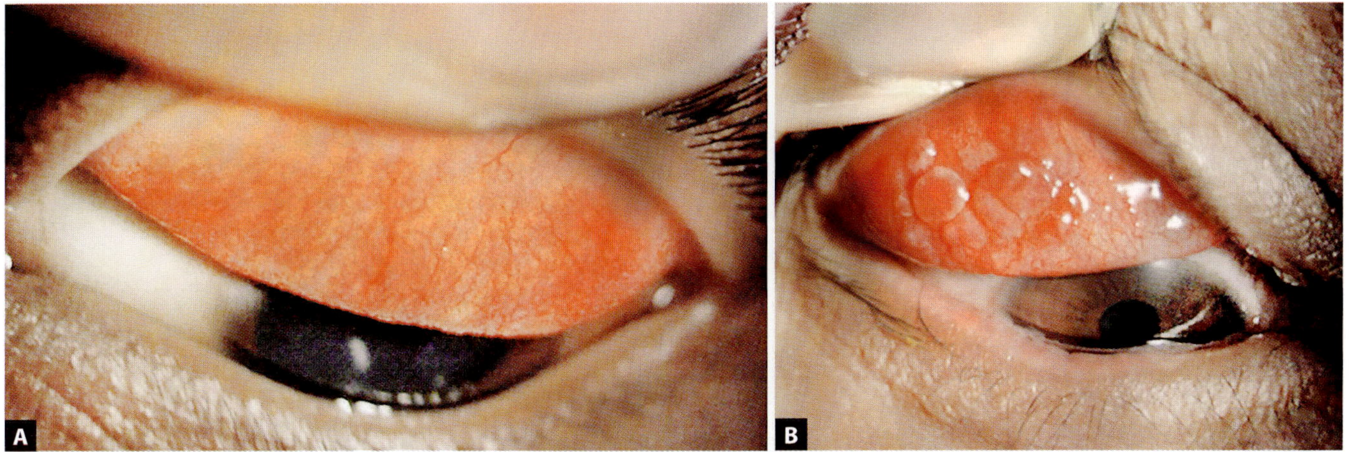

Figs. 1A and B: Clinical presentation of patients with allergic conjunctivitis. (A) Micropapillae on upper tarsal conjunctiva in patients with seasonal/perennial conjunctivitis and (B) Giant papillary reaction in a patient with chronic contact lens use in GPC.

trigged by allergen exposure or nonspecific stimuli like wind, sunlight, or dust.

Clinically, VKC presents with intense itching, tearing, redness, mucous discharge, photophobia, and sometimes blurred vision, often due to corneal involvement. Signs include conjunctival hyperemia, thick, ropy discharge which is a fibrinous secretion, transient limbal or conjunctival eosinophil-rich deposits (Horner–Trantas dots), and tarsal or limbal papillary reactions. In VKC, often giant papillae up to the size of 7–8 mm are seen in the severe grades and are termed as giant cobble stone papillae. Corneal involvement in moderate-to-severe grades often presents as superficial punctate keratitis and oval, sterile shield ulcers located in the superior cornea, which heal with varying degrees of subepithelial scarring. The development of shield ulcers is attributed to both inflammatory processes and mechanical trauma caused by giant papillae **(Figs. 2A to D)**. Other vision-threatening corneal complications, such as limbal stem cell deficiency and keratoconus in addition to shield ulcers, are considered disease-related manifestations in the chronic, persistent form of VKC. Treatment-related complications include steroid-induced cataract and glaucoma often resulting from inadvertent use of steroids. In the quiescent stage and in long-standing cases, additional features such as conjunctival pigmentation and pseudogerontoxon may be observed. Conjunctival pigmentation is often linked to chronic eye rubbing, particularly among Asian populations and pseudogerontoxon represents a peripheral corneal degenerative change caused by lipid deposition which closely resembles arcus senilis.

Atopic Keratoconjunctivitis

Atopic keratoconjunctivitis is a chronic, bilateral, and severe allergic inflammation of the ocular surface, commonly seen in adolescents and adults with AD. While rare in early childhood, it can develop in the context of long-standing eczema. Up to 40% of patients with AD show ocular involvement, often presenting with itching, burning, tearing, and persistent eyelid eczema.

Eyelid changes such as erythema, scaling, single or double infraorbital crease (Dennie–Morgan folds), and periorbital darkening ("allergic shiners") are characteristic. In older patients, absence of the lateral eyebrow (de Hertoghe's sign) may be seen because of constant rubbing. The conjunctiva is hyperemic, with papillary hypertrophy mostly involving the lower tarsal, and the cornea may show punctate epithelial erosions, neovascularization, and scarring, sometimes progressing to shield ulcers or vision loss **(Figs. 3A and B).** Secondary infections (e.g., *Staphylococcus* blepharitis, herpes simplex keratitis) are also common due to chronic skin breakdown. In advanced disease, cicatrizing conjunctivitis, fornix foreshortening, and symblepharon may develop, resembling ocular cicatricial pemphigoid. Meibomian gland dysfunction and reduced tear production are frequently observed.

A notable complication is keratoconus, reported in up to 16% of AKC patients, likely due to chronic eye rubbing. Atopic cataracts, typically anterior or posterior subcapsular, occur in 8–12% of severe AD cases, often developing within a decade of dermatitis onset. These cataracts may progress rapidly and have been linked

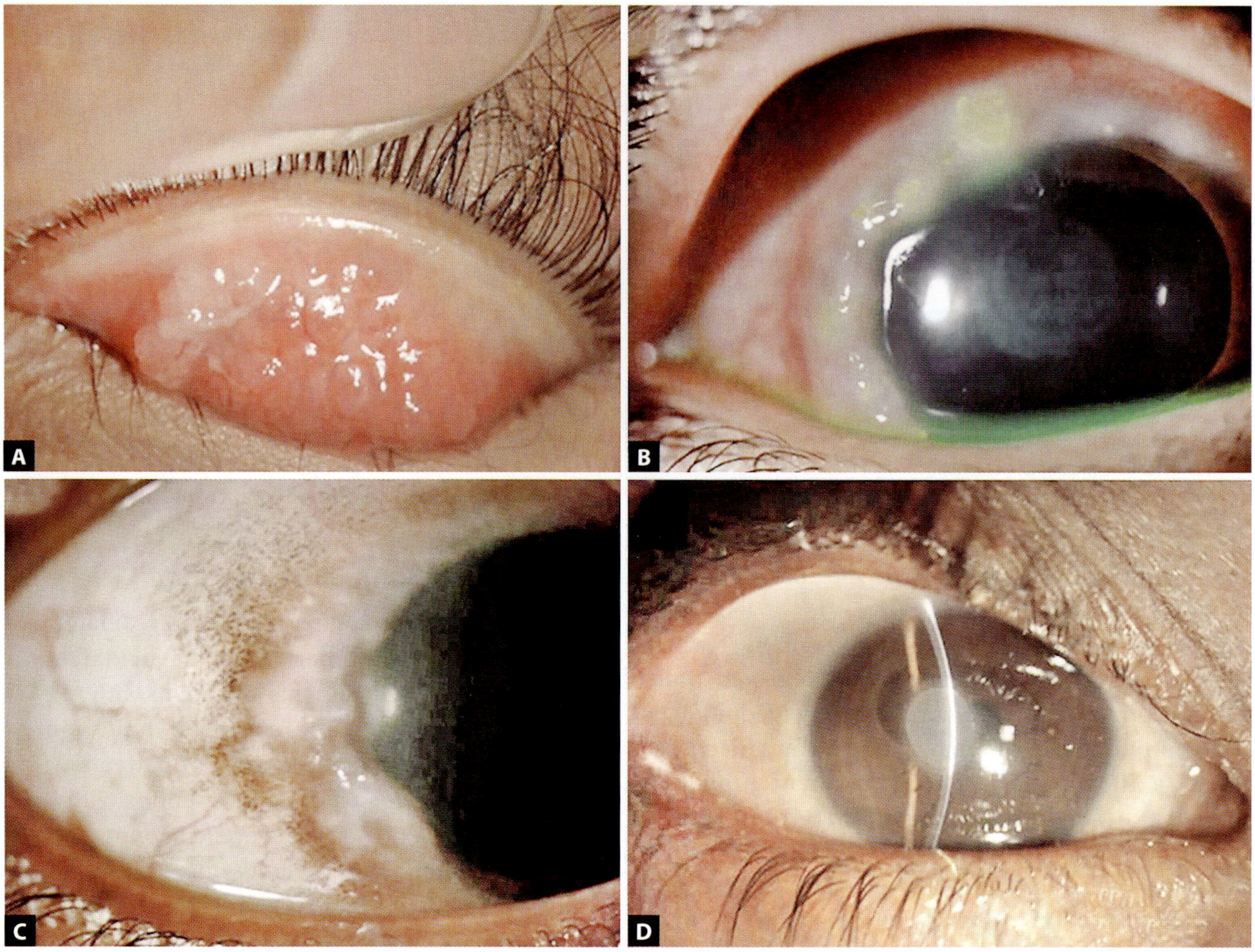

Figs. 2A to D: Clinical presentation in patients with vernal keratoconjunctivitis. (A) Giant papillae in upper tarsal conjunctiva with mucus discharge; (B) Horner–Trantas spots seen at the limbus; (C) Limbal hypertrophy with conjunctival pigmentation; and (D) Shield ulcer coated with fibrin plaque in the superior cornea caused by giant papillae in upper tarsal conjunctiva.

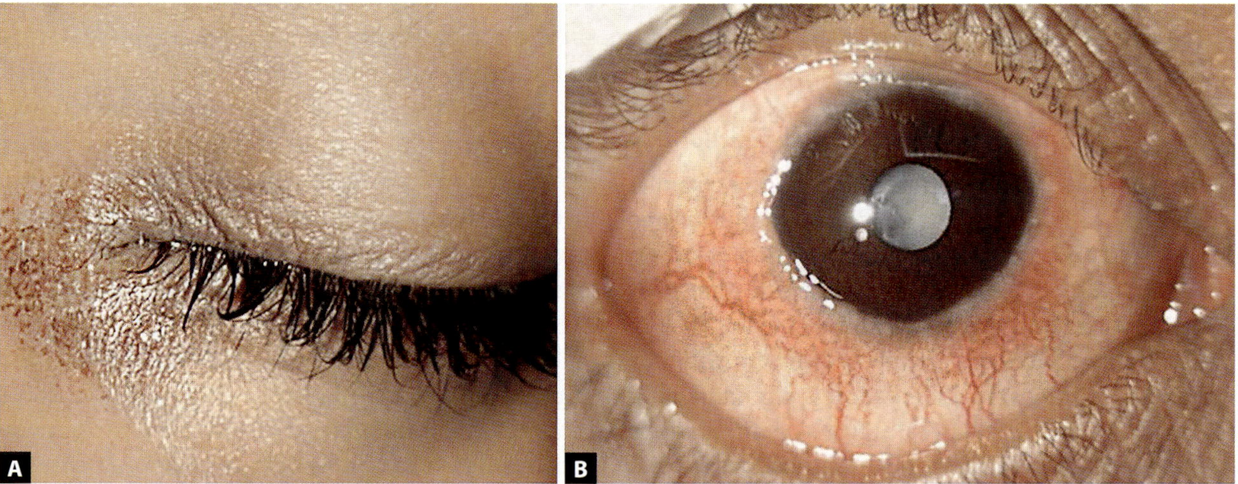

Figs. 3A and B: Clinical presentation of patients with atopic keratoconjunctivitis. (A) Eczematous lesions seen near the medial canthus of the eye indicating atopic dermatitis and (B) Bulbar conjunctival congestion with hypertrophied limbus and cataract.

TABLE 1: Differentiating features of allergic conjunctivitis types.

	SAC	*PAC*	*VKC*	*AKC*
Disease course	• Seasonal • Worse during summer/spring	• Perennial • All year-round, worse in autumn	• Seasonal/perennial • Worse during spring/summer	• Perennial • Worse in winter
Clinical presentation	Itching, hyperemia, watery discharge, mild papillary reaction	Itching, hyperemia, watery discharge, mild papillary reaction	Itching, hyperemia, ropy discharge, corneal involvement, papillary hypertrophy, Horner–Trantas dots	Itching, hyperemia, ropy discharge, corneal involvement, papillary hypertrophy, Horner–Trantas dots, conjunctival scarring, lid involvement
Age/gender	All ages/both sexes	All ages/both sexes	• 5–15 years of age • Occasionally adults • Male predominance	Peak 30–50 years Male predominance
Allergic mechanism	IgE-mediated	IgE-mediated	IgE and non-IgE-mediated	IgE and non-IgE-mediated
Treatment	• Topical antihistaminics • Mast cell stabilizers • Dual-acting agents	• Topical antihistaminics • Mast cell stabilizers • Dual-acting agents	• Topical dual-acting agents • Immunomodulators • On and off low-dose steroids	• Topical dual-acting agents • Immunomodulators • On and off low-dose steroids

(AKC: atopic keratoconjunctivitis; CDC: contact or drug-induced dermatoconjunctivitis; GPC: giant papillary conjunctivitis; PAC: perennial allergic conjunctivitis; SAC: seasonal allergic conjunctivitis; VKC: vernal keratoconjunctivitis)

to elevated serum IgE, food allergies, and chronic inflammation rather than steroid use alone.

Differences in the clinical presentation and mechanism of the varied AC are highlighted in **Table 1**. GPC and CDC though are considered as variants of AC, they are slightly different in their etiopathogenesis and hence are not included in the table.

Giant Papillary Conjunctivitis

Giant papillary conjunctivitis is a chronic inflammatory condition of the tarsal conjunctiva, primarily triggered by mechanical irritation from foreign bodies, most commonly contact lenses. It can also result from exposure to ocular prostheses, exposed sutures, scleral buckles, or surface irregularities such as filtering blebs or corneal deposits. The condition arises due to microtrauma caused by repeated friction of the upper eyelid against the ocular surface, leading to the development of giant papillae—papillary structures typically larger than 0.3 mm on the upper tarsal conjunctiva **(Fig. 1B)**. Though not a classic allergic condition, GPC shares morphological and immunological features with VKC. Patients often report itching, excessive mucus discharge, tearing, and discomfort, especially upon awakening. Symptoms may worsen during the spring pollen season, suggesting a secondary allergic component. Conjunctival hyperemia, mucous discharge, and occasionally limbal infiltrates or Trantas' dots may also be present. Contact lens deposits and poor lens hygiene are contributing factors. Prompt recognition and modification or discontinuation of contact lens use are essential for resolution.

Contact or Drug-induced Dermato-conjunctivitis

Contact dermatoconjunctivitis is a bilateral inflammatory condition of the eyelids and conjunctiva, more commonly seen in females. It typically presents with itching, burning, eyelid eczema, conjunctival hyperemia, follicular or papillary reactions, and punctate staining of the ocular surface. CDC may result from either irritant or allergic mechanisms. Irritant CDC is a nonspecific response to chemical exposure, leading to cytokine-mediated inflammation. Allergic CDC, on the other hand, is a delayed-type (type IV) hypersensitivity reaction involving Th1 lymphocytes and Langerhans cells, which present allergens to T cells and trigger local inflammation. Common triggers include topical medications (e.g., antibiotics, antivirals, glaucoma drops), preservatives, anesthetics, and cosmetic products such as mascara and fragrances. Symptoms of allergic CDC may develop 48–72 hours after exposure, whereas irritant reactions can occur within a few hours.

DIAGNOSIS OF ALLERGIC CONJUNCTIVITIS

Diagnosing OA can be challenging, as it is often underrecognized, misdiagnosed, or self-treated with over-the-counter medications. Most patients present first to primary care providers, such as pediatricians or family physicians, where ocular conditions like allergy, blepharitis, dry eye, or infection are frequently mistaken for one another, leading to suboptimal management.

A thorough clinical history is essential. Hallmark symptoms include itching, redness, tearing, burning, and occasionally blurred vision, often accompanied by nasal symptoms such as sneezing or congestion. Itching remains the most reliable distinguishing feature of AC. Seasonal variation or known exposure to allergens can further support the diagnosis.

On examination, findings may include conjunctival hyperemia, papillary hypertrophy, stringy mucous discharge, or other disease-specific features. OA is a clinical diagnosis and very rarely needs tear or systemic evaluation to confirm. However, in specialty settings, diagnosis can be refined with tests such as serum or tear-specific IgE testing, skin prick or patch testing or tear film analysis (e.g., osmolarity, inflammatory markers like MMP-9).

It is important to differentiate AC from other causes of red eye—such as infectious conjunctivitis, glaucoma, uveitis, or scleritis—with referral to an ophthalmologist.

TREATMENT

A multidisciplinary approach involving allergists, pediatricians, internists, ENT (ear–nose–throat) specialists, and eye care professionals is essential in managing AC. Management typically begins with allergen identification and avoidance, progresses through non-pharmacological strategies, and, when needed, includes pharmacologic therapies such as topical or oral antihistamines, mast cell stabilizers, corticosteroids, and immunomodulators. Immunotherapy may also be considered under specialist supervision.

Oral antihistamines provide symptomatic relief in OA but have a slower onset and might cause dryness of eyes in case of prolonged use. Since most patients present with both nasal and ocular symptoms, intranasal corticosteroids are often prescribed for both. Studies suggest no significant difference in ocular symptom control with use of intranasal steroids and oral antihistamines and therefore their role is limited in OA. Leukotriene antagonists, used alone or with antihistamines, are effective in allergic rhinitis. While they reduce conjunctival nitric oxide levels, their role in OA remains limited.

Topical Therapy

Topical therapy forms the cornerstone of management in AC, offering targeted relief from ocular symptoms while minimizing systemic side effects.

Artificial tears help flush out allergens from the ocular surface, reducing their impact by dilution and mechanical removal. Management of OA primarily centers on the use of topical anti-allergic medications, such as antihistamines, mast cell stabilizers, and dual-action agents with both antihistaminic and mast cell-stabilizing properties.

Topical decongestants alleviate redness and chemosis by vasoconstriction via α-adrenergic stimulation but do not address the underlying allergic response and prolonged use may lead to rebound hyperemia, thus limiting their role in AC.

Antihistaminics available are H1 antagonist and provide short-term relief from itching and redness by competitively and reversibly blocking histamine receptors but have no effect on other inflammatory mediators like prostaglandins and leukotrienes. Their limited duration of action requires frequent dosing and prolonged use may cause ocular irritation, making them less preferred for the treatment of AC. Combination antihistamine-decongestant drops offer synergistic relief, though their effect is short-lived and may carry decongestant-related side effects.

Mast cell stabilizers inhibit the release of inflammatory mediators, targeting both early and late allergic responses. They are most effective when used prophylactically, though some benefit may be seen within 24–48 hours after allergen exposure. These agents are generally safe but may cause transient stinging or irritation. Owing to their requirement for a loading period, limited effectiveness in alleviating acute symptoms, and the availability of dual-acting agents with antihistaminic, mast cell-stabilizing, and antieosinophilic properties, the clinical utility of mast cell stabilizers has become increasingly limited. Dual-acting agents exert a multifaceted therapeutic effect by combining antihistaminic action with mast cell stabilization, while also inhibiting eosinophil activation, leukotriene synthesis, and cytokine release. These agents provide rapid symptomatic relief—often within 30 minutes—and enhance patient compliance. Due to their proven efficacy and favorable safety profile, they represent the most commonly prescribed medications for the management of OA. Topical corticosteroids offer rapid and broad relief in all forms of OA due to their potent anti-inflammatory effects, typically within 6 hours. However, concerns over side effects such as glaucoma, cataracts, delayed healing, and infections limit their use. The low-dose steroids like fluorometholone or loteprednol are preferred and are primarily indicated during active episodes in a tapering manner. They should be used for the shortest effective duration under close monitoring.

Immunomodulating Agents

Topical immunomodulators like cyclosporin (0.05–2% drops) and tacrolimus (0.01–0.03% ointment) are T-cell inhibitors and are specially indicated in VKC and AKC as steroid-sparing agents. They exert their immunomodulatory effects primarily by targeting T lymphocytes and suppressing the production of lymphokines, notably IL-2, along with IL-3, IL-5, TNF-α, and interferon gamma (IFN-γ). They also inhibit mast cell degranulation and reduce the release of mast cell-derived cytokines such as IL-3 and IL-5 **(Table 2)**.

Allergen-specific immunotherapy is a long-term treatment aimed at reducing symptoms and preventing recurrence in patients with confirmed allergen-specific IgE. It enhances immune tolerance by lowering IgE levels and increasing IgG4 and IgA. It is indicated when symptoms are poorly controlled with standard therapy, require high medication doses, cause side effects, or when patients seek to minimize long-term drug use. The main aim is to induce clinical tolerance to sensitive allergens which can be identified with the help of skin prick testing or specific serum IgE levels. Both sublingual and subcutaneous immunotherapy have noted improvement in ocular sign and symptoms in patients with allergic rhinoconjunctivitis.

In patients with refractory or severe diseases, especially VKC and AKC, biologic therapies targeting key inflammatory pathways have emerged as promising options.

Omalizumab is a humanized monoclonal antibody that binds to circulating IgE, thereby reducing serum IgE levels and inhibiting IgE–FcεRI interactions on mast cells, basophils, and dendritic cells. Although not formally

TABLE 2: Topical antiallergics commonly used in allergic conjunctivitis.

Pharmacological drug	*Available medications (%)*	*Dose*	*Mechanism of action*	*Indication*
Antihistaminics	• Bilastine (0.6) • Levocabastine (0.5) • Emedastine (0.5)	Once or twice daily	H1 antagonist	SAC PAC
Mast cell stabilizers	• Cromolyn sodium (4) • Lodoxamide (0.1) • Nedocromil (2)	Twice—four times daily	Prevent mast cell degranulation	SAC PAC VKC
Dual-acting agents	• Olopatadine (0.1, 0.2, 0.7) • Alcaftadine (2.5) • Azelastine (0.5) • Bepotastine (1.5) • Ketotifen (0.025)	Twice daily	• H1 and sometimes H2 antagonist • Mast cell stabilization • Inhibits eosinophilic infiltration, leukotriene synthesis, and cytokine release	SAC PAC VKC AKC GCP CDC
Corticosteroids	• Loteprednol (0.5) • Fluorometholone (0.1)	Small pulsed dose with weekly tapering (stopped after limited period)	• Blocks phospholipase A2 • Inhibits mast cell degranulation, histamine release and T-cell activation	SAC PAC VKC AKC GPC CDC
Immunomodulators	• Cyclosporine (0.5, 1.2) • Tacrolimus ointment (0.01, 0.03)	Twice daily	Inhibit T-cell activity	VKC AKC

(AKC: atopic keratoconjunctivitis; CDC: contact or drug-induced dermatoconjunctivitis; GPC: giant papillary conjunctivitis; PAC: perennial allergic conjunctivitis; SAC: seasonal allergic conjunctivitis; VKC: vernal keratoconjunctivitis)

approved for the treatment of VKC, published reports on its use in refractory VKC and AKC have shown complete inflammatory control in most patients, partial response in some, and treatment failure in a few. Dupilumab (anti-IL4/IL-13) and mepolizumab (anti-IL-5) have also been reported in a few cases, however, long-term results are awaited.

CONCLUSION

Ocular AC encompasses a spectrum of disorders ranging from mild, self-limiting conditions like SAC/PAC to chronic, vision-threatening diseases such as VKC and AKC. Accurate diagnosis, identification of allergen triggers, and a stepwise, individualized treatment approach are essential for effective management. While conventional therapies—such as antihistamines, mast cell stabilizers, and corticosteroids—remain the mainstay, newer agents including dual-action drugs, immunomodulators, and biologics are expanding the therapeutic arsenal, especially for refractory cases. Allergen immunotherapy has also shown promise in select patients by providing long-term disease modification through immune tolerance. Given the systemic and often pediatric nature of these conditions, an interdisciplinary approach involving ophthalmologists, allergists, and pediatricians is vital for comprehensive care.

KEY POINTS

- Allergic conjunctivitis in children spans mild forms (SAC, PAC) to severe, vision-threatening disorders (VKC, AKC).
- *Itching is the hallmark symptom*, and diagnosis is largely clinical, supported by history and exclusion of mimics.
- *Dual-action topical agents* are the preferred first-line pharmacotherapy due to rapid relief and safety.
- *Immunomodulators (cyclosporin, tacrolimus)* are indicated for steroid-sparing treatment in severe or refractory VKC and AKC.
- *Biologics and allergen immunotherapy* represent emerging therapies for difficult-to-treat cases.

SUGGESTED READING

1. Bonini S, Leonardi A. The multifaceted aspects of ocular allergies: Phenotypes and endotypes. Ocul Surf. 2022;26:174-83.
2. Chandrasekar A, Agarwal S, Chauhan G, Srinivasan B, Chavda VB, Iyer G. Insights from 1096 clinical cases: pioneering a universal grading system for vernal keratoconjunctivitis management. Br J Ophthalmol. 2025;109(7):735-41.
3. Chauhan G, Mathimaaran S, Chandrasekar A, Chavda VB, Mugundhan R, Srinivasan B, et al. Unpacking VKC: How gender and age shape the clinical picture. Indian J Ophthalmol. 2025;73(4):594-8.
4. Fukuda K, Kishimoto T, Sumi T, Yamashiro K, Ebihara N. Biologics for allergy: therapeutic potential for ocular allergic diseases and adverse effects on the eye. Allergol Int. 2023;72(2):234-44.
5. Gupta Y, Tandon R, Vashisht P, Gupta V, Bhuyan J, Singh S, et al. Epidemiological insights into Childhood vernal keratoconjunctivitis in India: Unravelling clinical presentation and environmental influences - The EPIC VKC study - Fourth report of the ICMR EYE SEE study group. Ocul Surf. 2025;36:41-55.
6. Leonardi A, Castegnaro A, Valerio AL, Lazzarini D. Epidemiology of allergic conjunctivitis: clinical appearance and treatment patterns in a population-based study. Curr Opin Allergy Clin Immunol. 2015;15(5):482-8.
7. Leonardi A, Quintieri L, Presa IJ, LLoves JM, Montero J, Benítez-Del-Castillo JM, et al. Allergic Conjunctivitis Management: Update on Ophthalmic Solutions. Curr Allergy Asthma Rep. 2024;24(7):347-60.
8. Menta V, Agarwal S, Das US, Moksha L, Srividya G, Anandan AM, et al. Ocular surface sphingolipids associate with the refractory nature of vernal keratoconjunctivitis: newer insights in VKC pathogenesis. Br J Ophthalmol. 2023;107(4):461-9.
9. Ono SJ, Abelson MB. Allergic conjunctivitis: update on pathophysiology and prospects for future treatment. J Allergy Clin Immunol. 2005;115(1):118-22.
10. Villegas BV, Benitez-Del-Castillo JM. Current Knowledge in Allergic Conjunctivitis. Turk J Ophthalmol. 2021;51(1):45-54.

4 SECTION Skin, Drug, and Insect Allergies

***Section Editors:** Dipti Pujari, Rama Rajyam*

16 CHAPTER

Atopic Dermatitis

Dipti Pujari

INTRODUCTION

Atopic dermatitis (AD), also called eczema, is an inflammatory, chronically relapsing, noncontagious and extremely pruritic skin disease (World Allergy Organization).

According to European Academy of Allergology and Clinical Immunology *(EAACI)*, AD is defined as a complex interplay between skin barrier dysfunction, immune system dysregulation, and environmental factors.

Skin barrier dysfunction in AD causes thinner epidermis, with defective lipid and protein composition and function, leading to poor hydration, increased transepidermal water loss, causing extreme dryness and itchy skin. Filaggrin gene mutation is the underlying defect in most AD patients.

Immune system dysregulation in AD is thought to be T-helper cell type-2 (Th2) dominant pathway, with elevated immunoglobulin E (IgE), infiltration of mast cells, neutrophils, and increased biomarkers like interleukin 4, 13, 25, and 31.

Environmental triggers: AD is a chronically relapsing-remitting disease with flares triggered by viral, bacterial, or fungal infections, food allergens, cosmetics, fragrance, aeroallergens, irritants, and contact allergens.

The symptoms may vary, some of them are as follows:

- Dry, scaly or cracked skin
- Redness and inflammation
- Itching
- Oozing or crusting when scratched
- Thickened or scaly skin
- Darkened or discolored patches of skin

HANIFIN AND RAJKA DIAGNOSTIC CRITERIA FOR ATOPIC DERMATITIS

Major criteria: Three or more required (out of the four mentioned)

1. Pruritus
2. *Typical morphology and distribution*: Facial and extensor involvement in infants and children, flexural lichenification in adults
3. Chronic or chronically relapsing dermatitis
4. Personal/family history of atopy (asthma, allergic rhinitis, AD)

Minor criteria: Three or more required (out of the 23 mentioned)

1. Xerosis
2. Ichthyosis, keratosis pilaris, palmar hyperlinearity
3. Immediate (type 1) skin test reactivity
4. Elevated serum IgE
5. Early age of onset
6. Tendency towards cutaneous infections: herpes simplex, *Staphylococcus aureus*
7. Tendency toward nonspecific hand and foot dermatitis
8. Nipple eczema
9. Cheilitis
10. Dennie–Morgan folds
11. Recurrent conjunctivitis
12. Keratoconus
13. Anterior subcapsular cataract
14. Orbital darkening
15. Facial pallor
16. Pityriasis alba
17. Anterior neck folds
18. Itch when sweating
19. Intolerance to wool and lipid solvents
20. Perifollicular accentuation
21. Food intolerance
22. Course influenced by environmental and emotional factors
23. White dermographism, delayed blanch

AGEWISE DISTRIBUTION OF AD LESIONS

- *Less than 2 years:*
  - Commonly starts on face and scalp
  - Progresses to chest and extensor surfaces of limbs
  - Spares genitalia and diaper area
- *2 years to teenagers:*
  - Mostly involves antecubital fossa, popliteal fossa
  - Volar aspect of wrists, ankles, and neck

- *Adults:*
    - Continues on flexor surfaces and also on hands
    - Becomes leathery, rough, and lichenified

Severity of AD can be assessed by using various scoring systems. Eczema Area and Severity Score *(EASI)*, Patient Oriented Eczema Measures *(POEM)* and Scoring for Atopic Dermatitis *(SCORAD)* are some of them. Of these, SCORAD system is widely used to assess the control (and so decide the treatment) of AD.

SCORING FOR ATOPIC DERMATITIS

Area (A): Rule of 9: It is used to calculate the affected area **(Fig. 1)**. The total area affected is given *"A"*.

- Head and neck—9%
- Upper limbs—9% each
- Lower limbs—18% each
- Anterior trunk—18%
- Back—18%
- Genitals, palm, back of hand—1%

Intensity (B): Based on following signs **(Fig. 2)**, scores are added to give *"B"* (maximum 18).

Subjective symptoms (C): "Itch" and "sleeplessness", scored by the patient:

- 0 is no itch or sleeplessness.
- 10 is the worst imaginable itch or sleeplessness.

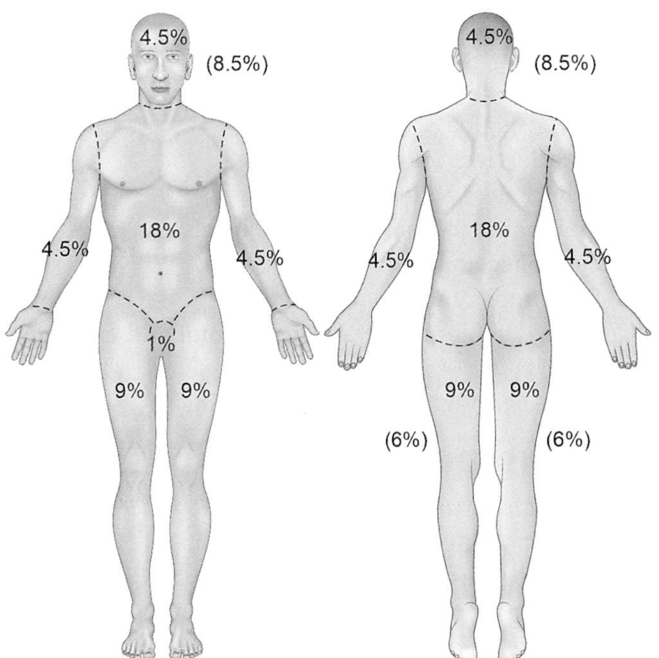

Fig. 1: Scoring for Atopic Dermatitis (SCORAD): Calculation of *area* affected in AD: "A".

These scores are added to give *"C"* (maximum 20).

Total score (SCORAD) for any individual is A/5 + 7B/2 + C.

- SCORAD is >50, it indicates severe disease.
- SCORAD 50–25, it indicates moderate disease.
- SCORAD is <25, it indicates mild disease.

DIAGNOSIS

- It is mostly a clinical diagnosis.
- History, morphology, and distribution of lesions with associated clinical signs help in clinching the diagnosis.
- No specific biomarkers are recommended for diagnosis and/or assessment of disease severity and monitoring of IgE levels or allergy testing is not recommended routinely.
- The decision to do allergy tests depends on the treating physician (if there is a clear history of aggravation of eczema on exposure to certain foods/allergens).

TREATMENT

Non-pharmacological Measures (Forms the Mainstay of Treatment)

Cleansing and Bathing

- Regular once-daily bathing with warm (27°–30°C) water of short duration (5–10 minutes) with low pH, hypoallergenic, and fragrance-free "syndets"
- Bleach baths with 0.005% *sodium hypochlorite* can be taken twice a week for 6–8 weeks, in children with repeated staphylococcal infections in moderate-to-severe cases of AD.

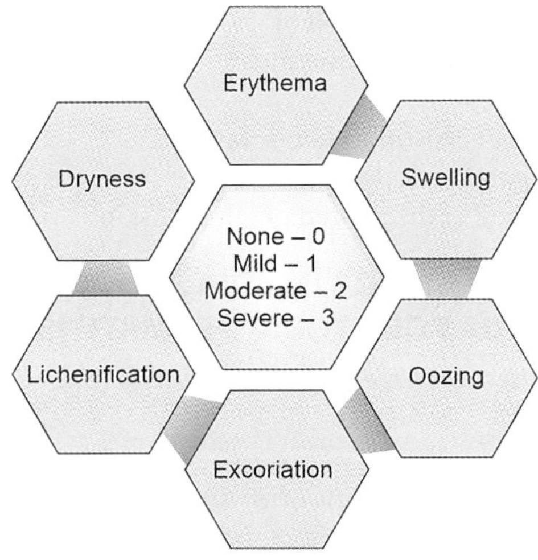

Fig. 2: SCORAD: Calculation of *intensity* of symptoms in AD: "B".

Moisturizers/Emollients

Liberal use of preservative and fragrance-free moisturizer is the key to good control in AD. At least 3 to 4 times daily application should be stressed upon. Application should be in the direction of hair growth. Various types of moisturizers are available:

- *Humectants:* They increase water absorption from deeper layers of the skin to stratum corneum and improve hydration of skin, such as urea, glycerol, lactic acid.
- *Occludents:* They reduce evaporation from skin, such as petrolatum and liquid paraffin.
- *Emollients:* They have the ability to instill small droplets of oil into the cracks between the desquamating corneocytes in the dry skin and ultimately improve the appearance of the skin. Examples are linoleic acid, linolenic acid, and oleic acid.

Wet Wrap Therapy

For localized, acute flare-ups, a layer of wet bandage can be applied on the active, oozing skin after application of moisturizer and mild steroid. Another dry cloth to be wrapped on this to keep the inner bandage wet. It can be used for several hours of a day depending on the patient tolerance.

Clothing

Smooth clothing, which is light weight, loose, and comfortable, like cotton, is recommended. Wool and synthetic clothing should be avoided.

Allergen/Trigger Avoidance (As They Increase the Skin Barrier Dysfunction)

- Aeroallergens like pollens and house dust mites should be avoided in allergen-sensitive individuals (proven on skin testing). Rooms should be well-ventilated with good sunlight, have comfortable temperature, and should be clutter-free and with minimal upholstery. One should avoid dry dusting and encourage wet mopping.
- Tobacco smoke avoidance, traffic exhaust, and volatile organic compounds exposure reduction (burning wood/essence sticks/mosquito repellents) helps in preventing the flare-ups.

Dietary Intervention

Dietary restriction is recommended in only those individuals with a known food allergy for specific food items. This should be proven by allergy test and clinically corelating to the flare-ups of the disease on consumption of the food items.

Pharmacological Measures

Pharmacological measures can be divided into two forms: topical medications and systemic medications.

Topical Medications

Topical corticosteroids (TCS): They are very effective, first line of management in controlling inflammation in atopic skin. The choice of TCS depends on the severity and extent of the disease, the age of the patient and the area of the body involved, and the type of steroid preparation and potency of steroids. One should always aim for lowest-potency steroids.

- *For acute flare-ups (reactive therapy):* Twice daily application, till active lesions subside (mostly 2–4 weeks); then should step down the potency of steroids.
- *For maintenance (proactive therapy):* Twice weekly application to prevent relapses (can be used up to 16 weeks) with liberal use of emollients; steroids should always be applied on well-hydrated skin.

Dose: One *fingertip unit* is enough to treat an area of skin twice the size of the flat of an adult's hand with the fingers together.

Concerns of TCS: Judicious use is warranted, address steroid phobia, avoid high potency on face and flexural areas, and try to step down to lower-potency steroids whenever possible.

Topical calcineurin inhibitors (TCI): Tacrolimus 0.03% (for children <15 years) and 0.1% (for >15 years) ointment; pimecrolimus 1% cream; they are steroid-sparing agents.

- *For acute flare-ups (reactive therapy):* Twice daily application (for 2–6 weeks); is very useful in sensitive skin areas like face, intertriginous sites, anogenital area as they do not cause skin atrophy, cataract, or glaucoma
- *For maintenance (proactive therapy):* Twice weekly application; has shown to be safe and effective for up to 1 year in reducing flare-ups

Concerns of TCI: Initial stinging and burning sensation (mostly resolves within a week); effective sun protection should be recommended when on TCIs.

Phototherapy: UVB, mostly narrowband (NB-UVB) of 311–313 nm and UVA of 340–400 nm has shown marked healing in AD skin due to its anti-inflammatory, immunomodulatory, and antimicrobial properties.

Topical phosphodiesterase-4 inhibitors (PDE-4):

Crisaborole: It is a topical PDE-4 inhibitor, effective in mild-to-moderate AD. 2% ointment is approved for use above 2 years of age.

Janus kinase (JAK) inhibitors: The JAK pathways are involved in signaling of various AD related cytokines like IL-4, IL-13, IL-31, IL-22, and IL-17. JAK inhibitors decrease AD severity and are found useful in moderate AD. Examples are *ruxolitinib and delgocitinib*. They are now licensed for children above 2 years.

Oral/Injectable Therapy

- *Antibiotics/antivirals/antifungals:* For superadded infections
- *Oral glucocorticoids:* Short course of low-dose steroids, 0.5 mg/kg/day up to 1 week can be used for acute flare-ups.
- *Immunosuppressive drugs:*
  - *Cyclosporine A:* For refractory, severe cases of AD, it is given at a dose of 5 mg/kg/day in two divided doses. It is mostly given for 6–12 weeks.
  - *Methotrexate, azathioprine, and mycophenolate mofetil* are some of the other immunosuppressive drugs that can be used in resistant cases.
- *Oral JAK inhibitors: Baricitinib, upadacitinib, abrocitinib, tofacitinib, cerdulatinib* are some of the available oral JAK inhibitors. These are mostly approved for children above 12 years.
- *Biologicals:* Biologicals are a new class of drugs, proving to be game-changers in AD.

Dupilumab: It is a human monoclonal antibody administered subcutaneously (SC) to inhibit the interleukin-4 receptor subunit α (IL-4Rα). IL-4Rα is a component common to both IL-4 and IL-13 receptor complexes which are the major culprits in AD.

Age approval for AD: Dupilumab is approved for children aged 6 months and above. It has to be given via SC injection.

Children aged 6 months to 5 years (no loading dose recommended):

- *5 to <15 kg:* 200 mg SC every 4 weeks
- *15 to <30 kg:* 300 mg SC every 4 weeks

Children aged 6–17 years:

- *<60 kg:* 400 mg SC once, and then 200 mg SC every other week
- *≥60 kg:* 600 mg SC once, and then 300 mg SC every other week

Some of the newer biologics currently in phase 2 and 3 clinical trials are lebrikizumab, tralokinumab, nemolizumab, tezepelumab, and ISB 830.

Flowchart 1: Stepwise management of AD according to SCORAD.

Step 1: Dry skin: Emollients, moisturizers

↓

Step 2: Mild AD (SCORAD <25): Emollients, moisturizers
+ Low potency topical steroids/topical CNIs

↓

Step 3: Moderate AD (SCORAD 25-50): Emollients, moisturizers
+ Proactive therapy: Medium potency topical steroids/topical CNIs/topical JAK inhibitors

↓

Step 4: Severe AD (SCORAD >50): Emollients, moisturizers
+ Proactive therapy: Medium/high potency topical steroids/CNIs/JAK inhibitors
+ Immunosuppressants: Cyclosporin A, methotrexate, azathioprine

↓

Step 5: Uncontrolled AD: Emollients, moisturizers
+ Proactive therapy: Medium/high potency topical steroids/CNIs/JAK inhibitors
+ Biologicals: Subcutaneous dupilumab

(CNIs: calcineurin inhibitors; JAK: Janus kinase)

STEPWISE MANAGEMENT OF ATOPIC DERMATITIS BASED ON SCORAD

Flowchart 1 provides stepwise management of AD based on SCORAD.

CONCLUSION

Atopic dermatitis is a chronic, relapsing inflammatory skin disease requiring long-term, holistic management. Effective care integrates barrier repair, trigger avoidance, targeted anti-inflammatory therapy, and patient education. Advances such as topical PDE-4 inhibitors, JAK inhibitors, and biologics have expanded treatment options for moderate-to-severe disease. By addressing both cutaneous and systemic contributors, clinicians can significantly improve symptoms, reduce flares, and enhance psychosocial well-being in children living with this condition.

KEY POINTS

- Atopic dermatitis is a chronic, relapsing, intensely pruritic inflammatory skin disease resulting from skin barrier dysfunction, immune dysregulation, genetic susceptibility, and environmental triggers.

- Diagnosis is primarily clinical, based on characteristic morphology, age-specific distribution of lesions, and Hanifin–Rajka criteria; routine allergy testing is not required.
- SCORAD is widely used to assess disease severity and guide treatment decisions.
- Skin barrier repair with regular emollient use, appropriate bathing practices, and trigger avoidance forms the cornerstone of management.
- Topical corticosteroids are first-line therapy for flares, while topical calcineurin inhibitors and newer agents (PDE-4 and topical JAK inhibitors) serve as effective steroid-sparing options.
- Systemic therapies and biologics, especially dupilumab, have transformed the management of moderate-to-severe and refractory atopic dermatitis, improving long-term control and quality of life.

SUGGESTED READING

1. Agache I, Akdis CA, Akdis M, Brockow K, Chivato T, Del Giacco S, et al. EAACI Biologicals Guidelines—dupilumab for children and adults with moderate-to-severe atopic dermatitis. Allergy. 2021;76(4):988-1009.
2. Axon E, Chalmers JR, Santer M, Ridd MJ, Lawton S, Langan SM, et al. Safety of topical corticosteroids in atopic eczema: an umbrella review. BMJ Open. 2021;11(7):e046476.
3. Eichenfield LF, Tom WL, Berger TG, Krol A, Paller AS, Schwarzenberger K, et al. Guidelines of care for the management of atopic dermatitis: Section 2. Management and treatment of atopic dermatitis with topical therapies. J Am Acad Dermatol. 2014;71(1):116-32.
4. Saeki H, Ohya Y, Arakawa H, Ichiyama S, Katsunuma T, Katoh N, et al. English version of clinical practice guidelines for the management of atopic dermatitis 2024. J Dermatol. 2025;52(2):e70-e142.
5. Silverberg JI, Barbarot S, Gadkari A, Simpson EL, Weidinger S, Mina-Osorio P, et al. Atopic dermatitis in the pediatric population. A cross sectional, international epidemiologic study. Ann Allergy Asthma Immunol. 2021;126:417-28.e2.

17 CHAPTER

Contact Dermatitis

Krishna Mohan R

INTRODUCTION

Contact dermatitis (CD) is an eczematous skin reaction triggered when the skin comes into contact with a substance that causes either irritation or an allergic response. While irritant forms may appear even in the first few months of life, allergic contact dermatitis (ACD) is relatively uncommon in infants. This is largely because the immune system's ability to mount a delayed hypersensitivity response is immature during early childhood, and because exposure to sensitizing agents tends to be low in infancy. As children grow, their risk of CD increases. Greater exposure to potential allergens—through accessories, piercings, cosmetics, and environmental changes associated with urbanization—all contribute to this rising incidence.

Beyond the physical discomfort, CD in children can lead to disturbed sleep, difficulty concentrating, and reduced academic performance. In some cases, it causes considerable morbidity. Recognizing the evolving patterns of exposure and sensitization in childhood is essential for timely diagnosis, management, and prevention.

Contact dermatitis in children is broadly classified according to pathogenesis into two major types—irritant contact dermatitis (ICD) and ACD. ICD results from direct damage to the skin by chemical, physical, or biological agents and does not involve the immune system. ACD, on the other hand, is an immune-mediated, type IV delayed hypersensitivity reaction that occurs in previously sensitized individuals after contact with specific allergens. **Table 1** outlines the key differentiating features between ACD and ICD.

IRRITANT CONTACT DERMATITIS

Irritant contact dermatitis arises when the stratum corneum (the skin's outermost layer) is directly damaged—by changes in pH, disruption of cellular lipase, or other insults. These changes activate skin cells, triggering inflammation,

TABLE 1: Differentiating features between ACD and ICD.

Feature	*Irritant contact dermatitis (ICD)*	*Allergic contact dermatitis (ACD)*
Pathogenesis	Direct cytotoxic effect of chemical/physical agents on skin barrier	Delayed-type (type IV) hypersensitivity reaction involving sensitization and re-exposure to allergen
Immune mechanism	Non-immunologic	Immunologically mediated (T-cell dependent)
Dose relation	Severity depends on concentration and duration of exposure	Even minute amounts can trigger reaction once sensitized
First exposure	Can occur with first exposure	Requires prior sensitization; reaction develops after repeated exposure
Eruption pattern	Sharply demarcated at sites of contact, often confined to exposed area	May extend beyond contact site, sometimes spreading to distant sites
Clinical features	Burning, stinging, erythema, edema, vesicles, fissures; chronic cases show lichenification and scaling	Pruritus predominant; erythematous papules, vesicles, oozing, crusting; later lichenification
Examples of causative agents	Soaps, detergents, saliva, urine, acids, alkalis, and disinfectants	Nickel, fragrances, rubber accelerators, hair dyes, topical antibiotics, and preservatives
Diagnosis	History and clinical correlation	Confirmed by patch testing

which may manifest as erythema (redness), blistering, or erosions. Importantly, anyone exposed to a sufficient dose of the same irritant can develop this reaction. ICD presents with a broad spectrum of clinical patterns, influenced by the nature of the irritant, concentration, duration of exposure, frequency of contact, and the individual's skin susceptibility. Recognizing these variations is important, as different subtypes have characteristic presentations, natural courses, and management considerations. Some of the distinct subtypes of ICD are described below.

Diaper Dermatitis

Diaper dermatitis is the most common form of ICD in infants. It typically affects the convex surfaces of the buttocks, genitalia, lower abdomen, and pubic area at sites of friction with the diaper, while characteristically sparing the skin folds.

The pathogenesis involves prolonged exposure to moisture, urine, and feces. Occlusion and maceration within the diaper increase enzymatic activity of fecal urease, protease, and lipase, leading to further skin irritation. Ammonia from urine, frequent cleansing with soaps, use of antiseptics or oils, and exposure to deodorants further aggravate the condition. Microbial factors also play a role, particularly urea-splitting organisms such as *Proteus*, *Escherichia coli (E. coli)*, *Staphylococcus aureus*, and *Candida albicans*.

Clinically, it manifests with erythema, edema, vesicles, and erosions. Extra-absorbent disposable diapers containing absorbent gelling material (AGM) are superior to cloth diapers as they reduce skin wetness and help maintain normal pH. Rare cases of contact allergy, referred to as "Lucky Luke dermatitis", have been attributed to rubber chemicals (mercaptobenzothiazole) and adhesives (p-tert-butyl phenol formaldehyde resin) present in some diapers.

The mainstay of management is frequent diaper change and use of barrier creams, particularly zinc oxide formulations. Use of topical corticosteroids should generally be avoided; however, short courses of low-potency steroids (1% hydrocortisone acetate for up to 2 weeks) may be used in severe cases. Potent or fluorinated steroids are contraindicated under the diaper due to risk of skin atrophy and systemic absorption. Rarely, erythematous nodular lesions may develop as a reaction to *Candida* infection, referred to as infantile gluteal granuloma (granuloma gluteale infantum).

Perianal Dermatitis

Perianal dermatitis presents with erythema, edema, and erosions in the perianal region, often described as Jacquet's erosive diaper dermatitis. It results from frequent exposure to feces, repeated washing with soaps, and mechanical irritation. Management includes avoidance of irritants such as soaps, detergents, and disinfectants, along with application of protective barrier creams (e.g., zinc oxide).

Cheilitis and Perioral Dermatitis

Cheilitis is common in children, particularly girls who engage in habitual lip licking, sucking, or biting. It presents as scaling and crusting of the lips and may extend beyond the vermilion margin in lip-lick cheilitis. Irritant reactions to food items such as fruit juices can worsen the condition. Perioral dermatitis is a benign eruption characterized by erythematous papules, pustules, and scaling around the mouth, sparing the lips and immediate vermilion border. It is often associated with the use of topical, nasal, or inhaled corticosteroids, which alter cutaneous microflora. Management includes discontinuation of corticosteroid exposure and treatment with topical metronidazole or calcineurin inhibitors.

Chemical Irritant Dermatitis and Burns

Children may also develop irritant dermatitis or chemical burns following exposure to household caustic substances. Immediate rinsing with copious water minimizes damage. Other irritants such as perfumed oils, toilet soaps, and disinfectants can cause dermatitis in skin folds. Lesions over the knees and shins may be seen in crawling infants due to contact with floor polishes and detergents.

ALLERGIC CONTACT DERMATITIS

Allergic contact dermatitis tends to emerge around ages 2–3 years once the immune system has matured. It becomes even more prevalent in children over 10 years old. Females are more commonly affected, likely due to greater exposure to sensitizing agents.

Unlike irritant dermatitis, ACD occurs only in predisposed individuals and requires an immunologic mechanism. There are two key phases:

- *Sensitization (induction) phase:* An allergen must first penetrate the skin and bind to a protein to form an immunogenic complex. This complex is taken up by Langerhans cells, processed, and presented via class II MHC molecules. Cytokines are released, and

Langerhans cells migrate to regional lymph nodes. There, specific effector and memory T lymphocytes are selected and proliferate. Once this process is complete, the individual is sensitized.

- *Elicitation phase:* On re-exposure to the allergen, the same antigen is again captured by Langerhans cells. The memory and effector T cells are recalled to the skin. They release cytokines that amplify inflammation, giving rise to the clinical signs of dermatitis.

Allergic contact dermatitis can be triggered by a wide range of allergens encountered in daily life and occupational settings. Among the most frequent culprits are metals such as nickel, cobalt, and chromium, which are found in jewelry, cosmetics, and industrial materials. Fragrances, preservatives, dyes, and hair colorants commonly cause reactions through personal care products. Rubber accelerators, adhesives, and leather chemicals are important allergens in footwear and occupational exposure. Topical medications such as neomycin and corticosteroids themselves may also provoke sensitization. Some of the common allergens associated with ACD are listed in **Table 2**, along with their sources.

Allergic contact dermatitis can involve virtually any area of the body, but certain sites are more frequently affected due to patterns of exposure, skin sensitivity, and local environment. Site-based classification is clinically useful, as it helps correlate allergen exposure with the typical distribution of dermatitis, thereby guiding targeted history-taking and allergen avoidance strategies. The following section outlines the common anatomical sites of ACD.

TABLE 2: Common allergens with their sources.

Nickel	Ear piercing, jewelry, eye glass frames, zippers and metal buttons, coins, belt buckles, and cell phones
Paraphenylenediamines	Hair dyes and henna tattoos
Cobalt chloride	Metal plated object and antiperspirants
Potassium dichromate	Cement and leather
Thiomersal	Vaccines and antiseptics
Balsam of Peru	Perfumes, lotions, soaps, shampoo, laundry and cleaning products, some foods, spices, and flavoring agents
Fragrance mix	Perfumes, lotions, soaps, shampoo, laundry and cleaning products, toothpaste, mouthwashes, and mints
Neomycin	Topical medication and soaps
Mercaptobenzothiazole (mercapto mix, black rubber mix for allergy to rubber)	Rubber slippers and shoes, watch straps, and elastic of diapers or clothing

Hand Dermatitis

Pediatric hand dermatitis commonly presents as fingertip eczema and apron eczema, involving the proximal parts of two fingers with adjacent skin over the metacarpophalangeal joints. Children frequently exposed to clay, colored toys, dyes, detergents, and soaps are susceptible. The dermatitis can extend proximally onto the arms. Allergens around the wrist often include nickel and cobalt found in metal watches **(Fig. 1)** and bangles, as well as p-tertiary butylphenol formaldehyde resin—an adhesive used in leather watch straps.

Dermatitis of the Feet

This is likely the most common ACD in school-aged children, primarily due to shoe-related allergens such as rubber, plastics, leather, glues, nickel, stockings, dyes, topical antibiotics, and antiperspirants. Foot dermatitis typically affects the dorsal surfaces **(Fig. 2)**, sparing interdigital spaces. Rubber allergens include thiuram, p-phenylenediamine, and p-tertiary butylphenol formaldehyde resins, while potassium dichromate sensitizes leather.

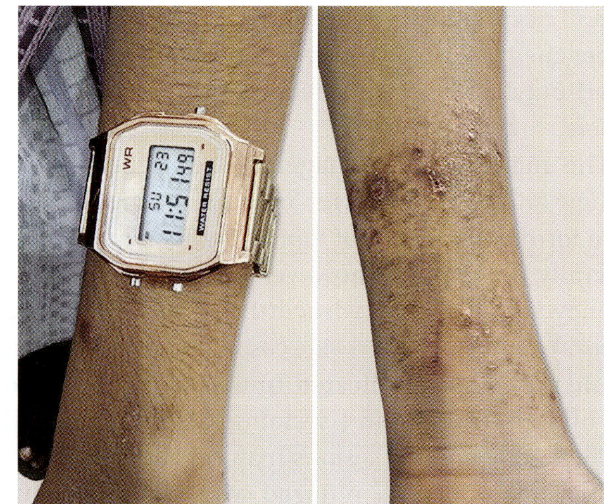

Fig. 1: Allergic contact dermatitis (ACD) due to nickel.

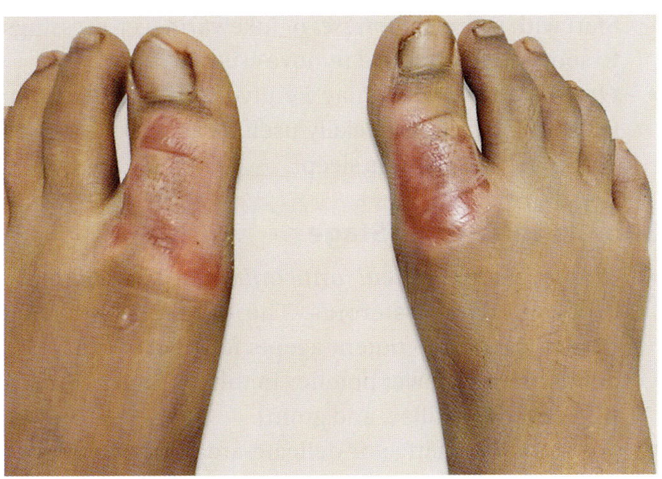

Fig. 2: Feet dermatitis.

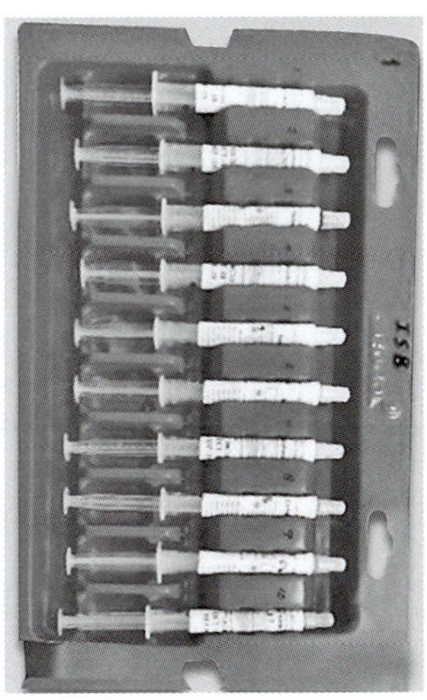

Fig. 3: Allergens in syringes.

Face Dermatitis

Facial dermatitis in children can be triggered by maternal perfumes, face powders, lipsticks, hair dyes, eyeliners, baby creams, and perfumes. Nail varnish may cause eyelid dermatitis. Forehead involvement may arise from sensitization to chrome in leather hats or hairbands. Ear lobe dermatitis often results from nickel-containing earrings. Lip dermatitis is associated with reactions to lip balms, lipsticks, flavoring agents, and toothpaste. A common allergen in dental care products is cinnamate.

Neck Dermatitis

Eruptions on the lateral neck commonly result from contact with nickel-containing jewelry or fabric irritation, particularly collars (collar dermatitis).

Waist Area Dermatitis

This can be linked to contact with colored waist strings or elastic materials in diapers or clothing that contact the waist.

Textile Dermatitis

The site of involvement varies depending on clothing style, typically affecting areas where clothing fits tightly, such as the axillae (with sparing of vault, thighs, and popliteal areas). Nickel buttons and belt fasteners are frequent allergens. Soaps, detergents, finishing agents, dyes, fabric softeners, and flame retardants contribute significantly to textile dermatitis.

Phyto Dermatitis

Contact with resins from trees and topical vapor rubs containing oils such as turpentine, eucalyptus, camphor, and menthol can cause ACD. Eczema may appear on the hands and perioral area after contact with raw mangoes and cashew nuts (Anacardiaceae family), with catechol as the allergen. Airborne CD can result from exposure to plants such as parthenium and chrysanthemum (Compositae family), containing sesquiterpene lactones. Coloring agents in henna used to enhance color intensity may provoke hand dermatitis. Aromatherapy with oils such as coconut, mustard, and gingelly, sometimes mixed with curcumin, jasmine, marigold, or sandalwood, used in body massage, can cause allergic dermatitis. Bergamot oil may induce phototoxic reactions.

Photodermatitis

Photodermatitis presents as eczematous reactions affecting the malar region, ears, V area of the neck, extensor forearms, and dorsal hands as a response to ultraviolet radiation. Plants containing psoralens, such as citrus fruits and celery, are well-known triggers of phototoxicity.

PATCH TESTING

Patch testing is widely recognized as the gold standard and the most scientifically validated method for pinpointing the causative allergen in cases of ACD. A set of allergens (baseline series and possibly additional ones based on exposure history) **(Fig. 3)** are applied onto the skin (usually the back) under occlusive patches **(Fig. 4)**. Avoid wetting, sweating, or disturbing the patches. Readings

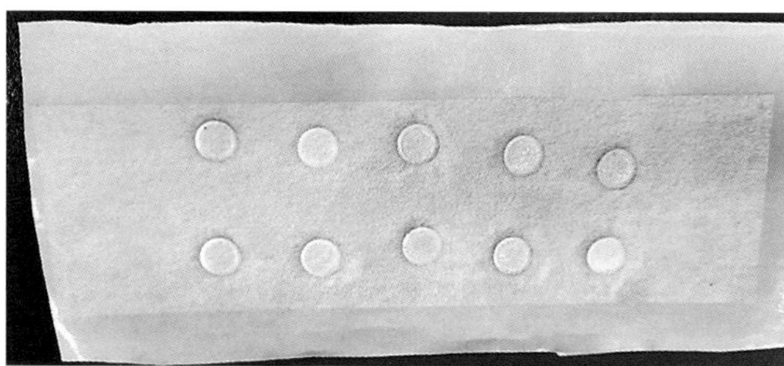

Fig. 4: Test Strip with wells.

TABLE 3: Grading of patch test reading.

0	No reaction	Negative patch test
+/-	Faint non palpable erythema only	Doubtful positive patch test
1+	Palpable erythema and possible papules	Weakly positive patch test
2+	Erythema, infiltration papules, and vesicles	Strongly positive patch test
3+	Intense erythema and infiltration and coalescing vesicles	Extreme positive patch test

are done first when patches are removed (~48 hours) and again after another 48 hours (i.e., around 96 hours) to detect delayed reactions. Sometimes later readings (day 5–7) may be required.

The selection of allergens includes common substances (metals such as nickel, preservatives, fragrances, topical medications, rubber accelerators, adhesives, resins, etc.). Baseline panels capture a majority of common allergens; additional ones are tailored depending on patient's history, occupation, suspected exposures.

Depending on the erythema, induration and blistering the positive reactions are graded in **Table 3.**

MANAGEMENT OF CONTACT DERMATITIS

The primary goal in managing CD is to *identify and eliminate* the offending allergen (or irritant). Equally important is awareness and avoidance of cross-reacting substances, which may trigger similar immune responses even if they differ chemically.

Acute Stage

- In the acute phase, when the skin is inflamed, edematous, or blistered, therapy should be gentle. Start with *saline compresses* or lukewarm wet-dressings to soothe irritation and remove crusts.
- *Oral antihistamines* may be given for symptomatic relief of pruritus, especially useful at night or in cases where itching disrupts sleep.

Sub-acute/Chronic Stage

- Transition to *topical anti-inflammatory therapy*, especially corticosteroids. The potency should be chosen carefully—potent agents for thicker skin (e.g., hands, palms), lower potency in thin or sensitive areas (face, eyelids, axillae, and groin).
- For steroid-sensitive or delicate areas, or when long-term daily steroids are undesirable, topical calcineurin inhibitors such as tacrolimus or pimecrolimus offer an alternative; they reduce inflammation without the risk of skin thinning.

Severe, Extensive, or Refractory Disease

- If the dermatitis involves a large surface area (for example, more than ~20% of body surface), or if there are intense acute inflammation and impaired function, a *short course of systemic corticosteroids* may be required. A regimen of 5–7 days or slightly longer, with tapering, is often adequate.
- Ensure that systemic therapy is judicious—only when topical therapy is insufficient or impractical and always combined with allergen avoidance.
- Prolonged or frequent application of topical steroids, particularly in occluded or thin skin areas, carries the risk of skin atrophy, striae formation, telangiectasia, pigmentation changes, and barrier impairment. Extensive or long-term use increases risk of systemic absorption, which can suppress the hypothalamic-pituitary-adrenal (HPA) axis, leading to systemic side effects. Monitor for signs if steroids are used over large areas or under occlusion.

CONCLUSION

Contact dermatitis in children is a significant clinical entity with both irritant and allergic forms contributing to morbidity. ICD arises from direct disruption of the skin barrier and can occur in any child exposed to sufficient irritants, while ACD is an immune-mediated, delayed type IV hypersensitivity reaction seen in sensitized individuals. Common pediatric presentations include diaper dermatitis, perioral and perianal dermatitis, as well as allergen-driven rashes from metals, cosmetics, footwear, textiles, and plant exposures. Patch testing remains the gold standard for diagnosing ACD, enabling precise allergen identification. Effective management hinges on allergen and irritant avoidance, supported by stage-appropriate therapy including barrier measures, topical corticosteroids, calcineurin inhibitors, and judicious systemic corticosteroids in severe cases. Early recognition, prevention, and education of families are essential to minimize chronicity and improve quality of life in affected children.

KEY POINTS

- Two main types of CD exist—ICD from direct barrier injury and ACD from T-cell mediated hypersensitivity.
- Clinical presentations vary by age and site, with diaper dermatitis, perioral cheilitis, and footwear dermatitis being particularly relevant in children.
- Common allergens in ACD include nickel, fragrances, preservatives, rubber chemicals, and topical medications.
- Patch testing is the diagnostic gold standard for ACD, allowing targeted allergen identification and avoidance strategies.
- Management is stepwise and stage-based barrier protection and compresses in acute lesions, topical steroids or calcineurin inhibitors in subacute/chronic disease, and short systemic steroid courses for severe widespread involvement.
- Education and preventive counseling are crucial, as strict avoidance of allergens and cross-reacting agents remains the cornerstone of long-term management in pediatric patients.

SUGGESTED READING

1. Dupuy E, Zug KA. What We Have Learned–Milestones in Pediatric Contact Dermatitis. Curr Dermatol Rep. 2022; 11(1):1-12.
2. Lazzarini R, Duarte I, Ferreira AL. Patch tests. An Bras Dermatol. 2013;88(6):879-88.
3. Mowad CM, Anderson B, Scheinman P, Pootongkam S, Nedorost S, Brod B. Allergic contact dermatitis: Patient diagnosis and evaluation. J Am Acad Dermatol. 2016;74(6): 1029-40.
4. Sharma VK, Asati DP. Pediatric contact dermatitis. Indian J Dermatol Venereol Leprol. 2010;76:514-20.

18 CHAPTER

Urticaria and Angioedema

Rama Rajyam Datti, Spurthi Chitta

INTRODUCTION

Urticaria and angioedema are commonly seen in pediatric practice and may either present with acute or chronic manifestations. While they are mostly benign, they can occasionally indicate serious systemic disease or anaphylaxis. Pediatricians must be able to distinguish these presentations in order to manage them effectively.

Urticaria, in either acute or chronic form, affects up to 20% of the population at some point during their life time. Acute urticaria is more common in children and is often triggered by infections like viral respiratory tract infections. Chronic urticaria has a prevalence of approximately 0.5–1% in adult population, whereas it is less common in children.

Definition: Urticaria is a clinical condition marked by the presence of *wheals (hives), angioedema,* or both. It is a cutaneous response to mast cell degranulation in the skin or mucosa.

Wheals are characterized by:

- *Sharply defined, superficial swellings* of variable size and shape, usually with a central pale area and surrounding *reflex erythema*
- *Itching,* occasionally accompanied by *burning* sensation
- A *transient nature,* typically resolving within *30 minutes to 24 hours* without residual skin changes

Angioedema involves deeper tissue layers and presents as:

- A *sudden, well-demarcated swelling* of the deep dermis, subcutaneous tissue, or mucosal membranes, with minimal or absent surface erythema and *absent pitting*
- A *tingling, burning, or tight sensation,* and sometimes *pain,* rather than pruritus
- A *slower course,* with swelling generally resolving *within 72 hours*

CLASSIFICATION OF URTICARIA

Urticaria is broadly classified based on *duration* and *triggers* into the following categories:

Duration-based Classification

- *Acute urticaria:*
  - Wheals, angioedema or both, that lasts <*6 weeks*
  - Spontaneous in onset, typically self-limited
- *Chronic urticaria:*
  - Wheals, angioedema, or both that occurs for *6 weeks or more*
  - Chronic urticaria may sometimes have almost daily symptoms or an intermittent/recurrent course. It requires further subdivision based on trigger presence.

Etiology-based Classification

Chronic spontaneous urticaria (CSU):

- It constitutes about 80% of chronic urticaria which presents as wheals and/or angioedema *without any identifiable external trigger.*
- It may involve autoimmune mechanisms, including functional autoantibodies against IgE or its receptor (FcεRI).
- It accounts for the majority of chronic urticaria in children and adults.

Chronic inducible urticaria (CIndU):

- It constitutes about 20% of chronic urticaria where symptoms are *reproducibly triggered* by specific physical or environmental stimuli.

Subtypes include:

- *Dermographism (symptomatic)*—induced by stroking/scratching the skin
- *Cold urticaria*—triggered by exposure to cold air, water, or objects
- Delayed pressure urticaria—swelling hours after sustained pressure (e.g., tight straps).
- Cholinergic urticaria—small wheals triggered by heat, exercise, or emotional stress, especially when the core body temperature goes up
- Solar urticaria—triggered by exposure to sun
- *Vibratory angioedema/urticaria, heat urticaria, aquagenic urticaria,* etc.

Note: A single patient may present with both spontaneous and inducible forms.

Morphology/Association-based Classification

- *Urticaria with angioedema*—both wheals and deeper swelling co-occur.
- *Urticaria without angioedema*—only wheals present.
- *Angioedema without urticaria*—suggestive of bradykinin-mediated processes like Hereditary angioedema (HAE) or angiotensin-converting enzyme (ACE) inhibitor-induced angioedema.

PATHOPHYSIOLOGY

- Urticaria is predominantly driven by the activation of mast cells. At the urticarial sites, mediators released from mast cells such as histamine, platelet-activating factor (PAF) and cytokines, cause vasodilatation, sensory nerve stimulation, and plasma extravasation.
- Histologically wheals are characterized by involvement of the upper and mid-dermis whereas in angioedema, lower dermis and subcutis is involved, though the changes are similar. "Vessel wall necrosis" is a hallmark feature of urticarial vasculitis which is not seen in urticaria.

Major mechanisms of activation are:
- Immunoglobulin E (IgE)-mediated (e.g., food allergy)
- Non-IgE [e.g., nonsteroidal anti-inflammatory drugs (NSAIDs)]
- Autoimmune (anti-FcεRI)
- Bradykinin pathway (e.g., HAE)

ETIOLOGY

Acute Urticaria

Acute urticaria is most commonly caused by identifiable factors:
- *Infections* (most frequent, especially viral upper respiratory infections in children, but also bacterial and parasitic)
- Food allergens, especially in younger children
- *Drugs,* particularly NSAIDs and antibiotics
- *Insect stings, contact allergens* (rare)

Chronic Urticaria

- *CSU:* In about 80% of chronic urticaria cases, the cause remains unknown with no identifiable trigger factor.
- *Autoimmunity:* Up to 30–45% of CSU cases are attributed to autoimmune mechanisms, with autoantibodies against the high-affinity IgE receptor (FcεRI) or IgE itself (type I or type IIb autoimmunity).
- Less commonly, associations exist with *chronic infections, stress, and rare systemic diseases* (autoimmune thyroid diseases, rarely malignancy).
- *CIndU:* It is caused by specific physical or environmental stimuli.

Complement-related and Kinin-mediated Angioedema

- *HAE:* C1-INH deficiency (type I/II/), type III
- Acquired angioedema
- ACE inhibitor-induced

DANGER SIGNS (RED FLAGS) IN URTICARIA

Certain clinical features in children with urticaria or angioedema should raise concern for potentially life-threatening conditions.

Airway and Breathing Compromise

- Swelling of the tongue, lips, or throat
- Stridor or hoarseness of voicc
- Wheezing or shortness of breath in respiratory distress
- Drooling or difficulty swallowing

Systemic Reactions or Anaphylaxis

- Rash that progress rapidly
- Hypotension or collapse
- Gastrointestinal symptoms like vomiting, diarrhea, or severe abdominal pain

Abnormal Skin Changes

- Wheals that are persistent and painful lasting >24 hours
- Purpura, bruising/post-inflammatory pigmentation, or fixed lesions suggesting urticarial vasculitis

Other Systemic Clues

- Fever, arthralgia, malaise, or lymphadenopathy
- Jaundice or hepatosplenomegaly
- Recurrent isolated angioedema, especially with multiple family members involved

Any child with these features requires urgent referral and evaluation to rule out systemic disease or anaphylaxis.

DIFFERENTIAL DIAGNOSIS OF URTICARIA

While urticaria is common and usually benign, there are several other conditions that may mimic or overlap with it. The following are important differentials to consider:

- *Urticarial vasculitis:*
  - Lesions last >24 hours, are often painful or burning, and may cause hyperpigmentation or bruising.
  - It may be associated with systemic symptoms like arthralgia, renal involvement, or low complement levels.
- *Maculopapular cutaneous mastocytosis (urticaria pigmentosa):*
  - Common in infants and young children
  - Presents as brownish maculopapular lesions that produce a wheal when stroked; this is called the positive Darier sign.
  - Cutaneous manifestation of *indolent systemic mastocytosis* in older patients should be considered.
- *Mast cell activation syndrome (MCAS):*
  - Characterized by episodic symptoms of mast cell mediator release with features such as flushing, urticaria, diarrhea, and hypotension
  - Occurs without increased mast cell numbers but with inappropriate activation
  - Distinguished by systemic involvement with often no identifiable trigger
- *Cryopyrin-associated periodic syndromes (CAPS):*
  - A group of auto-inflammatory diseases (e.g., familial cold auto-inflammatory syndrome, Muckle–Wells syndrome)
  - Urticarial-like rash, fever, arthralgia, and sensorineural hearing loss
  - Symptoms often start in early childhood and may have a genetic basis (*NLRP3* mutations).
- *Schnitzler's syndrome:*
  - Rare late-onset auto-inflammatory syndrome, usually around the age of 50–55 years
  - Presents with chronic urticaria-like rash (lasts >24 hours), fever, arthralgia, monoclonal gammopathy
  - Usually lacks pruritus and has systemic features
- *Gleich's syndrome:*
  - Recurrent episodes of angioedema with hypereosinophilia, periodic weight gain, and sometimes fever
  - Associated with elevated serum IgM levels
  - Symptoms mimic allergic angioedema but have distinct hematological findings.

TABLE 1: Differentials of urticaria.

Condition	*Key differentiators*
Viral exanthems	Often maculopapular/morbilliform, fixed, nonevanescent rash, often with systemic symptoms like fever, cough, and upper respiratory tract infection
Erythema multiforme	Fixed target lesions with mucosal involvement
Atopic dermatitis	Chronic, relapsing, scaly, lichenified lesions; typical distribution among various age-groups
Drug eruptions	Fixed drug eruptions or widespread serum sickness-like reactions
Vasculitis	Painful wheals lasting >24 hours, may leave pigmentation or bruises
Contact dermatitis	Localized, often vesicular; history of exposure to allergens or irritants

- *Well's syndrome (eosinophilic cellulitis):*
  - Presents with edematous plaques resembling cellulitis or urticaria
  - Lesions are itchy/painful, persistent, and relapsing that lasts for days to weeks.
  - Eosinophilia is often present in two-thirds of cases.
- *Bullous pemphigoid (early phase):*
  - May initially resemble urticaria before developing tense bullae
  - Pruritic, fixed lesions that evolve into blisters over time

Other Common Look-alikes

Other common look-alikes of urticaria are given in **Table 1**.

For practical pediatric practice and allergy care, *urticarial vasculitis, mast cell disorders, HAE, drug reactions,* and *viral exanthems* are the *most common and clinically relevant differentials* to rule out. Others, though rare, should be considered when patients present with *atypical features,* systemic symptoms, or poor treatment response.

EVALUATION AND INVESTIGATIONS

Acute urticaria:

- No tests needed unless history suggestive of food/drug allergy or clinical symptoms/signs suggestive of systemic disease

Chronic urticaria:

- *Focused workup guided by history:*
  - CBC, ESR/CRP, TSH, anti-TPO Ab (if autoimmune suspicion such as thyroid disease in family)
  - ANA (if systemic signs)
- *ASST (autologous serum skin test):* Research/laboratory-based autoimmune screening
- C4, C1-INH levels if angioedema without urticaria

MANAGEMENT

General

- Remove suspected triggers, avoid unnecessary testing.
- Reassurance about benign nature is crucial in most cases.

Pharmacologic Treatment

- *Nonsedating H1-antihistamines (first-line):*
  - Cetirizine, loratadine, levocetirizine, fexofenadine, bilastine, desloratadine
  - May increase dose up to 4× in CSU if inadequate control
- *Sedating antihistamines:*
  - Strongly recommended against its use because of its potentially serious side effects
- *H2 blockers*:
  - Ranitidine (limited pediatric evidence), not recommended
- *Leukotriene antagonists:*
  - *Montelukast:* Adjunctive role; particularly with coexistent asthma
- *Corticosteroids:*
  - Short courses (3–5 days) in acute severe urticaria/angioedema (very restricted measure in children)
  - Long-term use discouraged
- *Omalizumab:*
  - Approved ≥12 years; effective in antihistamine-refractory CSU
  - Used off-label in younger children with specialist guidance.
- *Cyclosporine:*
  - For refractory CSU, specialist use only

Stepwise management of CSU is given in **Flowchart 1**.

URTICARIAL ACTIVITY SCORE 7

Urticarial Activity Score 7 (UAS 7) is a patient-reported outcome measure used to assess disease activity in CSU. The scoring system is based on a sum of 7-day patient daily scoring of wheals and itch.

Wheals score from 0 to 3: 0—none; 1—mild (<20 wheals); 2—moderate (20–50 wheals); 3—severe (>50 wheals or confluent)

Itch severity score from 0 to 3: 0—none; 1—mild (minimal awareness); 2—moderate (bothersome but tolerable); 3—severe (hard to tolerate)

Disease activity is based on the following score:

- *0:* Complete control
- *1–6:* Well-tolerated
- *7–15:* Mild disease activity
- *16–27:* Moderate disease activity
- *28–42:* Severe disease activity

Flowchart 1: Stepwise management of chronic spontaneous urticaria.

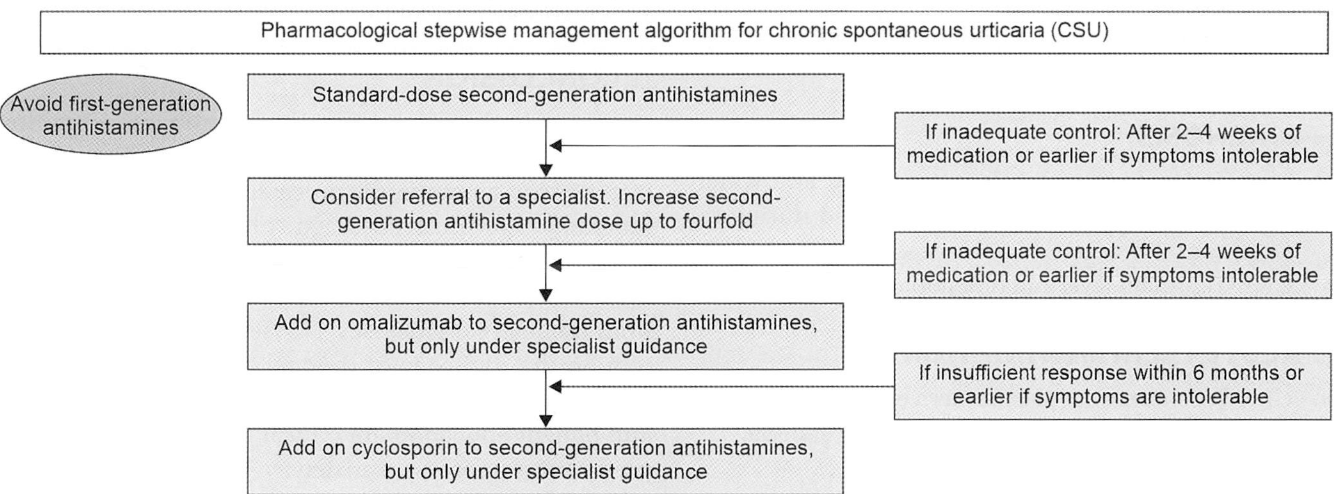

Source: Adapted from EAACI 2022 International guidelines.

A UAS (7) score of 7 or below indicates low or well-controlled disease, while higher scores reflect increasing severity.

SPECIAL CONSIDERATIONS

Angioedema without Urticaria

When angioedema occurs without urticaria and does not respond to antihistamines, corticosteroids, or adrenaline, it is likely mediated by bradykinin pathway rather than histamine-mediated pathway seen in urticaria. Further workup is needed.

Hereditary Angioedema

Most commonly inherited in an autosomal dominant pattern with a family history and multiple generations involved. But 20–25% may have de novo mutations and can pass the mutation to their children with 50% risk.

Most cases are caused by mutations in SERPING1 gene which encodes *C1 esterase inhibitor protein* or mutations in *factor XII*.

CLINICAL FEATURES

- Recurrent attacks of angioedema affecting skin, mucosa, and internal organs; edema is non pruritic, non-pitting, usually develops over several hours, and typically lasts for 2–5 days without treatment.
- *Gastrointestinal tract:* Abdominal attacks present with severe pain, nausea, vomiting, and diarrhea, and may mimic surgical abdomen.
- *Upper airway:* Laryngeal edema is potentially life-threatening.
- Attacks can occur spontaneous or may be triggered by trivial trauma, infections, emotional stress, dental/surgical procedures or hormonal changes.

DIAGNOSIS

- Low C4 (screening test, less expensive and widely available); it is almost always decreased during the attacks.
- C1-INH protein level and functional activity

ACUTE TREATMENT OPTIONS

- *C1-INH concentrate* (plasma-derived or recombinant); plasma-derived C1-INH is now available in India.
- *Fresh frozen plasma (FFP):*
    - FFP is used when specific therapies (e.g., C1-INH concentrate) are unavailable
    - FFP provides functional C1-INH but may theoretically exacerbate symptoms due to bradykinin substrate.

Dosage: 10–15 mL/kg IV (approximately 2 units in adults); may be repeated once after 4–6 hours if symptoms persist; administer with close monitoring for worsening of angioedema or volume overload.

- *Icatibant* (bradykinin B2 receptor antagonist)
- *Ecallantide* (kallikrein inhibitor)

Long-term prophylaxis (for frequent/severe episodes):

- *C1-INH prophylaxis (now available in India)*
- *Lanadelumab* (monoclonal antibody against kallikrein)
- *Attenuated androgens* (avoid in children due to adverse effects on growth and puberty)
- *Antifibrinolytics* in milder cases (safer in children and pregnant women when C1-INH is not accessible or affordable); they are not considered the first-line therapy because of their limited efficacy.

PROGNOSIS

- Acute urticaria resolves within 1–2 weeks.
- *Chronic urticaria* ~50% remission in 6–12 months; persistent in 10–20%; remission is defined as the absence of symptoms for 6 months without therapy.

PARENT/CAREGIVER EDUCATION

- Explain benign course of urticaria.
- Encourage adherence to antihistamines.
- Provide action plans for flare-ups or anaphylaxis.

CONCLUSION

Urticaria and angioedema in children are common presentations with diverse etiologies, ranging from benign infections to autoimmune processes and life-threatening reactions. A structured diagnostic approach—focused history, careful examination, and judicious investigations—helps distinguish acute from chronic and IgE-mediated from nonallergic processes. Nonsedating antihistamines remain the mainstay of therapy, with escalation steps reserved for refractory cases. Early recognition of red flags and patient education are critical to ensuring safety and preventing unnecessary anxiety.

KEY POINTS

- Acute urticaria is usually infection-related in children.
- Chronic urticaria is rarely due to allergy.
- Daily nonsedating antihistamines are cornerstone therapy.
- Urticaria with systemic signs needs further workup.
- HAE must be considered in angioedema without hives.

SUGGESTED READING

1. Bernstein JA, Lang DM, Khan DA, Craig T, Dreyfus D, Hsieh F, et al. The diagnosis and management of acute and chronic urticaria: 2014 update. J Allergy Clin Immunol. 2014;133(5):1270-7.
2. Chang J. Management of pediatric chronic spontaneous urticaria. Children (Basel). 2021;8(3):205.
3. Jindal AK, Sil A, Aggarwal R, Vinay K, Bishnoi A, Suri D. Management of hereditary angioedema in resource-constrained settings: A consensus statement from Indian subcontinent. World Allergy Organ J. 2023;16(6):100761.
4. Saini SS. Urticaria and angioedema. In: Burks AW, O'Hehir RE, Broide DH, Holgate ST, Bacharier LB, Khurana Hershey GK, et al. (Eds). Middleton's Allergy: Principles and Practice, 9th edition. Philadelphia: Elsevier; 2021.
5. Sánchez J, Pite H, Gómez RM, Ansotegui IJ, Canonica GW, Dávila I, et al. Chronic spontaneous urticaria remission definition and therapy stepping down: World Allergy Organization position paper. J Allergy Clin Immunol. 2025;155(3):1050-1056.e2.
6. Zuberbier T, Abdul Latiff AH, Abuzakouk M, Aquilina S, Asero R, Baker D, et al. The international EAACI/GA^{2}LEN/EuroGuiDerm/APAAACI guideline for the definition, classification, diagnosis, and management of urticaria. Allergy. 2022;77(3):734-66.

19 CHAPTER

Drug Allergy in Children

Jefferson Daniel

INTRODUCTION

Adverse drug reactions (ADRs) represent a major clinical hazard in pediatric practice, with unverified reactions to at least one drug reported in up to 16% of children visiting a hospital. However, true drug allergy, which is defined as specific immunologically mediated drug hypersensitivity reactions (DHRs), accounts for only a fraction of these reports. Most suspected reactions are Type A (predictable, dose-dependent) rather than Type B (unpredictable, immune-mediated) responses. The burden of incorrect and unverified drug allergy labels is substantial, leading to suboptimal alternative therapies, increased antibiotic resistance, higher medical costs, and significant parental anxiety. Accurate diagnosis through systematic evaluation is essential to prevent unnecessary drug avoidance while ensuring safety and optimal therapeutic outcomes in children.

EPIDEMIOLOGY

Adverse drug reactions account for 3–6% of hospital admissions globally, with DHRs representing <10% of all ADRs. True drug allergies occur in approximately 1–3% of children who are hospitalized. All who have allergy labels often do not have true allergies: the gap between suspected and confirmed cases is striking. Approximately 10% of children have confirmed drug allergies after a systematic allergy workup of those children with suspected allergies. Globally, β-lactam antibiotics are the most frequently implicated drugs, followed by nonsteroidal anti-inflammatory drugs (NSAIDs).

Epidemiological data specific to Indian children remain limited, but adult studies provide valuable insights into local patterns. A recent study from an Indian tertiary care center found drug allergy labels in 5.6% of hospitalized patients, with antibiotics being the most commonly implicated class, followed by NSAIDs. β-lactams dominated the antibiotic category, which is consistent with global patterns and reflects India's high antibiotic consumption rates. Anecdotal reports suggest patterns observed in Indian pediatric practice include frequent β-lactam hypersensitivity reactions, paracetamol-related reactions (often pseudoallergic rather than true allergy) and increasing reports of anticonvulsant reactions. The prevalent self-medication culture and easy over-the-counter availability of medications contribute to inappropriate drug exposure patterns. Additionally, genetic polymorphisms affecting drug metabolism, such as cytochrome P450 variants that are common in Indian populations, may influence individual susceptibility to specific drug reactions, particularly with anticonvulsants and sulfonamides.

ETIOPATHOGENESIS

Understanding drug allergic reactions requires familiarity with both their immunological classification and underlying molecular mechanisms. The Gell and Coombs classification provides a framework for understanding these mechanisms. Type I [Immunoglobulin E (IgE)-mediated] reactions occur within minutes to hours, manifesting as urticaria, angioedema, or anaphylaxis. β-lactams and antiepileptics are often the common culprits. Type II (cytotoxic) reactions involve complement-mediated cell destruction, causing hemolytic anemia or thrombocytopenia, typically a few days after exposure. Type III (immune complex) reactions result from prolonged high-dose therapy, producing serum sickness-like syndrome with fever and vasculitis. Type IV (T-cell mediated) reactions are delayed, subdivided into IVa (Th1-cell mediated), IVb (Th2-cell mediated), IVc (cytotoxic T-cells), and IVd (neutrophil-mediated).

Immunological Mechanisms

For the drugs to be treated as an allergen by the immune system, they must first be recognized as one. The following are some of the mechanisms by which the drugs are recognized and undergo allergic sensitization before manifesting clinical allergy symptoms. Hapten-carrier complex formation occurs when small molecular weight drugs bind covalently to host proteins. For example, in Penicillin, the β-lactam ring binds lysine residues, creating penicilloyl epitopes (major determinants) and other conjugates (minor determinants). Another mechanism is prohapten conversion, which involves the metabolic transformation of the drug into reactive intermediates (*Example:* sulfonamides forming nitroso metabolites). Pharmacological interaction (p-i concept) describes direct, reversible drug binding to human leukocyte antigen (HLA) molecules without covalent modification, triggering immediate T-cell responses even on first exposure.

Nonimmunological Mechanisms

Pseudoallergic reactions mimic allergic responses without immune involvement. Direct histamine release (morphine, vancomycin), MRGPRX2 receptor activation (fluoroquinolones), and cyclooxygenase-1 (COX-1) inhibition (NSAIDs, paracetamol) produce clinically similar but mechanistically distinct reactions. Children's immature immune systems may predispose them to different reaction patterns. Concurrent viral infections [Epstein–Barr Virus (EBV), cytomegalovirus (CMV)] can lower activation thresholds and increase drug reaction risk through danger signal activation and altered self-repertoire mechanisms.

Risk Factors for Drug Allergy

Drug-related risk factors include the drug's inherent immunogenicity (haptens like penicillins), route of administration (topical and parenteral routes carrying a higher risk), and pattern of exposure (intermittent administration being more sensitizing than continuous therapy). Patient-related risk factors encompass age-related immune system maturity, concurrent viral infections (particularly EBV infection, increasing amoxicillin rash risk), genetic predisposition, including HLA associations, and previous drug exposures that may enhance cross-reactivity patterns.

CLINICAL FEATURES

Immediate Reactions (Minutes to Hours)

Immediate DHRs typically manifest within 1–6 hours of drug administration. Urticarial rashes, pruritus, and erythema are the most common presentations, often accompanied by angioedema. Bronchospasm may occur, particularly with NSAIDs in children with underlying asthma. Anaphylaxis, though rare, is potentially fatal and presents with multisystem involvement, including cardiovascular collapse, respiratory distress, and gastrointestinal symptoms. In pediatric settings, urticaria, vomiting, and laryngeal edema represent the most common manifestations of anaphylaxis. Parenteral administration typically produces more rapid and severe reactions compared to oral routes.

Delayed Reactions (Days to Weeks)

Delayed reactions emerge 6 hours to several weeks after drug exposure and are predominantly T-cell mediated.

Mild cutaneous allergic reactions (MCAR): Maculopapular exanthema (MPE) is the most frequent delayed reaction, presenting as widespread erythematous macules and papules affecting the trunk and proximal extremities while sparing mucosae. MPE typically appears 5–7 days after drug initiation and resolves within 7–14 days after discontinuation. Importantly, most MPE occur during viral infections rather than representing true drug allergy. Fixed drug eruptions manifest as localized violaceous plaques that consistently recur at identical sites upon reexposure, often leaving persistent hyperpigmentation. Erythema multiforme presents with characteristic target lesions and variable mucosal involvement.

Severe cutaneous allergic reactions (SCAR): Stevens–Johnson syndrome (SJS) and toxic epidermal necrolysis (TEN) represent a spectrum differentiated by extent of skin detachment (<10% vs. >30%, respectively). These potentially fatal conditions frequently involve mucous membranes and systemic complications. DRESS (Drug Reaction with Eosinophilia and Systemic Symptoms) syndrome combines maculopapular rash with fever, eosinophilia, lymphadenopathy, and multiorgan involvement, particularly hepatitis. Acute generalized exanthematous pustulosis (AGEP) features widespread sterile pustules on erythematous skin, typically resolving within 15 days.

Noncutaneous presentations include hematological complications (thrombocytopenia, hemolytic anemia), hepatic injury, renal interstitial nephritis, and vasculitis. Drug-induced enterocolitis syndrome (DIES) is a recently described non-IgE-mediated reaction that primarily affects children, manifesting as severe vomiting, diarrhea, lethargy, and pallor. Amoxicillin and paracetamol are the most common triggers.

DIFFERENTIAL DIAGNOSIS

Viral Exanthems versus Drug Rashes

The most common diagnostic challenge in pediatric practice involves distinguishing viral-induced rashes from

TABLE 1: Comparison of clinical characteristics between viral exanthem and drug exanthem.

Feature	*Viral exanthem*	*Drug exanthem*	*EBV-viral interaction rash*
Onset timing	Concurrent with fever/illness onset	Days after drug initiation (5–7 days typical)	During/after viral prodrome
Clinical features	Face-to-trunk progression, viral-specific patterns, rarely pruritic	Symmetrical, trunk/proximal limbs, drug-dependent, centripetal spread, pruritic	Maculopapular rash involving trunk, extremities, palms, and soles. Palatal petechiae
Associated symptoms	Fever, malaise, respiratory/GI symptoms of viral illness	May have other allergic symptoms	May continue despite stopping the drug
Response to antipyretics	Improves with fever control	No relationship to fever management	No relationship to fever management
Recurrence pattern	May or may not recur	Consistent recurrence with drug reexposure	Infectious mononucleosis typically occurs once hence may not recur. However, other viral infections can act as cofactors
On drug challenge, when the child is stable	Negative test as the drug is not the culprit	A clear temporal relationship with drug exposure will elicit a positive drug challenge response	Negative drug challenge test, as EBV infection acts as a cofactor, and in its absence, the rash will not appear

(EBV: Epstein–Barr Virus; GI: Gastrointestinal)

DHRs, particularly when children receive medications during febrile illnesses **(Table 1)**.

Infectious mononucleosis particularly creates confusion. Recent studies show 15–33% of children with EBV infection develop maculopapular rashes when treated with ampicillin or amoxicillin. This non-IgE-mediated reaction resolves over time and does not preclude future β-lactam use. Viral infections combined with paracetamol administration frequently lead to incorrect "paracetamol allergy" diagnosis. The temporal association during febrile illness often misleads parents and physicians.

Inducible Laryngeal Obstruction

Patients reporting "allergies" to multiple inhalers may have inducible laryngeal obstruction (ILO). These patients develop cough, globus sensation, hoarseness, and throat tightness within minutes of inhaler use. Distinguishing features include normal oxygen saturation, absence of objective angioedema, stereotypical reactions to unrelated medications, and paradoxical worsening with epinephrine. Laryngoscopy during episodes confirms vocal cord dysfunction.

Multiple Drug Intolerance Syndrome

Patients reporting subjective reactions to three or more structurally unrelated medications warrant consideration of psychogenic etiology. These typically older, female patients develop symptoms such as metallic taste, brain fog, and fatigue without objective findings. Single-blind placebo-controlled challenges can be diagnostic when patients develop identical symptoms to placebo.

Serious Systemic Mimics

Hemophagocytic lymphohistiocytosis (HLH) can initially mimic DRESS syndrome with fever, rash, and multiorgan involvement, but carries higher mortality (40% vs. 10%). Distinguishing features include extremely elevated ferritin, cytopenias, and elevated soluble CD25. Neurological conditions like seizures from metastatic brain lesions may be erroneously attributed to contrast agents.

Nonallergic Drug Reactions

Gastrointestinal intolerance, central nervous system (CNS) effects, drug interactions, and vasovagal reactions during injections continue to be commonly mislabeled as allergies, creating unnecessary medication restrictions that compromise patient care.

DIAGNOSIS

Clinical History

Detailed history remains the cornerstone of drug allergy diagnosis. Key elements include a precise temporal relationship between drug exposure and symptom onset. Immediate reactions occur within 1–6 hours, while delayed reactions manifest days to weeks later. Document the exact drug name, dose, route, and duration of therapy. Assess concurrent medications and viral infections, particularly EBV, which predisposes to amoxicillin rashes. Family history of drug allergies and previous reactions guide risk assessment. Hospital records and photographs from the acute episode provide invaluable objective documentation.

Risk Stratification: Critical Clinical Decision Point (Alsulaiman 2024)

After a comprehensive history, classify the reaction risk to guide the management approach:

- *Low risk (likely nonimmunological reactions):*
  - Isolated nonspecific symptoms (vomiting, diarrhea, headache, dizziness)
  - Localized rash or itching without systemic features
  - Cough or runny nose without respiratory distress
  - Family history only
  - Unknown reaction many years ago without IgE-mediated features
  - Tolerated the same antibiotic since the index episode
- *High risk (potentially life-threatening IgE-mediated or severe reactions):*
  - Respiratory involvement (difficulty breathing, wheezing, stridor)
  - Cardiovascular symptoms (hypotension, tachycardia, collapse)
  - Facial, throat, or lip swelling (angioedema)
  - Severe cutaneous reactions (SJS, TEN, DRESS, AGEP, widespread blistering)
  - Anaphylaxis or systemic involvement
  - Organ-specific reactions (acute renal failure, hepatitis)

Physical Examination

Pattern recognition is crucial. Assess rash distribution, morphology, and mucosal involvement. Immediate reactions typically present with urticaria and angioedema, while delayed reactions show symmetric maculopapular patterns. System involvement evaluation includes lymphadenopathy (DRESS), hepatosplenomegaly, and vital sign instability, suggesting severe reactions.

Laboratory Investigations

Immediate Reactions

Serum tryptase measurement provides the strongest laboratory evidence. We must obtain samples within 30 minutes–2 hours of acute reaction and a baseline level 24 hours later. Elevated acute levels (>1.2 ng/mL + 20% of baseline) support an anaphylaxis diagnosis. Drug-specific IgE testing has limited availability in India, but it is useful when accessible. Complete blood count may reveal eosinophilia or other cytopenias.

Delayed Reactions

Liver function tests and renal function assessment are essential, particularly for DRESS and organ-specific reactions. Eosinophil count elevation supports delayed hypersensitivity. Patch testing for contact sensitization requires specialized allergy centers.

Drug-specific Diagnostic Approaches

β-lactams

Skin testing hierarchy begins with skin prick tests, followed by intradermal tests using standardized concentrations when available. Cross-reactivity depends on R1 side chain similarity. Several international guidelines provide cross-reactivity charts for penicillins and cephalosporins that enable careful selection of alternative drugs. Cefaclor and cefadroxil share high cross-reactivity with penicillins, while cefuroxime and ceftriaxone show minimal cross-reactivity.

Nonsteroidal Anti-inflammatory Drugs

Challenge testing remains the gold standard. Distinguish between selective reactions (single drug) and cross-intolerant reactions (multiple NSAIDs via COX-1 inhibition). Aspirin challenge helps define cross-intolerance patterns.

Anticonvulsants

Delayed intradermal testing and patch testing are preferred for mild reactions. High cross-reactivity (40–80%) exists among aromatic anticonvulsants (carbamazepine, phenytoin, phenobarbital).

Drug Provocation Tests: Gold Standard

Graded challenge protocols provide definitive diagnosis when safely performed. Start with one-tenth therapeutic dose, escalating to full dose over 2–4 hours. Contraindications include SCAR, anaphylaxis, and organ involvement. Tests should be performed 4–6 weeks postreaction in controlled settings with resuscitation equipment available.

When to Refer to an Allergist

Immediate referral is warranted for severe/life-threatening reactions, unclear temporal relationships, need for essential drug continuation, and suspected multiple drug hypersensitivity syndrome. Specialized testing requirements or complex cross-reactivity assessments also necessitate expert consultation. Most importantly, refer when an accurate diagnosis would significantly impact therapeutic options or when safer alternatives are unavailable **(Fig. 1)**.

MANAGEMENT

Acute Management

Immediate Reactions

Discontinue the suspected drug immediately upon recognition of allergic symptoms. For anaphylaxis, administer adrenaline 0.01 mg/kg intramuscularly (maximum 0.5 mg) as first-line treatment, repeated every 5–15 minutes if needed. Antihistamines (H1 and H2 blockers) and corticosteroids provide adjunctive support but never replace adrenaline. Ensure airway patency, establish intravenous access, and provide supportive care with fluid resuscitation and oxygen as needed. Monitor vital signs continuously for at least 4–6 hours postreaction.

Delayed Reactions

Immediate drug discontinuation is paramount. For SCAR (SJS, DRESS, AGEP), initiate systemic corticosteroids early and consider specialist dermatology consultation. Monitor closely for progression—DRESS can evolve over weeks with multiorgan involvement requiring liver function monitoring, complete blood counts, and renal assessment.

Long-term Management

Documentation and Communication

Create comprehensive documentation, including reaction details, temporal relationship, and photographic evidence when available. Provide medical alert bracelets/cards with specific drug names and reaction types. Patient and parent education must include written instructions about drug avoidance, emergency management, and when to seek medical care.

Drug Avoidance and Alternative Selection

Understanding cross-reactivity patterns guides safe alternative selection.

- *β-lactam allergies:* Noncross-reactive cephalosporins (cefuroxime, ceftriaxone) can be administered to most penicillin-allergic patients under the supervision of an experienced allergist. Carbapenems and monobactams show minimal cross-reactivity and represent safe alternatives.
- *NSAID intolerance:* Paracetamol at doses <15 mg/kg is often well-tolerated even in COX-1 sensitive patients. Selective COX-2 inhibitors (nimesulide from age 12, etoricoxib from age 16) provide alternatives for older children.
- *Anticonvulsant allergies:* Avoid aromatic anticonvulsants (carbamazepine, phenytoin, phenobarbital) due to high cross-reactivity (40–80%). Select structurally different alternatives like levetiracetam or valproate.

Desensitization Protocols

Desensitization creates temporary tolerance through graded dose escalation when essential drugs have no safe alternatives. Indications include life-threatening infections requiring specific antibiotics, cancer chemotherapy, or insulin allergy in diabetics.

Strict contraindications include SCAR, type II/III hypersensitivity reactions, organ involvement, and hemolytic reactions. The procedure requires specialist supervision in intensive care unit (ICU) settings with resuscitation equipment immediately available.

Protocol basics involve starting with 1/1,000–1/100 of the therapeutic dose, with dose doubling every 15–20 minutes until the full therapeutic dose is achieved. Common pediatric scenarios include β-lactam desensitization in cystic fibrosis patients and chemotherapy desensitization in oncology.

Drug Label Reassessment and "Delabeling"

Regular reassessment of drug allergy labels is crucial—up to 90% of reported penicillin allergies are not confirmed

Flowchart 1: Practical management algorithm for the general pediatrician.

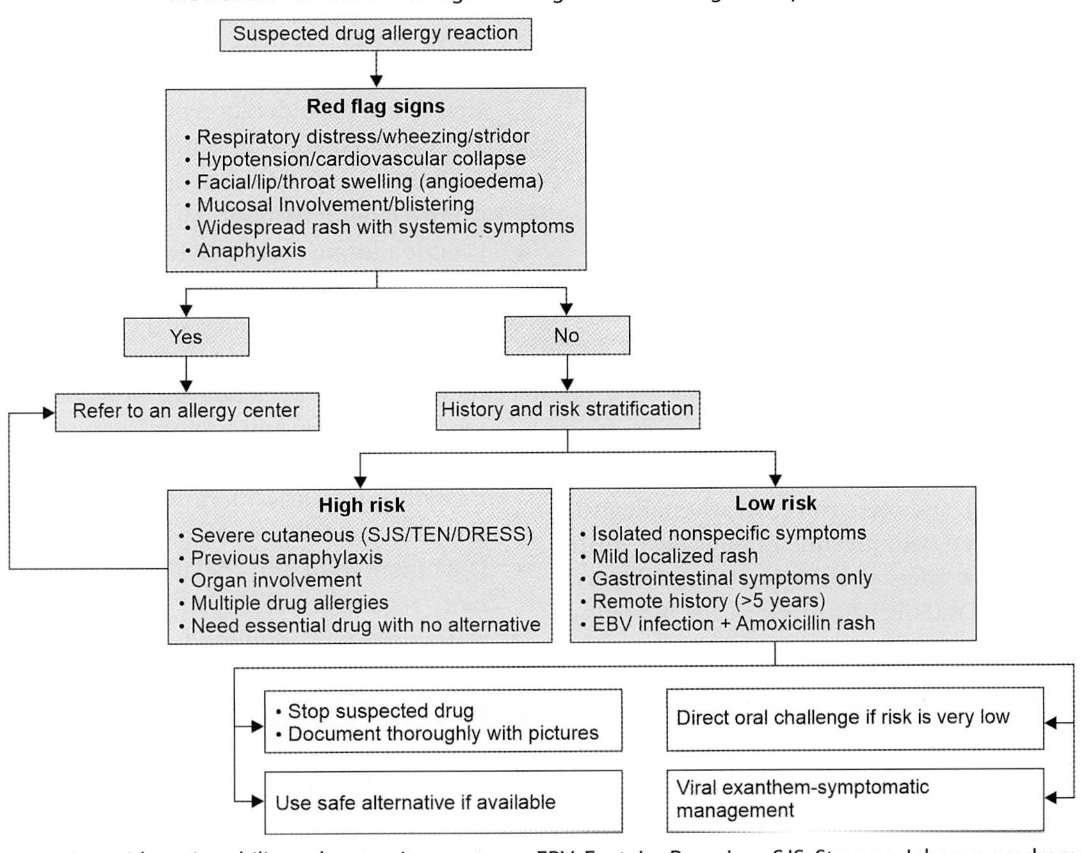

(DRESS: Drug reaction with eosinophilia and systemic symptoms; EBV: Epstein–Barr virus; SJS: Stevens–Johnson syndrome; TEN: Toxic epidermal necrolysis)

upon proper evaluation. "Delabeling" through systematic allergy evaluation prevents unnecessary use of broader-spectrum, more expensive, and potentially more toxic alternatives.

For benign cutaneous reactions (maculopapular rash, urticaria) occurring >5 years ago, consider direct drug challenges without prior skin testing when the drug is needed. This approach safely restores access to first-line therapies while reducing antimicrobial resistance risks.

COMMON DRUG ALLERGIES IN CHILDREN

β-lactam Antibiotics

Standard penicillin skin testing kits are unavailable in India, so historical risk assessment is the practical first step. True penicillin allergy is rare. Only 2.8% of Danish children with suspected penicillin allergy had positive drug challenges, with isolated rashes unlikely to represent true allergy (Krusenstjerna-Hafstrøm 2020). Low-risk cases (isolated maculopapular rash, distant history) can undergo direct oral amoxicillin challenge, but we strongly recommend performing such challenges in tertiary care settings with allergy expertise.

High-risk cases (anaphylaxis, severe cutaneous reactions) often require cross-reactivity assessment using available charts. Safe alternatives include noncross-reactive cephalosporins (cefuroxime, ceftriaxone), carbapenems, or aztreonam, administered with caution. Sulfonamides (trimethoprim-sulfamethoxazole) carry SJS risk, particularly in slow acetylators, requiring immediate discontinuation if skin reactions develop.

Nonsteroidal Anti-inflammatory Drug and Analgesic Reactions

NSAID hypersensitivity in children manifests through two distinct mechanisms: cross-intolerant reactions (multiple NSAIDs via COX-1 inhibition leading to excessive leukotriene production) and selective reactions (IgE-mediated, affecting single drugs). Ibuprofen causes the majority of confirmed reactions.

Cross-intolerant reactions typically present within 1–6 hours as facial angioedema (most common), often without urticaria, progressing to generalized urticaria/angioedema. Children <10 years frequently develop "blended reactions" combining cutaneous and respiratory symptoms (laryngospasm, bronchospasm), while older children show distinct phenotypes: NIUAA (urticaria/angioedema/anaphylaxis in healthy children), NECD (exacerbation of chronic urticaria), and NERD (respiratory symptoms in asthmatics). Selective reactions present as isolated urticaria/angioedema or anaphylaxis to single NSAIDs, typically IgE-mediated with consistent, reproducible symptoms.

Safe alternatives for cross-intolerant patients include selective COX-2 inhibitors such as nimesulide (>12 years), etoricoxib (>16 years), and celecoxib (≥12 years). Registry data from 274 children with juvenile idiopathic arthritis demonstrates similar safety profiles between celecoxib and traditional NSAIDs (Sobel 2014). However, individual pediatricians must carefully weigh risk-benefit ratios, particularly in very young children, where alternative management strategies should be prioritized.

Paracetamol reactions represent a special subset of NSAID pseudoallergy. Most suspected "paracetamol allergies" are pseudoallergic responses. Confirmation rate is only 13% (Cavkaytar 2022). Clinical findings are characteristically inconsistent. Rashes occur intermittently, reflecting dose-dependent precipitation during febrile infections when paracetamol's weak COX-1 inhibition triggers inflammatory responses. Paracetamol <15 mg/kg is often tolerated even in cross-intolerant patients.

CONCLUSION

Drug allergies are frequently suspected but infrequently confirmed in pediatric practice. Over-diagnosis can lead to avoidance of first-line therapies, antimicrobial resistance, and increased healthcare burden. Structured evaluation **(Flowchart 1)**—including risk stratification, appropriate skin or in-vitro testing, and drug provocation tests—remains essential to accurate diagnosis. Management focuses on immediate safety, long-term documentation, and patient counseling. Strengthening awareness and availability of specialist services will help reduce the prevalence of incorrect drug-allergy labels and ensure safe, effective treatment choices.

KEY POINTS

- Most suspected drug allergies in children are not, genuine immunological reactions—careful history and viral illness consideration prevent over-diagnosis.
- Temporal relationship is the most important diagnostic factor—a detailed drug and symptom timeline trumps laboratory tests.
- Pseudoallergic reactions (especially to paracetamol and NSAIDs) are common—these do not require complete drug avoidance, just dose modification.
- Cross-reactivity patterns guide safe alternatives—understanding β-lactam R1 side chains and NSAID mechanisms prevents unnecessary restrictions.
- SCAR (SJS, DRESS, AGEP) require immediate recognition—early identification and drug discontinuation can be life-saving.
- Documentation and "delabeling" are equally important—regular reassessment prevents unnecessary drug restrictions into adulthood.

SUGGESTED READING

1. Alsulaiman JW, Kheirallah KA, Alrawashdeh A, Saleh T, Obeidat M, Alawneh YJ, et al. Risk stratification of penicillin allergy labeled children: A cross-sectional study from jordan. Ther Clin Risk Manag. 2024;20:505-14.
2. Ashok N. Drug allergy–Review article. Karnataka Paediatric Journal. 2023;37(4):111-6.
3. Kathuria PC, Rai M. Management of drug allergy-clinical update. Indian J Allergy, Asthma Immunol. 2022; 36(1):4.
4. Krusenstjerna-Hafstrøm T, Rubak S. The use of direct oral challenge to confirm allergies to penicillin class antibiotics in Danish children. BMC Pediatr. 2020;20:523.
5. Park JS, Suh DI. Drug allergy in children: What should we know? Clin Exp Pediatr. 2020;63(6):203-10.
6. Piccorossi A, Liccioli G, Barni S, Sarti L, Giovannini M, Verrotti A, et al. Epidemiology and drug allergy results in children investigated in the allergy unit of a tertiary-care paediatric hospital setting. Ital J Pediatr. 2020; 46(1):5.
7. Sobel RE, Lovell DJ, Brunner HI, Weiss JE, Morris PW, Gottlieb BS, et al. Safety of celecoxib and nonselective nonsteroidal anti-inflammatory drugs in juvenile idiopathic arthritis: results of the Phase 4 registry. Pediatr Rheumatol Online J. 2014;12:29.
8. Waldron JL, Glennon CM, Kroshinsky DA, Khan DA, Wolfson AR. Drug Allergy Mimics. J Allergy Clin Immunol Pract. 2024;12(5):1122-29.e1.

20 CHAPTER Insect Venom Hypersensitivity

S Narmada Ashok

INTRODUCTION

Insect venom hypersensitivity is an under-recognized yet clinically significant allergic condition capable of causing reactions ranging from large local swelling to life-threatening anaphylaxis. Although systemic reactions are less frequent in children compared to adults, the anxiety provoked by insect stings in families often leads to medical consultations. In India, sensitization to common insects such as bees, wasps, and ants is increasingly documented, with regional variations in prevalence. Advances in diagnostics—including skin testing, serum-specific immunoglobulin E (IgE) assays, and component-resolved diagnostics—have improved our ability to identify sensitization patterns and guide management. Venom immunotherapy (VIT) remains the most effective preventive treatment for patients with systemic reactions, drastically reducing the risk of recurrence. With rising awareness and research interest in India, this field offers opportunities for improved diagnosis, standardization of care, and preventive strategies in pediatric allergy practice.

EPIDEMIOLOGY

Insect sting allergy has a prevalence that varies from 0.4 to 7.5% of adults. However, some studies report that around 15–25% of the general population exhibit venom specific IgE antibodies. In a study in India in West Bengal, 450 patients seeking treatment at Allergy and asthma center for insect bite 82% of them had sensitization to any one of the tested insect allergen. The predominant insect they showed sensitivity was to common black ant, fire ant, honeybee, mosquito, and wasp. This was one of the first studies that investigated the sensitization pattern among Indians.

COMMON INSECTS IMPLICATED

The common insects in Hymenoptera order implicated in India the Hymenoptera basically has three main family—Apidae, Vespidae, and Formicidae. Understanding the order of insects is important as there can be significant cross reactivity among members of the same family.

Apidae family mainly encompassed the Apis (honeybees), Bombus (bumble bees) and Xylocopa (carpenter bees). The commonest species in India are Apis mellifera and they are usually domesticated. Occupational exposure or disturbing the nest of the honeybees intentionally can lead on to multiple bites. The bite of the honeybees can be recognized with the stinger left behind at the site of the bite **(Fig. 1)**. Bumble bees are usually not common in India and because of cross reaction can lead to severe symptoms **(Fig. 2)**.

Vespidae family comprises of yellow jackets, hornets and wasps **(Fig. 3)**. They are aggressive and are usually

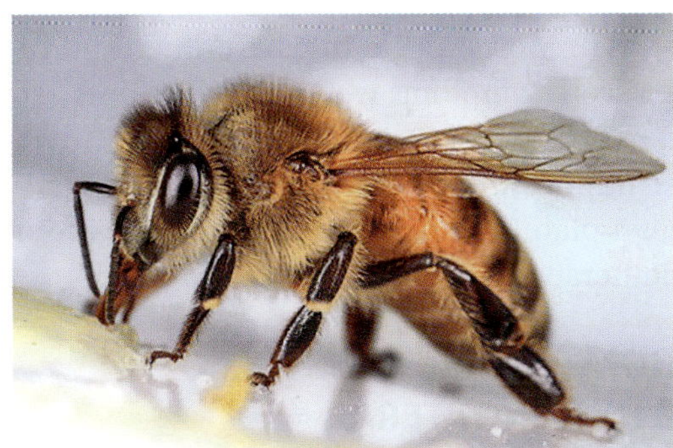

Fig. 1: Honeybees with the stinger.

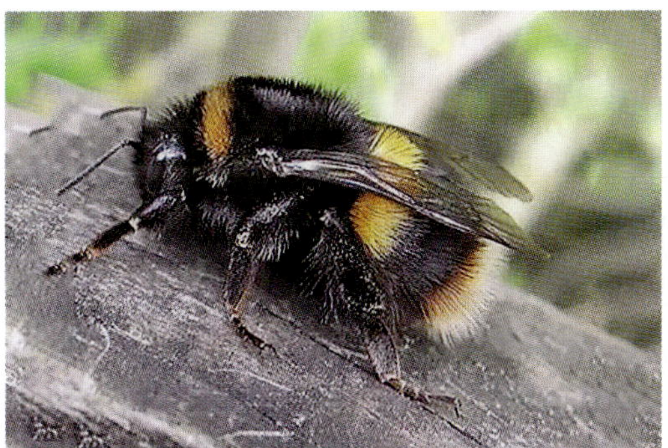

Fig. 2: Bumble bees.

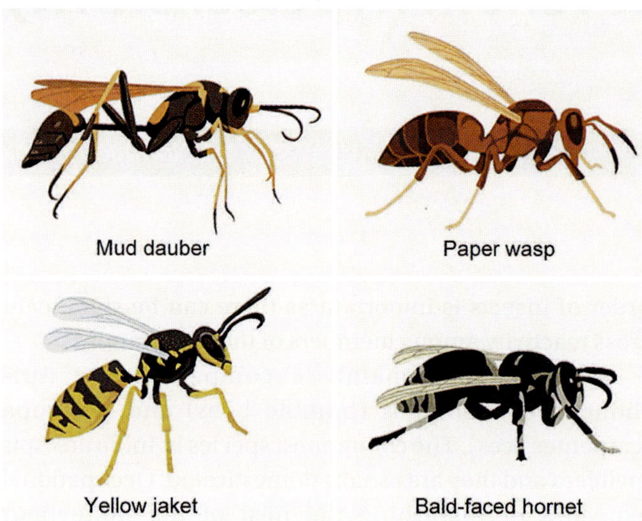

Fig. 3: Vespidae family.

attracted to sweet foods and grilled foods and found near garbage cans, leftover foods or in outdoor events. The nests of the Vespidae are also in the ground level that can be easily disturbed by children. Studies in India have shown wasp bites are more common than bees.

Formicidae family contains ants especially the fire ants which is the most important cause of systemic reactions. Most of the reports of the bites are due to ant species causing severe symptoms where from fire ants especially in USA.

It is important to identify the insects as we can help them plan immunotherapy in places where single immunotherapy is practiced.

VENOM CHARACTERISTICS OF THE HYMENOPTERA

The venom of Hymenoptera is a complex mixture of compounds, primarily peptides and proteins that can cause pain, inflammation, and allergic reactions. The recent techniques in bioinformatics have helped us to understand the characteristics of Hymenoptera venoms. The most bioactive compounds are the peptides and proteins. The most prominent honeybee venom (HBV) allergens include phospholipase A2, hyaluronidase and 26 amino acid peptide melittin. Yellow jacket venom is also chemically similar—phospholipase A2, hyaluronidase, and antigen 5, however, antigenically different due to the specific protein component. The various peptides and proteins by themselves can cause mast cell degranulation, chemotaxis, cell lysin, hemolysis, and chemotaxis of inflammatory cells. However, these proteins are also capable of triggering sensitization and cause immunological reaction. The ant venom has 50% of proteinaceous toxins.

TYPES OF REACTION DUE TO INSECT BITES

Insect bites can cause immunological responses that manifest as either local or systemic reactions. Large local reactions are defined as those exceeding 10 cm in diameter or extending beyond two joints. Common symptoms include red ness, swelling, itching, and pain. Systemic reactions may involve areas of the body separate from the sting site and can range in severity. Cutaneous systemic reactions are confined to skin symptoms, while anaphylaxis involves two or more organ systems. Possible systemic manifestations include bronchospasm, upper airway obstruction, cardiac arrhythmias, coronary artery spasm, hypotension, shock, nausea, or vomiting. Management is aggressive when systemic reactions occur.

INSECT HYPERSENSITIVITY BEYOND HYMENOPTERA

In contrast to bees and wasps, there are certain insects which are not discussed in allergological practice, because their bites primarily cause no systemic reactions but only cutaneous manifestations. The insect saliva secreted contains biogenic amines and vasoactive peptides capable of producing immediate cutaneous reaction. Sometimes indurated papule can persist for several days developing after 12–24 hours (late reaction). In rare cases there may be delayed swellings up to >10 cm in diameter with blisters or necrosis are also found. Papular urticaria is seen in tropical regions following usually mosquito bites. If the same is accompanied by fever and generalized lymphadenopathy it is called skeeter syndrome. Most hematophagous insects causing allergic reactions belong to either mosquitoes or flies. Further investigation of the same is individualistic. Topical antihistamines are widely used for cutaneous immediate reactions.

MANAGEMENT OF INSECT STINGS

Most insect stings can cause mild local reaction, and no specific treatment is required.

- Some local reactions can be managed by cold compresses.
- If still worse, then antihistamines (systemic) can be given.

- Oral steroids do not have definite proof of efficacy and can be used where there are large local reactions.
- Mostly it requires only symptomatic management.

Large local reactions rarely create systemic reactions but 10% might eventually have a systemic reaction if they had subsequent stings.

Systemic reaction involving multisystem causing anaphylaxis will involve stabilization of airway, breathing and circulation. Epinephrine intramuscular (i.m.) to be given as soon as the patient starts developing symptoms. Further oxygen, ventilatory care, systemic steroids, and bronchodilators may be needed. The patient has to be observed for a period of 24–48 hours as there may be delayed reaction.

Intramuscular epinephrine is the first and most important corner stone of management of systemic reactions.

FURTHER MANAGEMENT OF THE PATIENT

Once stabilized the patient should be referred to allergologist/immunologist for further assessment. Epinephrine injector to be given for home care and the patient to be evaluated for further preventive management and the feasibility of immunotherapy should be evaluated in patients. If the patient has had only cutaneous reaction, it may not be essential to start immunotherapy.

INVESTIGATIONS NEEDED FOR FURTHER MANAGEMENT

- Paired serum tryptase sample—serum tryptase taken at the time of the episode and 48–72 hours later may help to rule out systemic mastocytosis or hereditary tryptasemia.
- Skin test with the venoms or specific serum IgE levels against potentially relevant sensitivities with all commercially available bees, vespid venoms and fire ant venoms is to be done. This is essential as even if the culprit insect is identified it is essential to identify future reactions to other venoms. In any event the skin test reactivity is negative still it is essential to repeat the skin testing or use new modalities such as basophil activation test (BAT) before concluding venom immunotherapy (VIT) is not essential.
- Cross sensitization and extensive immunologic cross reactivity have been demonstrated between hornet and yellow jacket venom, and it is less among honeybee and vespid venoms. Fire ant has less cross-reactivity than other venoms. The use of component resolved diagnostics can help us to understand the phenomenon in greater depth. Component-resolved diagnostics (CRD) help us to understand the specific venom proteins which the patient is sensitized to:

Venom Immunotherapy

Venom immunotherapy (VIT) greatly reduces the risk of systemic reactions in patients with stinging insect sensitivity. The efficacy can range up to 98% and all patients who have had a systemic reaction and have demonstrable venom specific IgE are candidates for immunotherapy.

Venom immunotherapy is usually given once a week in the routine schedule beginning with doses of 0.1 μg and increased slowly to a maintenance dose of 100 μg of each venom to which they show sensitivity. It is essential that they give a written consent to the same and ask to wait for 30 minutes after receiving the immunotherapy. The dosing intervals and increments are based on the patient's need and physician discretion.

The dosage schedule for build-up phase can be done within 72 hours in ultra rush or within a week in rush therapies and maintenance dose can be given once a month or 2 months once.

Venom immunotherapy should be continued for minimum of 3–5 years and can be stopped if there are no high-risk factors such as occupational exposure, mastocytosis, lifestyle factors, and history of relapse during the treatment.

FUTURE DIRECTIONS

Though India has several cases of insect allergy, it is imperative to have studies with standardized diagnostic protocols to understand the sensitization patterns, the incidence of anaphylactic reactions for insect venom and standard of care available for the same. We further need to concentrate on standardization of the tests available to confirm the sensitization. There is also a need to develop biomarkers for the diagnosis and to understand the response to treatment. The availability of component resolved diagnostics in India needs to be utilized for better management of the above condition.

CONCLUSION

Insect venom allergy, though less common in children, can lead to significant morbidity and anxiety. Differentiating local from systemic reactions and identifying high-risk patients is crucial. Diagnostic modalities including skin testing, serum-specific IgE, and CRD guide appropriate decisions regarding VIT. VIT remains the only proven long-term preventive therapy for systemic reactions and offers excellent efficacy. Education on avoidance strategies and emergency preparedness further enhances safety.

KEY POINTS

- *Clinical spectrum:* Insect venom hypersensitivity ranges from mild local reactions to severe systemic anaphylaxis, necessitating early recognition and intervention.
- *Common culprits:* Bees, wasps, and fire ants are the most important insects implicated in systemic allergic reactions, while mosquitoes and other insects usually cause localized cutaneous reactions.
- *Diagnostic approach:* Confirmation of sensitization relies on skin testing and serum-specific IgE; advanced tools such as CRD and basophil activation tests provide deeper insights.
- *Cornerstone therapy:* Intramuscular epinephrine is the first-line treatment in systemic reactions, while *VIT* offers long-term protection with up to 98% efficacy in preventing severe recurrence.
- *Future directions:* There is an urgent need in India for standardized diagnostic protocols, epidemiological studies, and biomarker development to optimize patient care and outcomes in insect venom allergy.

SUGGESTED READING

1. Ashok N. Insect Venom Hypersensitivity. In: Gupta N, Moitra S, Nagarajan S (Eds). Comprehensive Textbook of Allergy: Striking the right balance. New Delhi: Jaypee Brothers Medical Publishers(P) Ltd; 2024. pp. 396-407.
2. Floyd ML, Adams KE, Golden DBK. Updates and Recent Advances on Venom Immunotherapy. Curr Treat Options Allergy. 2023:1-19.
3. Golden DBK, Demain J, Freeman T, Graft D, Tankersley M, Tracy J, et al. Stinging insect hypersensitivity. Ann Allergy Asthma Immunol. 2016;118(1):28-54.
4. Laha A, Sarkar T, Dey D, Mondal P, Bhattacharya S, Moitra S, et al. Assessment of Hymenoptera and Non-Hymenoptera Insect Bite and Sting Allergy Among Patients of Tropical Region of West Bengal, India. J Med Entomol. 2020;57(1):1-7.

21 CHAPTER Anaphylaxis

Jijo Joseph John, Vikram Patra

INTRODUCTION

Anaphylaxis is a sudden, severe, and potentially life-threatening systemic allergic reaction that demands immediate recognition and treatment. It is characterized by rapid onset, multi-organ involvement, and a high risk of fatality if not promptly managed. In children, food allergens are the most frequent triggers, though drugs and insect stings also play significant roles. Pediatric presentations often differ from adults, with behavioral changes and subtle cardiovascular signs sometimes preceding full-blown collapse. Early diagnosis is purely clinical, as delaying treatment to await confirmatory tests may prove disastrous. Adrenaline remains the cornerstone of therapy, supported by comprehensive post-event observation, education, and preventive strategies. A strong emphasis on awareness, timely intervention, and caregiver preparedness is vital to reducing morbidity and mortality associated with pediatric anaphylaxis.

EPIDEMIOLOGY

Worldwide Trends

Reported annual cases of anaphylaxis among children vary widely, with estimates ranging from one up to 761 per 100,000 person-years. Prevalence rates fluctuate between 0.04 and 1.8%, with food-induced anaphylaxis more frequent in children below 4 years of age. Hospital admissions among adolescents have also shown a rising trend. Cumulatively, 0.3–5.1% of the general population may experience anaphylaxis during their lifetime. Boys predominate at younger ages; however, sex differences in outcomes tend to disappear after puberty.

Indian Data

Data from Indian studies suggest annual anaphylaxis rates of 4–100 per 100,000 population, with lifetime risk estimates reaching up to 2%. Common triggers include antibiotics, analgesics, and anesthetic agents, especially in adults aged 20–40 years. Certain studies indicate a female predominance. Severe anaphylaxis is frequently characterized by cardiovascular compromise, significantly impacting prognosis.

Etiopathogenesis

Anaphylaxis results from an acute hypersensitivity reaction of the immune system, categorized into:

- *Immunoglobulin E (IgE)-mediated:* Common in children; often due to foods (e.g., milk, peanuts), drugs, or insect stings. Cross-linking of IgE on mast cells/basophils leads to the release of mediators such as histamine.
- *Non-IgE-mediated:* Agents such as contrast dyes and some medications directly activate mast cells.
- *Idiopathic:* No clear trigger is identified.

Release of vasoactive substances causes vasodilation, capillary leak, bronchospasm, and mucosal edema—resulting in the classical symptoms of anaphylaxis.

CLINICAL FEATURES

Children with anaphylaxis commonly present with:

- *Skin:* Urticaria, angioedema, and itching (seen in ~70–90% of cases).
- *Respiratory system:* Wheezing, stridor, cough, and voice changes (60–80).
- *Gastrointestinal tract:* Vomiting, cramps, and diarrhea (~30%).
- *Cardiovascular system:* Hypotension, syncope, and altered sensorium (~15–20%).
- *Behavioral changes:* Inconsolable crying and lethargy in young children.

See **Table 1** for a summary of common pediatric anaphylaxis symptoms.

TABLE 1: Common pediatric anaphylaxis symptoms.

System	*Signs/symptoms*	*Frequency (%)*
Cutaneous	Urticaria, angioedema, and itching	70–90
Respiratory	Wheeze, cough, and stridor	60–80
GI	Nausea, vomiting, and diarrhea	30
CV	Hypotension, dizziness, and syncope	15–20

TABLE 2: Differential diagnosis.

Condition	*Key features*
Angioedema	Localized swelling without urticarial—slower onset
Asthma	Isolated respiratory symptoms; usually no skin/GI involvement
Carcinoid syndrome	Flushing, diarrhea, bronchospasm but slower onset
Medullary thyroid carcinoma	Flushing diarrhea and no allergen exposure
Systemic mastocytosis	Recurrent episodes; elevated baseline tryptase
Panic attack	Tachycardia, dyspnea, no urticarial, and GI symptoms uncommon
Vasovagal syncope	Pallor, hypotension, recovery on lying down, and no urticaria

DIAGNOSIS

Clinical Identification

Diagnosis is clinical. Key diagnostic criteria include:

- Acute onset of symptoms involving skin/mucosa and respiratory compromise or hypotension.
- Rapid involvement of *two or more* systems (e.g., skin + GI + cardio) after allergen exposure.
- Drop in blood pressure after known allergen exposure (without other causes).

Laboratory/confirmatory tests: These tests support but do not confirm the diagnosis:

- *Serum tryptase:* Peaks at 1–2 hours post-onset; may remain elevated for up to 6 hours.
- *Histamine levels:* Peak early (5–15 minutes); rarely practical.
- *Specific IgE tests:* For trigger identification during follow-up (blood tests or skin prick) if IgE mediated reaction is suspected.
- *Emerging markers:* Platelet-activating factor under research.

MANAGEMENT

Indian Guidelines [Indian Academy of Pediatrics (IAP)/National Health Mission (NHM)]

- *Immediate actions:*
  - Cease exposure to suspected allergen.
  - Activate emergency medical support.
  - Assess and support airway, breathing, and circulation.
  - Place the child supine (unless contraindicated).
- *Drug therapy:*
  - *Adrenaline (epinephrine):* 0.01 mg/kg IM (maximum 0.5 mg) into the thigh; repeat every 5–10 minutes if necessary.
  - *Oxygen:* Administer via mask or nasal cannula.
  - *Fluids:* IV boluses for hypotension.
  - *Bronchodilators:* Inhaled salbutamol or nebulized adrenaline for respiratory symptoms.
- *Observation:*
  - Monitor for *minimum 4 hours* post-reaction.
  - Extend to *12–24 hours* if severe features or biphasic symptoms are present.
- *Adjunct medications:*
  - Antihistamines and corticosteroids (do *not* delay adrenaline administration).
- *Discharge planning:*
  - Educate parents/caregivers on trigger avoidance.
  - Prescribe and demonstrate *adrenaline auto-injector* use.
  - Provide a *written action plan* and consider allergy specialist referral.

International Best Practices

- Rapid intramuscular adrenaline administration is *non-negotiable.*
- Supine posture post-injection is critical to prevent sudden circulatory collapse.
- Monitoring recommendations are similar to Indian guidelines.
- *Auto-injector dosing:* 0.15 mg for 7.5–20 kg; 0.3 mg for >20 kg.

Stepwise Approach (Adapted to Indian Clinical Practice)

1. Suspect anaphylaxis based on clinical criteria.
2. Call for help and assess ABC (airway, breathing, and circulation).

3. Remove suspected allergen (if applicable).
4. Administer intramuscular *adrenaline immediately.*
5. Provide oxygen, fluids, and nebulized therapies as needed.
6. Observe for 4–24 hours depending on severity.
7. *At discharge*: Educate, prescribe auto-injector, and refer if needed.

CONCLUSION

Anaphylaxis is a pediatric emergency that demands immediate recognition and prompt intramuscular adrenaline administration. Because diagnosis is entirely clinical, clinicians, and caregivers must maintain high vigilance for subtle presentations in children. Post-event observation, education, and provision of an adrenaline auto-injector are vital to preventing future morbidity and mortality. Strengthening awareness among families, schools, and healthcare providers remains a critical step toward reducing anaphylaxis-related deaths and improving long-term outcomes.

KEY POINTS

- *Clinical diagnosis first:* Anaphylaxis is primarily a clinical diagnosis; treatment must not be delayed for investigations.
- *Adrenaline saves lives:* Intramuscular adrenaline is the first-line therapy and should be administered immediately, with repeat dosing if required.
- *Food as the leading trigger in children:* Particularly in younger age groups, food allergens (milk, peanuts, eggs, etc.) remain the most common culprits.
- *Risk of biphasic reactions:* Children must be monitored for at least 4 hours post-reaction, and up to 24 hours in severe cases, to detect delayed recurrence.
- *Preparedness and education:* Discharge planning must include parental education, prescription of adrenaline auto-injectors, and provision of a written action plan to prevent future morbidity and mortality.

SUGGESTED READING

1. Brown SG. Diagnosis and management of anaphylaxis in children. Pediatr Allergy Immunol. 2023.
2. Choudhury N, et al. Incidence, triggering factors, symptoms, and treatment of anaphylaxis. J Adv Med. 2022.
3. Gupta S, et al. Pediatric Anaphylaxis: Etiology and Predictive Factors in an Emergency Setting. Indian J Pediatr. 2021.
4. Lee S, et al. The global incidence and prevalence of anaphylaxis in children. World Allergy Organization J. 2019.
5. Medscape Reference. Anaphylaxis Differential Diagnoses. 2025.
6. Muraro A, et al. The 2020 update on anaphylaxis in paediatric population. Eur J Allergy Clin Immunol. 2021.
7. RCH Australia. Clinical Practice Guidelines: Anaphylaxis. 2020.
8. Shah A, et al. Drug-induced anaphylactic reactions in Indian population. Indian J Med Res. 2004.
9. Simons FE. Anaphylaxis in Children: Current Understanding and Key Features. Allergy Asthma Clin Immunol. 2012.
10. Turner PJ, et al. Diagnosis and management of anaphylaxis. Br Med J. 2020.

5 SECTION Special Considerations

Section Editors: Nandana Bala, Nayan Mani Deka

22 CHAPTER

Allergen Immunotherapy in Children

Nandana Bala, S Karthikeyan

INTRODUCTION

Allergic diseases affect 25% of children worldwide with prevalence rates continuing to increase. These conditions can significantly impact quality of life, academic performance, and healthcare utilization. Conventional pharmacotherapy offers symptomatic treatment but does not address the underlying immunological dysfunction driving allergic diseases.

Allergen immunotherapy (AIT) is an allergen tolerance inducing treatment for allergic diseases. It is the only specific and disease modifying treatment for allergic conditions. AIT limits allergic inflammation and in turn reduces disease severity, symptoms, medication requirements, and prevents new sensitizations. It can induce specific tolerance beyond the duration of the treatment.

Allergen immunotherapy is a safe and clinically effective treatment in carefully selected patients with aeroallergen induced immunoglobulin E (IgE)-mediated disease such as allergic rhinitis (AR)/conjunctivitis and allergic asthma and in insect venom allergy. The strongest evidence supports AIT for respiratory allergies including pollen and dust mite sensitivities while food AIT remains an emerging field with higher risks.

Treatment mainly involves either subcutaneous immunotherapy (SCIT) as the gold standard or sublingual immunotherapy (SLIT) which offers improved safety and convenience for home administration. Both require careful patient selection, comprehensive treatment safety protocols, and 3–5 years of treatment duration.

DEFINITION

Allergen specific immunotherapy (AIT or SIT) or allergen vaccination is the practice of administering to allergic subjects increasing amounts of allergens (allergenic extract or vaccine), to achieve hyposensitization, that is, to reduce the symptoms occurring due to the natural exposure to the allergen(s) itself.

BRIEF HISTORY

Allergen immunotherapy began in the first years of the twentieth century, through the subcutaneous route, based on the idea of vaccination against infectious agents. It was found to be effective in reducing symptoms of hay fever and SCIT remained standard practice. Subsequently other routes of administration were proposed to find a more convenient and safer route, and in 1986, the first randomized control trial of sublingual route (SLIT) was published and has since been extensively studied.

MECHANISM OF ACTION OF ALLERGEN IMMUNOTHERAPY

Allergy is caused by a hypersensitive immune reaction to a normally harmless substance, e.g., house dust mite or pollen. AIT works through complex immunological mechanisms to induce tolerance, modulating both innate and adaptive immune responses. It involves coordinated shift from Th2 dominated responses toward Th1 and regulatory T-cell responses accompanied by changes in tissue resident immune cells and epithelial barrier function.

Primary mechanism involves the induction of regulatory T-cells (Tregs) specifically those expressing the transcription factor FoxP3. These produce anti-inflammatory cytokines including interleukin-10 (IL-10), interleukin-35 (IL-35), and transforming growth factor-beta (TGF-β) which suppress the Th2 dominated allergic response. Tregs also suppress basophils and eosinophils and induce allergen specific regulatory B cells (B-reg cells). Breg, natural killer regulatory cells (NKreg cells) and regulatory innate lymphoid cells (ILCreg cells) contribute to induction and maintenance of allergen specific tolerance **(Fig. 1)**.

Allergen immunotherapy also promotes changes in antibody production patterns (antibody switching), inducing the production of allergen specific IgG4 antibodies, which act as blocking antibodies that compete with IgE for allergen binding, effectively reducing the allergic response. AIT influences mast cell and basophil

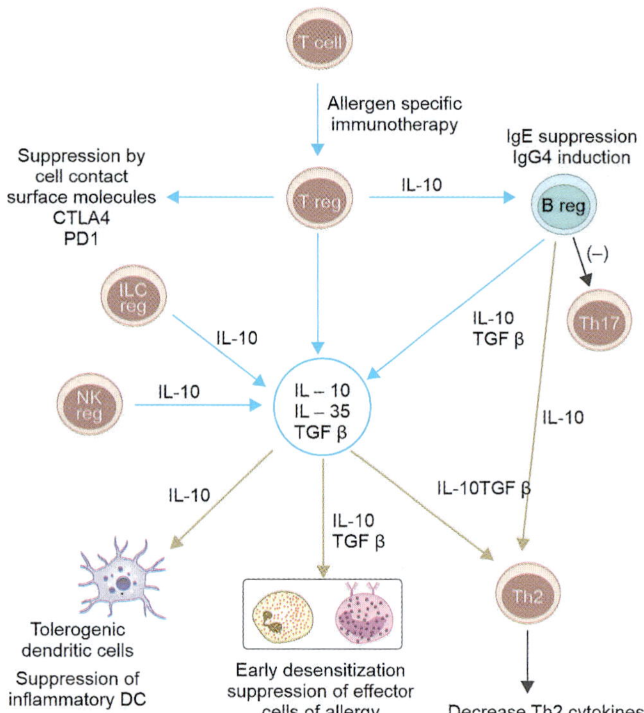

Fig. 1: Immune regulation as a consequence of AIT. (AIT: allergen immunotherapy; Treg: regulatory T cells; Breg: regulatory B cells; ILCreg: regulatory innate lymphoid cells; IL-10: interleukin 10; TGFβ: transformation growth factor β; Th2: helper T cells type 2; Th17: helper T cells type 17)

reactivity reducing their propensity to degranulate on allergen exposure.

In SLIT, the allergens are captured by antigen presenting cells in the oral mucosa and migrate to local lymph nodes where they induce regulatory responses.

The developing immune system in children pose both opportunities and challenges in AIT. Immune tolerance may be more readily achieved in younger patients whose immune systems retain greater plasticity. Children demonstrate superior long-term outcomes to AIT compared to adults.

TYPES OF ALLERGEN IMMUNOTHERAPY

Subcutaneous immunotherapy remains the most extensively studied modality with the most safety and efficacy database. It is administered via injection in a clinical setting and hence requires regular clinic visits. It uses lower allergen doses compared to SLIT.

Sublingual route has emerged as an attractive alternative to injections, particularly in children. It can be administered at home after initial supervision and has an excellent safety profile. Doses of allergens are higher.

Oral immunotherapy (OIT) is used in certain food allergies. Other modalities under investigation include epicutaneous immunotherapy, intralymphatic immunotherapy, nasal immunotherapy, and bronchial immunotherapy.

CLINICAL INDICATIONS OF ALLERGEN IMMUNOTHERAPY

The strongest evidence base for AIT is for allergic rhinoconjunctivitis, controlled allergic asthma, and insect venom allergy.

Respiratory Allergies

The strongest evidence base for pediatric AIT exists for AR with or without asthma or conjunctivitis. Pollen allergy constitutes the most well studied indication for pediatric AIT. Tree pollen, grass pollen, and weed pollen all have established efficacy profiles. Perennial allergy like house dust mite allergy has shown excellent response to AIT in children.

Atopic Dermatitis

AIT may benefit children with clear aeroallergen triggers, but evidence is still developing. The best results are seen in children with concurrent respiratory allergies.

Food Allergy

Food AIT represents an emerging field. Food AIT carries inherently higher risk due to the systemic nature of food allergic reactions and the potential for severe anaphylaxis. However, the profound nature of food allergy on children's quality of life has driven intense research interest. OIT, epicutaneous immunotherapy (EPIT), and SLIT each present distinct risk-benefit profiles. While not yet standard clinical practice in many countries, food AIT shows promise in reducing reaction severity and increasing tolerance thresholds. The Food and Drug Administration (FDA) has approved an oral immunotherapy powder for peanut OIT for children 4–17 years of age.

Ocular Allergy

Allergen immunotherapy is effective for moderate-to-severe seasonal or perennial allergic conjunctivitis, reducing symptoms and medication use, with stronger evidence for SCIT. The disease modifying benefits of AIT also help prevent progression to asthma in children with AR and conjunctivitis.

Insect Venom Immunotherapy

It is recommended after systemic reaction with insect stings like honey bee, wasp, and yellow jacket, as avoidance of stings is unpredictable. It is generally given as SCIT. It is highly effective with success rates of >95%.

SUMMARY: MAIN INDICATIONS OF ALLERGEN IMMUNOTHERAPY

Proven IgE-mediated diseases (positive skin prick test spIgE with clinical correlation) such as:

- Allergic rhinoconjunctivitis—moderate-severe intermittent or persistent
- Controlled allergic asthma
- Systemic reaction to insect bite
- Atopic dermatitis with aeroallergen sensitivity (low-level evidence)
- *Additional requirements:*
    - Symptoms of sufficient duration and severity.
    - Pharmacotherapy has been optimized.
    - Allergen avoidance is not possible or inadequate.
    - Availability of standardized allergen extracts.
    - Proven efficacy of the planned AIT for the indication and age group.

CONTRAINDICATIONS OF ALLERGEN IMMUNOTHERAPY

- *Absolute contraindications:*
    - Uncontrolled severe asthma [forced expiratory volume in 1 second (FEV_1) <70% despite treatment].
    - Malignancy
    - Children <2 years
    - Significant cardiovascular disease
    - Severe immunodeficiency
    - Active severe systemic autoimmune disease
- *Relative contraindications:*
    - β-blocker therapy
    - Cardiovascular disease
    - Human immunodeficiency virus (HIV) (asymptomatic or symptomatic; CD4 >200/μL).
    - Children 2–5 years
    - Psychiatric disorders
    - Chronic infections
    - Systemic autoimmune disorders in remission
    - Children on immunosuppressive therapy

PATIENT SELECTION CRITERIA

Appropriate patient selection is a critical determinant of AIT success and safety **(Flowchart 1)**.

- Age—5 years and older are preferred (young children may be unable to report adverse symptoms accurately). Individual circumstances may warrant earlier initiation.
- Clear demonstration of IgE-mediated sensitization [through skin prick test (SPT) and/or serum specific IgE measurement].
- Sensitization must be clinically relevant, demonstrated through controlled allergen exposure (provocation testing) or convincing clinical history.

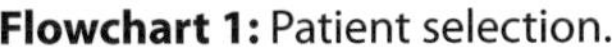

Flowchart 1: Patient selection.

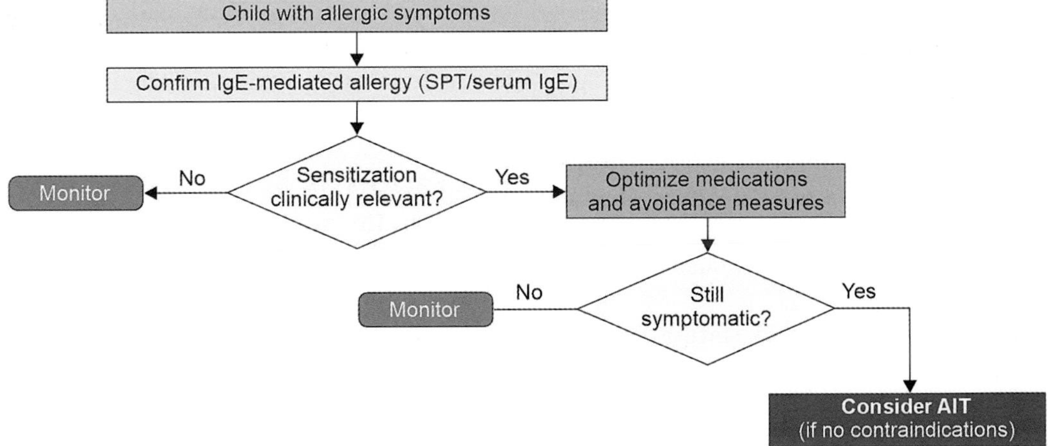

(AIT: allergen immunotherapy; SPT: skin prick test)

- Patient remains symptomatic despite optimizing pharmacotherapy and avoidance measures, interfering with sleep or daily activity.
- May be considered in less severe AR where patient wishes to take advantage of the long-term effect on AR and potential to prevent asthma, particularly with grass pollen AIT.

TREATMENT MODALITIES AND PROTOCOLS: SUBCUTANEOUS IMMUNOTHERAPY AND SUBLINGUAL IMMUNOTHERAPY

Subcutaneous Immunotherapy

Subcutaneous immunotherapy protocols typically involve a buildup phase (3–6 months), during which doses are gradually increased weekly, and a maintenance phase (3–5 years) where a stable dose is administered regularly. Gradual escalation allows immune system to develop tolerance, minimizing the risk of severe reactions. Maintenance therapy involves monthly injections for a period of 3–5 years. It is important to follow the manufacturers' instructions regarding dosing schedule.

High sensitivity cases: If local/systemic reactions occur with standard dilution, restart at higher dilution.

Accelerated updosing protocols are used for hypoallergenic extracts. Maintenance is achieved in 4 weeks. Safety and tolerability are comparable to conventional dosing.

Faster routes of reaching maintenance dose such as cluster immunotherapy and rush immunotherapy are not generally preferred in children due to the higher rates of systemic reactions.

Sublingual Immunotherapy

Systematic analysis of pediatric AIT efficacy has demonstrated comparable therapeutic benefits SCIT and SLIT. It involves placing allergen extract (drops/disintegrating tablet) under the tongue where they are absorbed. SLIT tablets have been standardized for several allergens including grass, ragweed, and house dust mites (HDM).

Advantages include improved safety profile, elimination of injection related anxiety, and convenient daily home administration. SLIT drops regimens use gradual dose escalation protocols in contrast to SLIT tablets which come as a standard dose. Total dose of allergen extract used in SLIT may be 50–100 times or more than the SCIT dose.

For children with pollen allergy, preseasonal initiation allows for immune tolerance development before natural allergen exposure.

Safety Considerations and Risk Management

Both SCIT and SLIT have been thoroughly evaluated in the pediatric population and are safe and well tolerated in children with AR and well controlled asthma.

Subcutaneous Immunotherapy

Most SCIT reactions are local in the injection site—redness, itching, swelling. Local measures such as cooling, topical corticosteroids, and oral antihistamines are helpful. Systemic reactions (asthma, angioedema, generalized urticaria, and anaphylaxis) have been described in about 0.2% of SCIT patients. Near fatal or fatal reactions are rare. SCIT injections should be administered by trained and experienced healthcare professionals in a healthcare setting equipped to treat severe anaphylaxis and patient is observed for at least 30 minutes after the injection.

Sublingual Immunotherapy

High frequency of local adverse reaction has been reported with SLIT, usually limited to the oral mucosa. Side effects such as asthma, urticaria, abdominal pain, and eosinophilic esophagitis have been reported. Anaphylaxis has been anecdotally reported and no fatality has been reported in over three decades of its use. Patients are observed for 30 minutes after administration of first dose, in a setting equipped to treat anaphylaxis. Following this, SLIT can be administered at home. Parents and caregivers must be educated regarding recognition of reactions and emergency management. SLIT is withheld during sickness like asthma exacerbation, febrile illness, gastroenteritis, and oropharyngeal infections.

Risk Factors for Systemic Reactions during Allergen Immunotherapy

- Current allergy symptoms and potential allergen exposure
- Current infections
- Mast cell disease
- Previous systemic reaction to SCIT or SLIT
- Uncontrolled or severe asthma (contraindication for AIT)

- High degree of sensitization
- β-blocker use (relative contraindication)
- High intensity physical exercise

Emergency Management Protocol

Correct and early recognition of anaphylaxis is crucial. Immediate management involves standard anaphylaxis treatment protocol, that includes injection epinephrine 0.01 mg/kg IM (maximum 0.5 mg). It is important to stop the allergen administration immediately in case of reaction.

Prevention Strategies

- *Pretreatment assessment:*
  - Confirm asthma is well-controlled
  - Check for concurrent illness
  - Review any new medications
  - Assess recent allergen exposure
- *During treatment:*
  - Use proper dilution and dosing
  - Never rush dose escalation
  - Maintain 30-minute observation period
  - Have emergency equipment readily available
- *Patient education:*
  - Recognize early warning signs
  - When to delay SLIT dosing (illness, severe asthma)
  - Proper medication technique
  - Emergency contact information

Comparison between SCIT versus SLIT is given in **Table 1**.

TABLE 1: Comparison between SCIT versus SLIT.

	SCIT	*SLIT*
Efficacy	Proven, extensive data	Comparable to SCIT
Dose requirement	Lower allergen dose	Requires about 50–100 times more allergen for equivalent efficacy; low dose SLIT ineffective
Visit requirement	Requires regular clinic visits; 30 minutes observation postinjection	First dose under supervision, followed by home administration. Supervised initiation of new vial with increased concentration of allergen during updosing
Premedication	Not routinely required	Antihistamines recommended before initiation for some products
Adverse reaction	• Mild injection site swelling or local reactions • Very safe with proper precautions • Higher risk of systemic reaction compared to SLIT	• Excellent safety profile • Local oral reactions—oral itching, tingling, mild swelling; usually resolve within 30 min–1 hour
Advantages	• Wide range of preparations • Lower dose requirement	Noninvasive home administration

(SCIT: subcutaneous immunotherapy; SLIT: sublingual immunotherapy)

Factors that Increase Clinical Efficacy of Allergen Immunotherapy

- Short duration of disease
- Early age of initiation
- Good compliance and adherence with 3–5 years of AIT
- Minor or no involvement of lower airways
- A high cumulative AIT dose.

Follow-up Schedule

- *During build-up phase:*
  - Weekly for SCIT
  - Monthly for SLIT after initial supervised period
  - As needed for concerns or reactions
- *During maintenance phase:*
  - Every 3–4 months minimum
  - Before each injection for SCIT
  - Quarterly clinical assessments for SLIT
  - Annual comprehensive reviews

Assessing Response to Allergen Immunotherapy

Primary clinical measures:

- Primary efficacy endpoints using combined symptoms and medication scores
- Standardized visual analogue scores for symptom assessment
- Validated quality of life instruments

Additional tests mainly in research: Immunological biomarkers including SPT, specific IgE, IgG4, and cytokine profiles.

Note: These may not always correlate with clinical improvement.

When to Modify Treatment

- *Dose reduction indications:*
  - Frequent large local reactions
  - Mild systemic reactions
  - Concurrent illness
  - Moving to higher allergen concentration period
- *Treatment discontinuation considerations*
  - No improvement after 12–18 months of appropriate therapy
  - Repeated severe systemic reactions
  - Development of contraindications
  - Patient/family request after thorough discussion

Duration of Allergen Immunotherapy

- Usual period of 3–5 years.
- Decision to discontinue if no clinical response by 1 year.
- Sustained clinical benefits documented up to 12 years after discontinuation.
- Persistence of benefits influenced by type of allergen extract used.

Key Considerations for Clinical Practice

- Have knowledge of aeroallergen epidemiology in your area.
- Make sure child is treated with appropriate pharmacotherapy and avoidance measures.
- Confirm allergic status by history and investigations (SPT/SpIgE).
- Careful patient selection for AIT based on indications and contraindications criteria.
- Consider AIT only for clinically relevant allergic sensitizers.
- If possible, use single allergen vaccines.
- Where there are >1 clinically relevant allergens, use maximum of three allergens.
- Select products with documented clinical evidence (safety/efficacy).
- Robust emergency preparedness protocols to be established and followed.
- Maintain treatment for at least 3 years with regular follow-up.

Long-term Clinical Effects

- Sustained clinical effect extending >10 years posttreatment.
- Reduced development of new allergen sensitization.
- Lower rates of asthma development and progression.
- Significant reduction in lifetime healthcare utilization.
- Lower rates of emergency department attendance and hospitalization.
- Reduced school absenteeism.

EMERGING THERAPEUTIC APPROACHES AND PRECISION MEDICINE

The field of AIT continues to evolve, with novel formulations and delivery methods showing promise for improved safety and efficacy profiles.

Allergoid preparations, which involve chemical modification of native allergens to reduce IgE binding while maintaining T-cell stimulation, may offer improved safety.

Recombinant allergen technology allows for standardized, consistent allergen preparations with defined molecular compositions.

Alternative delivery routes, including epicutaneous patches and intranasal administration, offer potential advantages for children.

Component-resolved diagnostics may enable more precise patient selection and personalized treatment protocols. The development of biomarkers to predict treatment response, guide dosing decisions, and determine optimal treatment duration represents a major research priority.

The future of pediatric AIT lies in personalized medicine approaches that optimize treatment selection based on individual patient characteristics. The potential for AIT to prevent the development of allergic diseases represents an exciting research frontier, with primary prevention studies targeting high-risk children before allergen sensitization occurs.

SCENARIO OF IMMUNOTHERAPY IN INDIA

India presents unique challenges and opportunities for pediatric AIT implementation.

- *Challenges:*
  - Limited availability of standardized allergen extracts

- Batch-to-batch variability in current preparations
- SLIT not yet approved by DCGI (except HDM tablet)
- Few allergologists who are trained comprehensively in AIT
- Cost considerations
- Variable healthcare infrastructure across regions

- *Opportunities:*
  - Growing awareness of allergic diseases
  - Increasing specialist training programs
  - Recent introduction of standardized HDM SLIT tablet
  - Ongoing discussions about SLIT approval pathway
  - Rising healthcare access in urban areas
- *Future directions:*
  - Anticipated approval of additional SLIT preparations
  - Development of India-specific allergen extracts
  - Quality assurance protocols

CONCLUSION

Allergen immunotherapy in children represents a therapeutic approach that extends beyond symptomatic improvement to alter the natural history of allergic disease. Current evidence strongly supports the role of SCIT and SLIT as safe and effective interventions in appropriately selected patients. SLIT offers advantage in terms of safety profile and patient acceptance. The integration of precision medicine approaches and novel delivery systems promises to further enhance the therapeutic potential of AIT. The evidence available so far clearly demonstrates that AIT can provide long-term benefits, making it an important component of pediatric allergy management.

KEY POINTS

Allergen immunotherapy represents the only disease-modifying treatment for allergic diseases. They demonstrate the following.

- *Efficacy:* Both SCIT and SLIT show significant symptom reduction and medication sparing effects.
- *Safety:* Well-established safety profiles when administered appropriately.
- *Mechanisms:* Clear understanding of tolerance induction through T-cell and B-cell modulation.
- *Real-world effectiveness:* Validation beyond controlled trial settings.
- *Future directions:* Novel approaches for enhanced safety and efficacy.

SUGGESTED READING

1. Alvaro-Lozano M, Akdis CA, Akdis M, Alviani C, Angier E, Arasi S, et al. Allergen immunotherapy in children User's Guide. Pediatr Allergy Immunol. 2020;31 Suppl 25:1-101.
2. Canonica GW, Ansotegui IJ, Pawankar R, Schmid-Grendelmeier P, van Hage M, Baena-Cagnani CE, et al. A WAO - ARIA - GA^{2}LEN consensus document on molecular-based allergy diagnostics. World Allergy Organ J. 2013; 6(1):17.
3. Durham SR, Shamji MH. Allergen immunotherapy: past, present and future. Nat Rev Immunol. 2023;23(5): 317-28.
4. Gaur SN, Kumar R, Singh AB, Agarwal MK, Arora N. Guidelines for practice of allergen immunotherapy in India: 2017 – An update. Indian J Allergy Asthma Immunol. 2017;31(1):3-33.
5. Kristiansen M, Dhami S, Netuveli G, Halken S, Muraro A, Roberts G, et al. Allergen immunotherapy for the prevention of allergy: A systematic review and meta-analysis. Pediatr Allergy Immunol. 2017;28(1):18-29.
6. Mahesh PA, Samajdar SS, Nagarajan SA, Murthy GMV, Moitra S. Immunotherapy: Current indications and recommendations in the management of ocular allergy. Indian J Ophthalmol. 2025;73(4):526-36.
7. Pajno GB, Fernandez-Rivas M, Arasi S, Roberts G, Akdis CA, Alvaro-Lozano M, et al. EAACI Guidelines on allergen immunotherapy: IgE-mediated food allergy. Allergy. 2018;73(4):799-815.
8. Pandit GS, Balachandra BV. Allergen immunotherapy practice in India. J Pediatr Pulmonol. 2023;2(Suppl 2):S129-S134.
9. Roberts G, Pfaar O, Akdis CA, Ansotegui IJ, Durham SR, Gerth van Wijk R, et al. EAACI Guidelines on Allergen Immunotherapy: Allergic rhinoconjunctivitis. Allergy. 2018;73(4):765-98.
10. Valovirta E, Petersen TH, Piotrowska T, Laursen MK, Andersen JS, Sørensen HF, et al. Results from the 5-year SQ grass sublingual immunotherapy tablet asthma prevention (GAP) trial in children with grass pollen allergy. J Allergy Clin Immunol. 2018;141(2):529-38.e13.

23 CHAPTER

Pollution and Allergy in India

Shebna A Khader

INTRODUCTION

Air pollution is a pressing public health concern in India, with significant implications for pediatric populations. According to the World Air Quality Report 2024, Indian cities continue to dominate the list of the most polluted locations globally, with Delhi being the most polluted city in 2024. Exposure to air pollution—both outdoor and indoor—poses severe risks to children's respiratory and immune health, reducing overall life expectancy by approximately 5.2 years. The complex interplay between environmental pollutants and allergic disorders has led to increasing cases of allergic rhinitis, chronic sinusitis, and other immune-mediated conditions in Indian children. This chapter explores the sources of pollution, mechanisms linking pollution to allergic diseases, and evidence-based strategies to mitigate these threats.

SOURCES OF POLLUTION

51% of India's air pollution is caused by industrial pollution, 27% by vehicles, 17% by crop burning, and 5% is indoor pollution. Indoor air pollution is a complex mixture of outdoor pollutants migrating indoor and pollutants generated indoor **(Flowchart 1)**.

Outdoor Pollutants

With fast urbanization, outdoor pollutants in India are on the rise.

Flowchart 1: Types of pollutants.

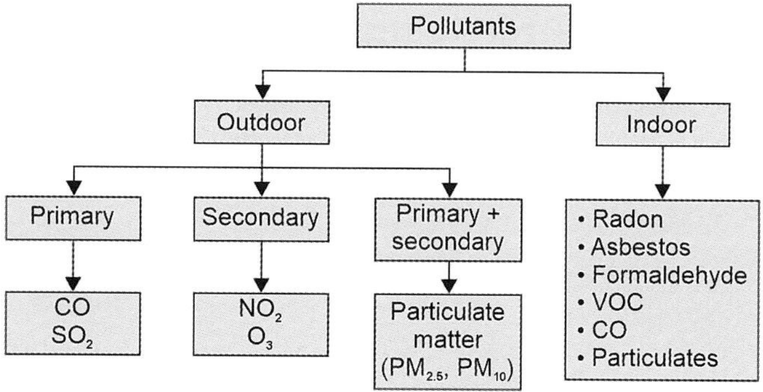

- *Industrial combustion:* CO, NO_2
- *Vehicles:* CO, PM, SO_2
- *Thermal power plant:* NO_2, SO_2, CO

Indoor Pollutants

Due to urbanization, many materials that we use indoors have been found to release pollutants.

- *Construction material:* Radon
- *Insulation:* CO, CO_2, NO_2, VOC
- *Wood compounds:* Formaldehyde
- *Air fresheners:* Fluorocarbons
- *Cleaning liquids:* VOC

There is a high level of indoor pollutants in residential areas of India from:

- Cooking using biomass fuels
- Indoor smoking
- Burning of mosquito coils (equivalent to 100 cigarettes)
- Usage of incense sticks (equivalent to 10–15 cigarettes)
- Burning of firecrackers in festival days [release black carbon, particulate matter 2.5 ($PM_{2.5}$), trace gases]
- Allergens from dust mites, fungi, cockroaches, pollens, pet dander, rodents are
- common in households.

PARTICULATE MATTER

According to Lancet Planetary Health Survey published in 2024, about 1.5 million deaths in India every year from 2009 to 2019 were potentially linked to $PM_{2.5}$ exposure. PM is a key indicator of air pollution and major determinant of indoor air quality.

Effects on human body depend on the size of PM. US Environmental Protection Agency (USEPA) has differentiated PM to three categories.

- *Course particles:*
  - PM_{10} - <10 μm
- *Fine particles:*
  - $PM_{2.5}$ - <2.5 μm
- Capable of reaching alveoli

- *Ultrafine particles:*
  - $PM_{0.1}$ - <0.1 μm
  - Can enter the circulation reaching the organs.

Particulate matter 2.5, because of its small particle size and prolonged suspension time, is mainly associated with respiratory allergies.

Sources

90% of outdoor pollution in urban areas is from diesel exhaust particles producing $PM_{2.5}$

- *Indoor sources:*
  - Biomass fuels for cooking
  - Mosquito coils
  - Smoking
- *Outdoor sources:*
  - Vehicle emission
  - Coal combustion
  - Construction emission
  - Firecrackers
  - Burning of biowaste, incineration

Effects

Particulate matter 2.5 has both biological and non-biological components. Biological components include pollen dust mite, and spores. Non biological components include carbonaceous fractions and inorganic ions (SO_4, NO_3, and NH_4 ions).

$PM_{2.5}$ affects body in multiple ways:

- Disrupts barrier function
- Alters immune balance
- Increases oxidative stress
- Synergistic sensitization effects-pollen

Particulate matter 2.5 has been found to have effects on all types of allergies because of its multiple effects on immune mechanism. It has been found to increase the risk of asthma, allergic conjunctivitis, allergic rhinitis, and urticaria in short-term exposure itself. Long-term exposure has shown to increase airway inflammation, hyperreactivity, airway remodeling. Ultrafine particulate matter has been found to enter the systemic circulation resulting in cardiovascular risks and malignancy. This health effects further stress upon the need for controlling particulate matter, both indoors and outdoors.

EFFECTS OF POLLUTION ON ALLERGY

Air pollution has been found to have a direct effect on respiratory allergies, especially in pediatric age group. The factors that make pediatric population the most vulnerable group are:

- Increased respiratory rate
- Higher minute ventilation
- Ineffective nasal filtering capacity
- Immature metabolic pathways
- In smaller kids, higher concentration of pollutants in the lower layer air they breath
- More outdoor play activities

Air Pollution Exposure on Adolescent Lungs (APEAL) study is a longitudinal prospective cohort study conducted on adolescents from four cities across India categorized by $PM_{2.5}$ levels—Delhi (very high), Mumbai, Bangaluru (high), Mysore (moderate). It has been found that symptomatic bronchial hyper responsiveness affects a substantial proportion of urban Indian adolescents and is associated with age, undernutrition, and $PM_{2.5}$ exposure.

Bronchial Asthma

Exposure to particulate matter, ozone, NO_2 can induce eosinophilic and neutrophilic inflammation resulting in onset of asthma and progression. $PM_{2.5}$ can specifically lead to asthma exacerbation due to oxidative stress, airway remodeling, and inflammation.

Allergic Rhinitis

Prenatal pollution exposure is associated with early onset of allergic rhinitis. Short-term exposure to $PM_{2.5}$, NO_2, ozone has been found to have association with emergency visits for allergic rhinitis.

Chronic Sinusitis

Recurrent or chronic exposure to particulate matter and NO_2 results in impaired epithelial barrier, oxidative stress leading on to increase in prevalence of chronic sinusitis.

Atopic Dermatitis

Particulate matter, VOC, gaseous components, and heavy metals are related to early onset atopic dermatitis and its severity.

Urticaria

Short-term exposure of ozone and particulate matter is associated with increased risk of acute urticaria, and emergency visits and chronic exposure has been found to have cumulative effect.

Food allergy: Early life exposure to pollutants results in epithelial barrier damage, increased allergen sensitization leading on to high risk for food allergy in late infancy and early childhood.

CLIMATE CHANGES AND ALLERGY

Increased prevalence of allergic airway diseases can be partially attributed to global environmental changes. The mechanism by which climate changes and air pollution impacts respiratory allergies is complimentary and interactive. Increase in CO_2, methane, and nitrous oxide, which are the important contributors of greenhouse gases are the largest drivers of global warming. Changing climate has major implications on incidence, prevalence, and severity of allergic disorders.

Mode of Impact of Climate Changes on Allergy (Fig. 1)

- Extreme rise in temperature—damages the respiratory tract epithelium and induces allergic respiratory illness.
- Thunderstorms—fragmentation of pollens and increase allergenicity.
- Flood—increase humidity and mold exposure.
- Increase in temperature and CO_2_prolonged pollination time, mold growth.
- More tendency for migration of humans and animals—exposure to new allergens.
- *Effects of climate on pollen allergy:*
  - Increase in concentration of atmospheric CO_2 may boost plant growth and pollen production.
  - Earlier flowering and prolongation of pollen season.
  - More chances for pollen dehiscence.
  - Climate changes along with pollution increase the allergenicity of pollen groups.
  - Boosts up proinflammatory and immune modulatory effects resulting in more clinical symptoms.

Various studies have been conducted in India to assess the impact of climate on pollen. A recent study in Chandigarh showed a statistically significant correlation with temperature and pollen concentration of *Parthenium* and Poaceae. A similar study was conducted comparing allergenicity of aeroallergenic plant, Cassia in industrial area, and residential area of Nagpur. It showed change in pollen morphology resulting in increased allergenicity.

As global temperature continues to rise, there is an urgent need to make population aware the effects of climate change on allergy. In addition, government agencies responsible for making policies should plan adaptation and mitigation measures.

AIR QUALITY INDEX

Air quality index (AQI) is an index developed by government agencies to indicate how polluted the air is. It transforms complex air quality data of various pollutants to a single number, commendatore and color for easy understanding of general population. It is primarily aimed to make people aware of potential health hazards, preventive measures, and pollution control. The air quality indices are different for different countries.

In India, NAQI (National Air Quality Index) was launched in New Delhi on 17 September 2014 after operation National Air Monitoring Program (NAMP) in 240 cities of the country. Continuous monitoring systems that provide data on near real time basic are installed in five cities New Delhi, Mumbai, Pune, Kolkata, and Ahmedabad.

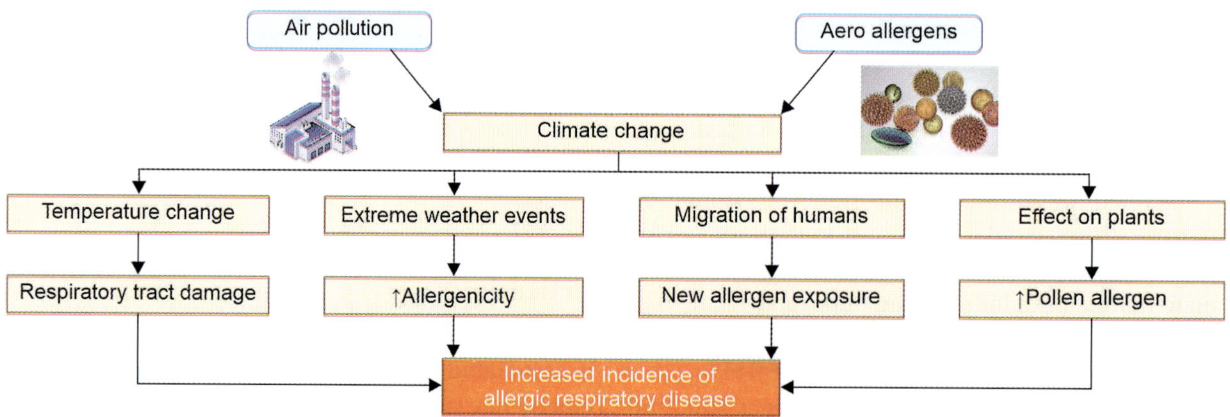

Fig. 1: Effects of climate change on allergy.

TABLE 1: National Air Quality Index (NAQI) categories.

NAQI	*Color code*	*Remarks*	*Health impact*
0–50	Green	Good	Minimal impact
51–100	Light green	Satisfactory	Minor breathing discomfort to sensitive people
101–200	Yellow	Moderate	Breathing discomfort to the people with lungs, asthma, and heart diseases
201–300	Orange	Poor	Breathing discomfort to most people on prolonged exposure
301–400	Red	Severe	Respiratory illness on prolonged exposure
401–500	Purple	Hazardous	Affects healthy people and seriously impacts those with existing diseases

National Air Quality Index has six categories (good, satisfactory, moderately polluted, poor, very poor, and severe). These categories are based on sub-index evolved for eight pollutants PM_{10}, $PM_{2.5}$, NO_2, SO_2, CO, O_3, NH_3 and Pb). Subindex is calculated for each pollutant based on short-term average values (24 hours average values for PM_{10}, $PM_{2.5}$, NO_2, SO_2, NH_3, Pb, and 8 hourly values for CO and O_3) NAQI is also presented as a remark, color code and possible health impacts for public awareness **(Table 1)**.

AIR POLLUTION CONTROL MEASURES

Indoor Air Pollution Control

According to State of Global Air (2019) report, about 846 million people of India (60% of population) were exposed to Indoor Air Pollution, Strategies for lowering indoor pollution include (1) source control, (2) increase the ventilation, (3) humidity control measures, and (4) Pollution control equipment.

Among pollution control equipment, air purifier is the best solution to improve indoor air quality.

Air Purifiers

Indoor air filtration is recommended environmental control measure of contaminants of biological and nonbiological origin. It can be done either as whole house filtration via centralized air conditioning system or potable air cleaners or a combination of the two.

The key attribute to any our filter is a balance of these three points—(1) Air flow to assure adequate ventilation; (2) efficiency to filter out small particle sizes; (3) cost-effectiveness. There are various types of air-purifiers.

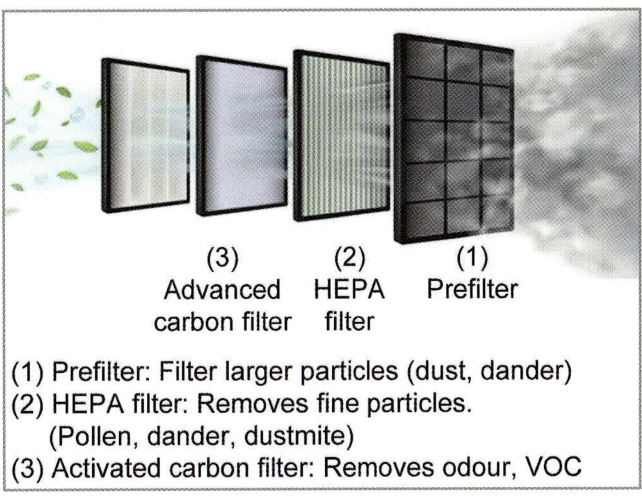

Fig. 2: Air purifier filters.

High efficiency particulate air filters: High efficiency particulate air filter (HEPA filter) can filter 0.3 μm particles. Very effective in filtering 99.97% particles if of good quality and certified. Effective against dust mite, pollen, fungus, and dander.

Activated carbon filters: Removes odor, VOC, gases by absorbing onto the surface of filters.

*Combination purifiers **(Fig. 2)**:* Most commonly available with combination of Prefilter (removing large dust), activated carbon filters, and HEPA filters.

Other types are UV light purifiers, ionizers, ozone generators which are not currently used alone for indoor pollution.

Air purifier efficiency depends on:

Clear air delivery rate (CADR): Volume of filtered air delivered by an air purifier per unit time usually measured as cubic feet/min (CFM). It is typically measured for three types of pollutants—dust, pollen, and tobacco smoke. Filtering efficacy of purifier is directly proportional to CADR value. CADR value should be equal to or >2/3 of room area in square feet.

Minimum efficiency reporting value (MERV): It means the filter's ability to capture and remove particles of various sizes from air. MERV values range from 1 to 20 and value of 14 is ideal for a clean room. MERV 13–16 is ideal for hospitals and clean rooms for allergic individuals, but moderate filtration for residential area can be achieved by MERV 5–8.

Selection of air purifier based on:

- Size of room
- Indication of using purifier (allergy or pollution)
- Cost effectiveness
- CADR
- MERV
- Noise level
- Energy efficiency
- Filter replacement

Disadvantages:

- Noise
- Not useful for some pollutants—dust mite fecal pellets, sticky cat dander
- Not useful for deposited allergens or pollutants
- Energy consumption
- Cost

Where to keep air purifier:

- Keep closer to the area where you need cleaner air
- Avoid corners of room or near walls.
- Ensure at least some space around air purifier for optimal air flow-ideal will be a central location.
- Keep the purifier elevated if it is a small unit as it helps circulate air more effectively.
- Higher fan setting improves air circulation but increases energy consumption.
- Keep windows closed or keep open only intermittently.

Plant Air Purifiers

Indoor plants have some effect in reducing air pollution by absorbing.

For example,

- Money plant (ozone)
- Cacti (VOC)
- Rubber palm (formaldehyde)
- Spider plant (carbon monoxide)

Other Measures to Reduce Indoor Pollution

- Choosing furniture with less chemical emissions
- Evaluating home systems regularly
- Ventilating home frequently
- Avoid biomass fuels
- Improve efficiency of gas stoves
- Dust mite, mold, and cockroach control measures

Measures to Reduce Outdoor Pollution

- Close fitting particulate respirators/N95 masks
- Reduce motorized transport
- Optimize driving style
- Check air quality and periodic adoption of preventive measures

Most sources of outdoor pollution are well beyond the control of individuals and demand local, regional policymakers in sectors such as energy, transport, waste management, urban planning, and agriculture. Government agencies responsible should introduce preventive measures which are crucial to limit the environmental changes as it is the right of each human being to breath clean air.

NATIONAL CLEAN AIR PROGRAM

Multisectoral public health approach is essential in controlling air pollution. National Clean Air Program (NCAP) is program launched by Government of India in 2019. It emphasizes a multi-sectorial approach, city-specific action plane with collaboration between central, state government agencies, local bodies, and other stakeholders. The target on initial introduction was to deduce $PM_{2.5}$ and PM_{10} in cities by 20–30% by 2024. This has been now revised to 40% reduction of PM_{10} by 2025–26. NCAP is a continuous effort, and success depends on sustained commitment.

CONCLUSION

Air pollution is to be considered as a public health emergency. It has effects on triggering allergic response, progression of allergic symptoms and increases the chances of long-term complications. $PM_{2.5}$ is a key indicator of air pollution. It affects human body in multiple ways directly and indirectly. Indoor air pollution is a major cause of allergic respiratory symptoms especially in India. National air quality index has to be monitored, and policies made to control air pollution thereby improving the quality of life and life expectancy of Indian population.

KEY POINTS

- *India's cities among the most polluted globally:* In 2024, 13 out of the world's 20 most polluted cities are in India, highlighting the severe impact of air pollution on public health, especially children.
- *Sources of pollutants:* Outdoor pollutants such as industrial combustion generate gases such as carbon monoxide (CO) and nitrogen dioxide (NO_2), while indoor sources—construction materials, air fresheners,

and particulate matter ($PM_{2.5}$)—significantly contribute to household air pollution.

- *Particulate matter and health effects:* Fine particles ($PM_{2.5}$, diameter <2.5 µm) penetrate deeply into the lungs, disrupting epithelial barrier function and altering immune balance. These changes have been associated with increased prevalence of allergic rhinitis and chronic sinusitis in children.
- *Impact on allergy patterns:* Pollution leads to earlier flowering and prolongation of pollen seasons, aggravating allergy symptoms and increasing the burden of allergic diseases among Indian pediatric patients.
- *Mitigation and monitoring:* Initiatives such as the NAQI launched in 2014, along with technological interventions such as HEPA filters and continuous air quality monitoring systems in major cities (Delhi, Mumbai, Pune, Kolkata, and Ahmedabad), support primary prevention and management of pollution-induced allergies.

SUGGESTED READING

1. Dubey S, Rohra H, Taneja A. Assessing effectiveness of air purifiers (HEPA) for controlling indoor particulate pollution. Heliyon. 2021;7(9):e07976.
2. Kurmi OP, Adhikari TB, Tyagi SK, Kallestrup P, Sigsgaard T. Addressing air pollution in India: Innovative strategies for sustainable solutions. Indian J Med Res. 2024;160(1):1-5.
3. Lai A, Owens K, Patel S, Nicholas M. Impact of air pollution on atopic dermatitis; A comprehensive review. Curr Allergy Asthma Rep. 2023;23(8):435-42.
4. Mahesh PA, Kaleem Ullah M, Greeshma MV, Patil S, Samdarshi P, Veerabhadraiah H, et al. Prevalence of Asymptomatic Bronchial Hyperresponsiveness in Indian Adolescents: Insights From the APEAL Study. Clin Exp Allergy. 2025;55(9):795-807.
5. Singh AB, Mathur C. Climate change and pollen allergy in India and South Asia. Immunol Allergy Clin North Am. 2021;41(1):33-52.
6. Zhang ZQ, Li JY, Guo Q, Li YL, Bao YW, Song YQ, et al. Association between air pollution and allergic upper respiratory diseases; a meta-analysis. Eur Respir Rev. 2025;34(176):240256.

24 CHAPTER Climate Changes and Allergies

R Prasanna

INTRODUCTION

Over the past 60 years, there has been a significant global rise in the prevalence of asthma. There are 300 million asthmatics worldwide, with 37.9 million living in India. 10% of people aged 0–18 develop asthma and allergic rhinitis (AR), according to a national epidemiological survey. In 2022, the report by Intergovernmental Panel on Climate Change Sixth Assessment confirmed that climate change poses a direct threat to respiratory health, especially asthma.

Since 1950, the world has been seeing an increase in global temperatures and so has global warming. Greenhouse gases namely carbon dioxide (CO_2), methane and other gases such as nitrous oxide, and fluorinated gases have increased since the industrial revolution. More excess heat is being trapped in the atmosphere as a result of these industrial activities. The current temperature is about 1°C warmer than it was before the industrial revolution. They are on the increase and they pose a constant threat.

HOW CLIMATE CHANGES AFFECT ALLERGIC BARRIER

Over the years, heat waves are more intense and prolonged in Europe, Africa, Australasia, and Americas and have been responsible for causing extreme temperatures. Apart from heat waves, air pollution; sand, dust storms, and wildfires are considered as a risk for respiratory and skin allergies from the young to old age uniformly. This increase in temperature can disrupt the epithelial barriers of the skin and respiratory tracts, both directly and indirectly through climatic exposures.

When epithelial cells are damaged, they release alarmins that trigger a type 2 immune response, leading to inflammation. Additionally, cytokines and chaperones that become active in this process stimulate cholinergic responses. These immune and environmental interactions contribute to the rising incidence of asthma, AR, and atopic dermatitis (AD).

Evaporation is reduced, and the temperature feels higher than it actually is when high temperatures and high humidity are combined; this phenomenon is known as the "wet-bulb temperature". Generally speaking, 35°C is regarded as the minimum temperature required for human survival. Mortality and morbidity will rise as a result of the human body's inability to adjust to wet-bulb temperatures above 35°C. Increasing data shows that heat waves, cold spells, dust storms, hurricanes, floods, and storm surges increase asthma-related outcomes.

The respiratory epithelial barrier is a very thin physical barrier that has antibacterial and mucociliary cleansing properties. A pseudostratified columnar ciliary epithelium with goblet and basal cells lines the conductive portion of the nasal cavity that extends from the nasal cavity to the bronchi, while stratified squamous epithelium lines the anterior portion of the nasal cavity. Clara cells, also known as nonciliary cubic cells, cover the terminal bronchi. The two main cell types—(1) type 1 pneumocytes (thin, flattened simple squamous cells) and (2) type 2 pneumocytes (cuboidal cells) that line the alveoli are responsible for gas exchange. The respiratory tract of humans therefore contains a diverse representation of epithelial cells.

Secretory goblet cells join ciliated cells to form a physical barrier against outside agents by adhering to one another through tight junctions (TJ). They make up the zonula adherens, along with the adherens junctions beneath them. This is how the coordinated action of cilia mediates the cephalic propulsion of tracheobronchial secretions. Here, epithelial cells express neural transient receptor potentials (TRPs), which control barrier permeability. In certain clinical condition, the integrity of the epithelial barrier is compromised by increased expression of a specific TRP known as TRP vanilloid 1 (TRPV1) **(Fig. 1)**.

Atopic dermatitis patients have a compromised skin barrier, which makes it possible for allergens and air

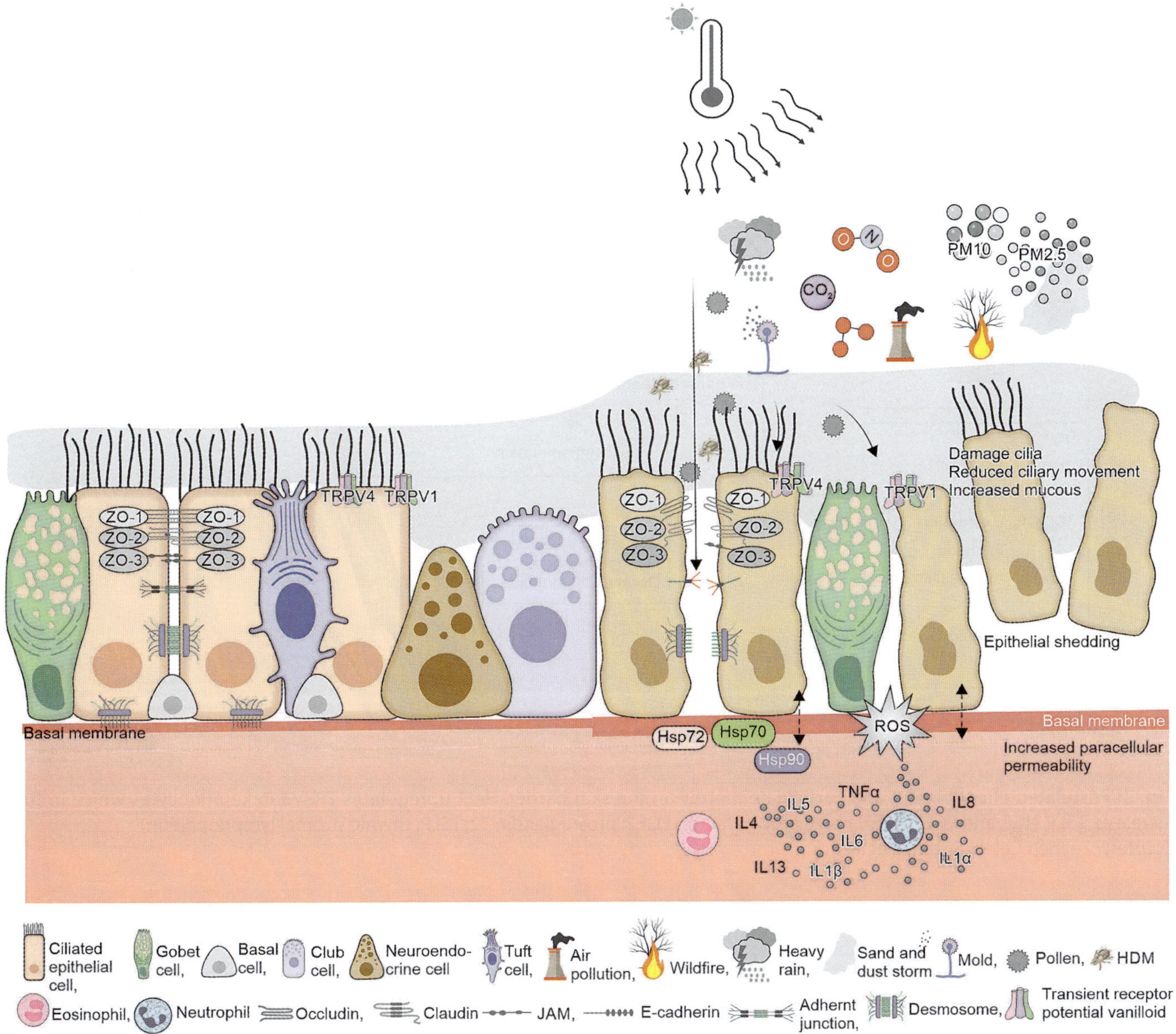

Fig. 1: The left side of the figure illustrates the airway epithelial barrier and how its integrity is maintained by tight junction proteins (ZO-1, occludin, claudin, and JAM), adherens junctions (E-cadherin), and desmosomes along the basal membrane. Right side of the diagram represents the respiratory epithelium on exposure to environmental insults, leading to loss of ciliary function, epithelial shedding, increased mucus secretion, and disruption of paracellular permeability. Stress proteins (Hsp70, Hsp90, and Hsp72) and inflammatory mediators including TNF-α, IL-6, IL-8, IL-13, IL-33, and IL-1β are released, leading to recruitment of eosinophils and neutrophils. (IL: interleukin; TNF-α: tumor necrosis factor-alpha)
Courtesy: Zeynep Çelebi Sözener et al.

pollutants to enter the body and sets off a classical type 2 immune response. Heat triggers keratinocytes to activate thymic stromal lymphopoietin 3 (TRPV3), which raises thymic stromal lymphopoietin (TSLP) and nerve growth factor (NGF). In AD, TRPV3 expression and function are elevated.

There are multiple hypothesized effects of particulate matter (PM) in AD **(Fig. 2)**:

- Modified expression of TJ and stratum corneum proteins
- This gene variant of aldo-keto reductase 1C3 (AKR1C3) is overexpressed.

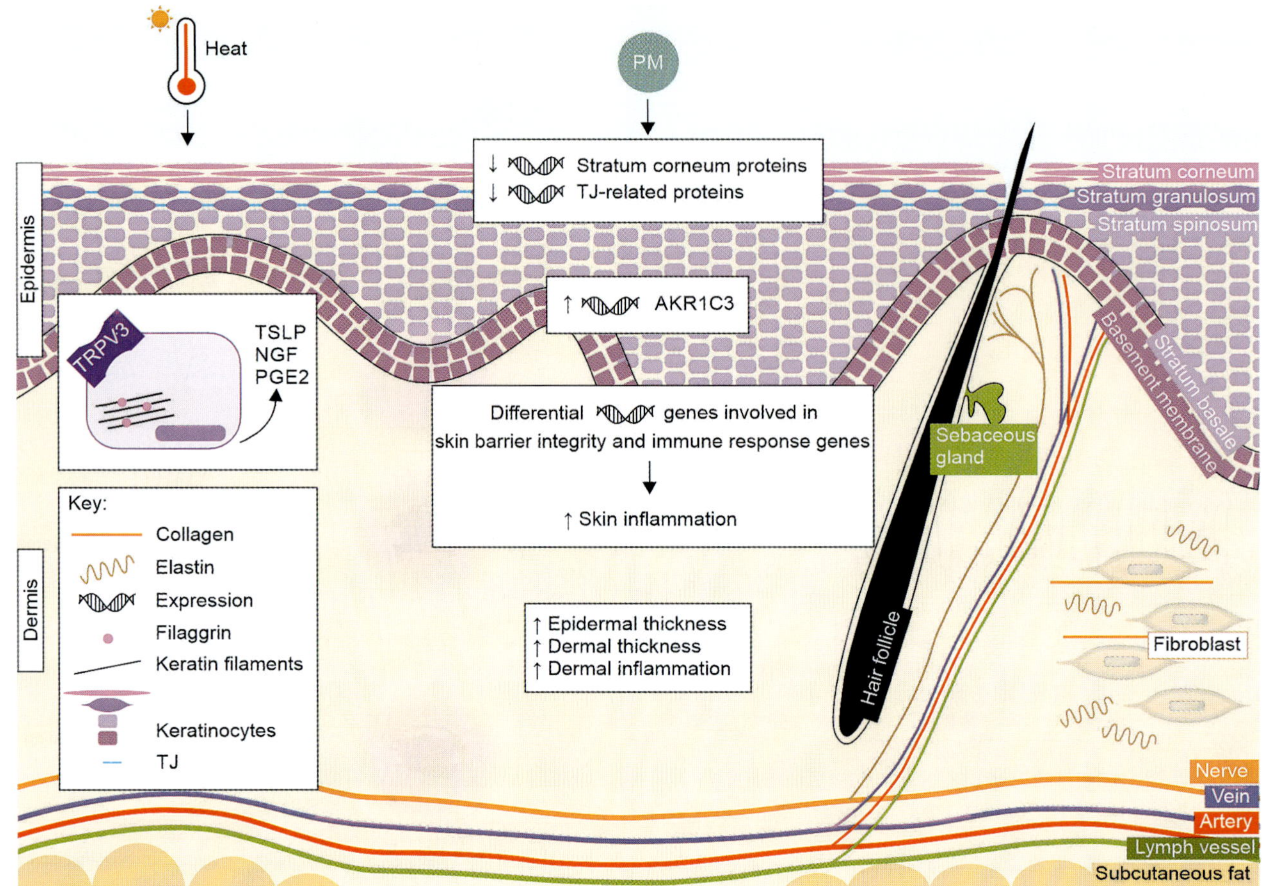

Fig. 2: Postulated effect of heat and particulate matter on the skin barrier. Heat upregulates TRPV3 in keratinocytes which in turn increases TSLP, NGF, and PGE2. (NGF: nerve growth factor; PGE2: prostaglandin E2; TSLP: thymic stromal lymphopoietin)
Courtesy: Zeynep Çelebi Sözener, et al.

- Differential expression of other genes controlling skin barrier integrity and immune response, causing an increase in skin inflammation
- This leads to increased epidermal and dermal thickness and increased dermal inflammation. *NGF*, *PGE2*, and TRPV.

Heat Wave

Excessive heat impairs the thermoregulatory system, by raising tidal volume, respiratory rate, and the systemic inflammatory response. According to animal models, heat stress directly affects the epithelial barrier by raising TJ permeability, downregulating the functional protein zonula occludens, and upregulating the structural protein occludin. In ciliated respiratory epithelial cells, it was discovered that a rise in temperature increased the ciliary beat. According to another study, the cilia in the airway cells exhibited normal motility between 20°C and 45°C, but decreased motility above 45°C. According to a recent meta-analysis, extreme heat has a major impact on asthma flares. Sensory fibers of vagal nerves, composed of unmyelinated afferent fibers expressing neural TRP channels, innervate the respiratory tract. The TRP receptors, which are particularly sensitive to high temperatures (TRPV1 and TRPV4) are activated when hot air is inhaled. Patients in AR and asthma have overexpressed TRPV1 which are activated by chemical mediators during chronic airway inflammation. Hot and humid air when inhaled, increased the risk of developing AR and asthma because it activates bronchopulmonary vagal C fibers, which upregulates TRPV1 and TRPV4, enhancing cholinergic responses, and increases airway resistance and thereby causing reflex bronchoconstriction **(Fig. 3)**.

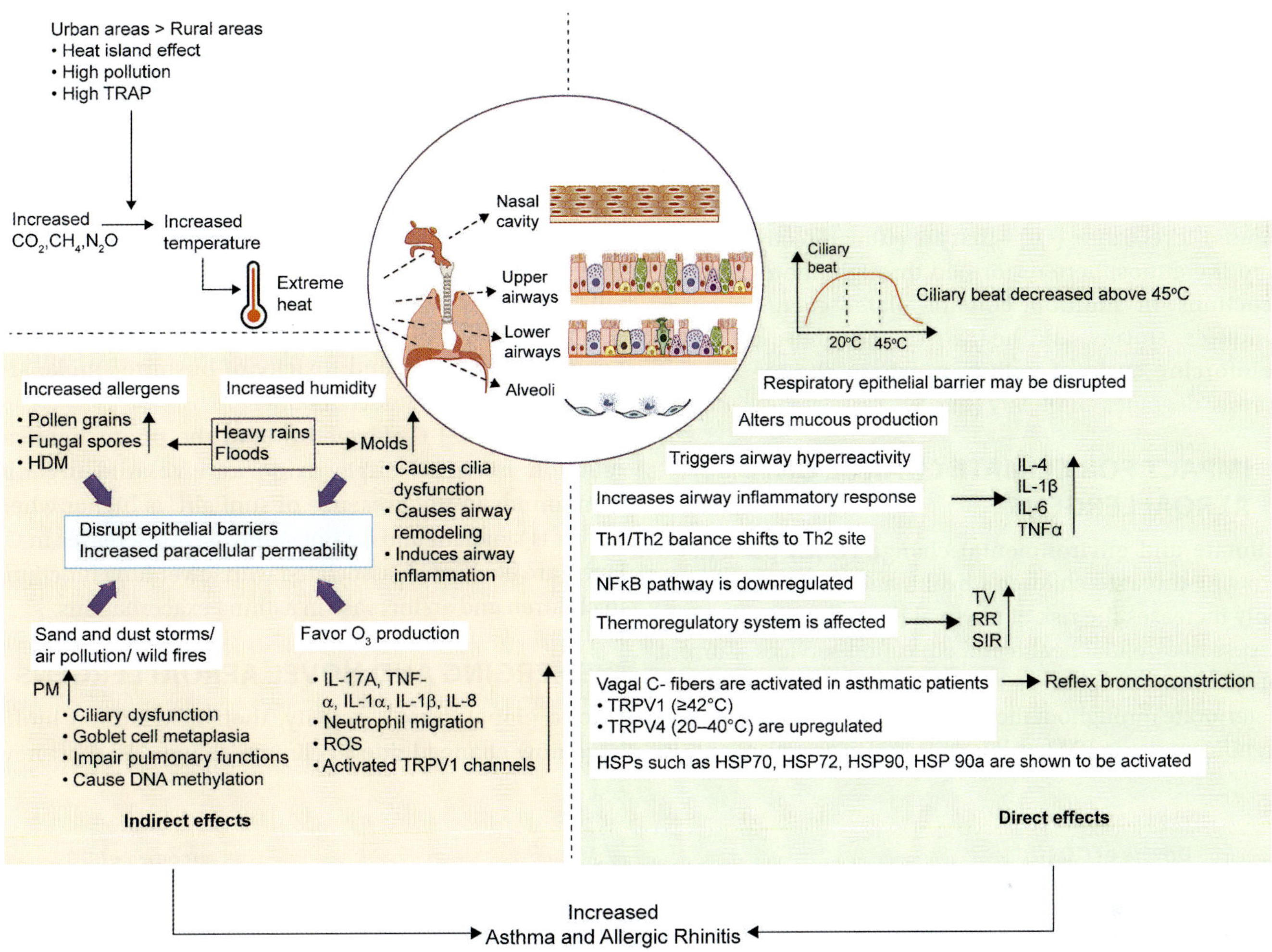

Fig. 3: Indirect and direct effects of extreme heat on respiratory epithelial barrier.
Courtesy: Zeynep Çelebi Sözener et al.

Air Pollution, Sand and Dust Storms, and Wildfires

Air pollution and climate change have an impact on allergic disease morbidity and mortality. The effects of smaller particles of size 2.5 mm or less (PM2.5) are amplified by increased solar activity, which results in decreased forced vital capacity (FVC) and forced expiratory volume (FEV1). Certain DNA methylation patterns in nasal epithelial cells caused by wildfires can impact the TH1 and TH2 pathways. Because wildfires absorb CO_2 from the atmosphere and produce particulate substances such as dust storms, they can also devastate ecosystems. Extremely powerful winds known as "dust storms" expose large areas to particles. Both immediate and long-term consequences resulting from these storms have large-scale and localized impacts on air quality.

Following three studies showed the effects of PM on the skin:

1. In animal models, it has been found that exposure to PM (<10 mm) worsens skin inflammation via the differential expression of genes controlling skin barrier integrity and immune response.
2. Several stratum corneum and TJ-related protein expression levels are decreased by PM in a mouse model of oxazolone-induced AD of skin and human keratinocyte cells.
3. In the GINIplus/LISA birth cohort, a gene variant of AKR1C3 is highly expressed. This manifests in human skin occurs as a result of exposure to PM.

CLIMATE CHANGE AND POLLUTION INHALATION—A NEXUS

The increasing concentration of greenhouse gases and continued reliance on fossil fuels has led to worsening air quality and accelerated climate change **(Fig. 4)**. Air pollution refers to a mix of particles and gases—such as ground-level ozone (O_3)—that are either directly released into the atmosphere or formed through photochemical reactions. In addition, climate-related events such as wildfires, storms, and heatwaves contribute to a self-reinforcing cycle of pollution, where climate change further degrades air quality **(Fig. 5)**.

IMPACT FOR CLIMATE CHANGE ON AEROALLERGENS

Climate and environmental change (CEC) presents a growing threat to children's health and well-being. It not only increases the risk of physical harm but also disrupts access to essential health and education services. Current projections suggest that air quality will continue to deteriorate throughout the 21st century. Notably, the most significant rise in PM levels is expected to occur not only in densely populated regions, but also in areas near 60° south latitude—raising concerns about the global reach and impact of air pollution linked to environmental change.

In equatorial regions, specific humidity rises, whereas in densely populated areas, nitric oxide levels rise. In many countries, bushfire smoke is being inhaled by a growing percentage of the population. With forecasts indicating that the dense smoke haze over the capital cities during recent devastating fire seasons will become the norm, CEC is likely to make this worse. The harmful health mechanisms and toxicity of bushfire smoke are surprisingly poorly understood.

Surface level O_3 formed due to the photochemical reaction between nitric oxide and volatile organic compounds in the presence of sunlight, is higher when the air is stagnant and on hot sunny days. Increases in O_3 levels are likely to be associated with lower lung functions in children and an increase in asthma exacerbations.

EMERGING AND NOVEL AEROALLERGENS

Due to global human activity, their distribution limits have now changed due to climate change. In their new

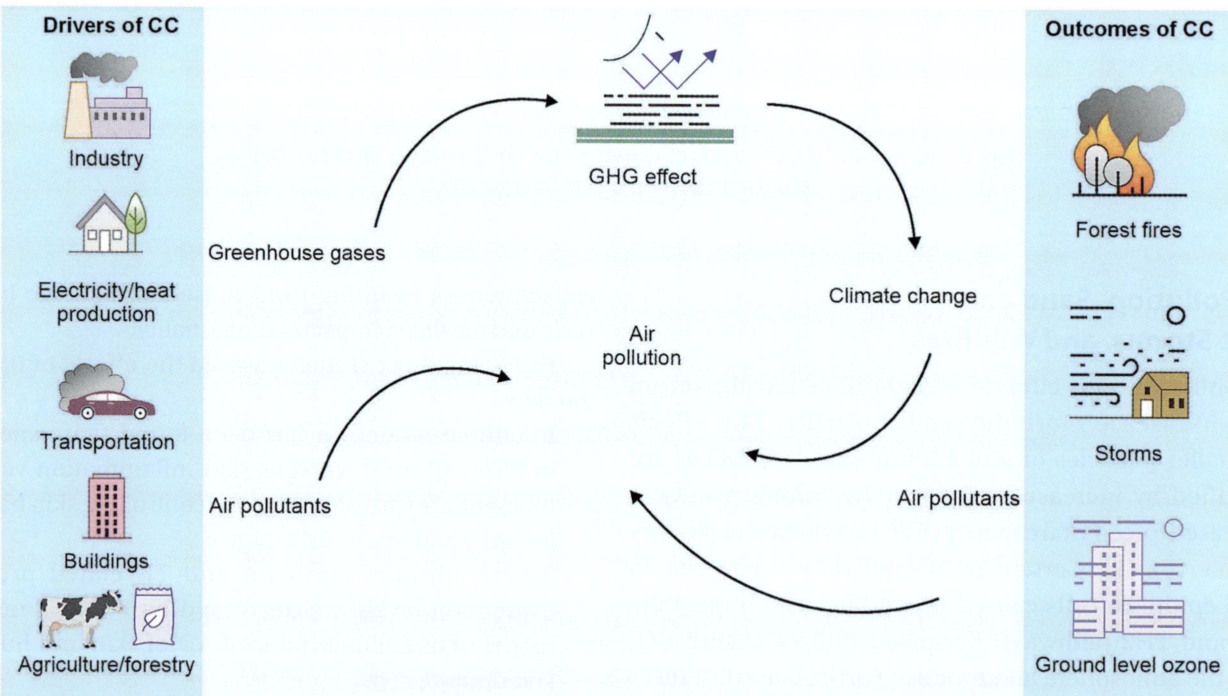

Fig. 4: Relationship between climate change and air pollution.
Source: Pacheco SE, Guidos-Fogelbach G, Annesi-Maesano I, Pawankar R, D' Amato G, Latour-Staffeld P, et al. Climate change and global issues in allergy and immunology. J Allergy Clin Immunol. 2021;148(6):1366-77.

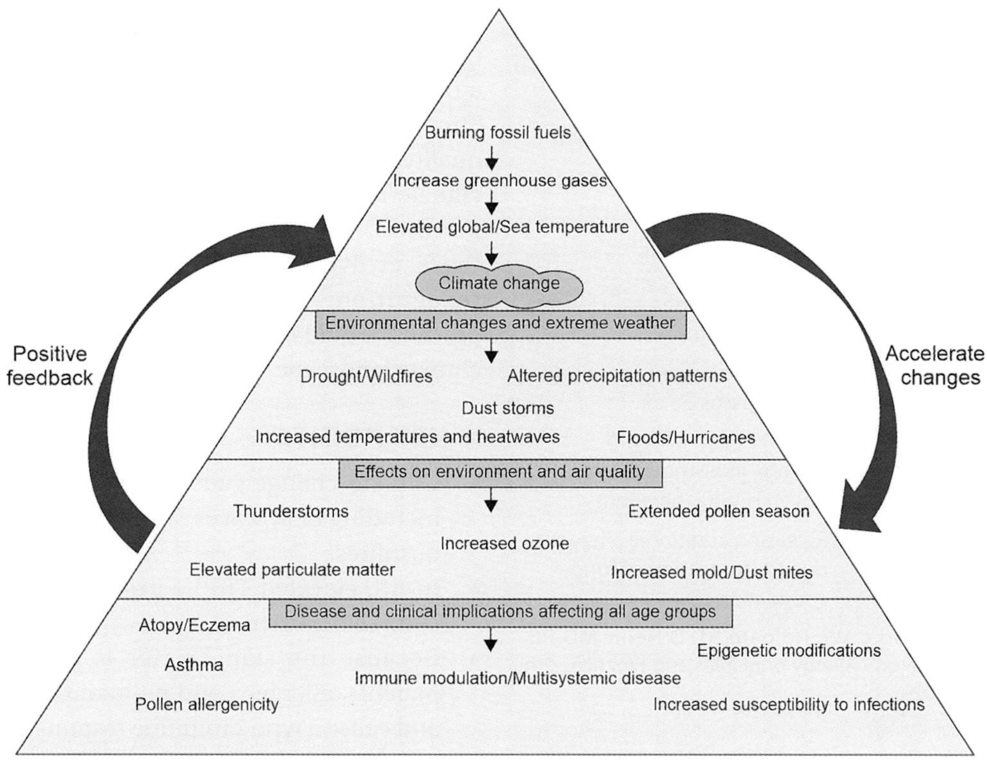

Fig. 5: How ripple effect from climate change causes disease and its clinical consequence.
Source: Pacheco SE, Guidos-Fogelbach G, Annesi-Maesano I, Pawankar R, D' Amato G, Latour-Staffeld P, et al. Climate change and global issues in allergy and immunology. J Allergy Clin Immunol. 2021;148(6):1366-77.

environments, many plants are now able to reproduce freely, primarily by seed dispersal or artificial planting. *Ambrosia, Ailanthus, Broussonetia, Cupressus arizona,* and *Cannabis,* for instance, may have pollen that is a novel or developing aeroallergen in the area. The pollen of a number of these species has been introduced to various regions of the world and has been identified as allergenic. Pollen grains and fungal spores are examples of aeroallergens that have been shown to be bioindicators of climate change. For prompt identification and the application of suitable mitigation techniques, focused research and the development of easily accessible databases on these novels or developing aeroallergens are crucial. The pollen taxa *Olea* and *Quercus* in southern Europe, *Betula* and *Poaceae* in central and northern Europe, and *Ambrosia* and Cupressaceae in North America have all been the subject of research. According to studies, a variety of stimuli, including rising temperatures and pollutants—specifically, NO_2 for Betula and CO_2 for *Ambrosia*—can raise the expression of aeroallergens. Additionally, microorganisms such as fungi and bacteria increase the pollen grains' ability to produce airborne allergens. Numerous studies indicate that pollen seasons are generally getting longer, which lengthens the time that allergy sufferers may be at risk from pollen.

The **Table 1** summarizes the overview of the effects of climate change and pollution on allergen and pollen-related allergenicity.

IMPACT OF GLOBAL WARMING ON AERO-ALLERGY—INDIAN SCENARIO

Due to the growing urbanization, air pollution, and global warming, development of new aeroallergens is emerging in recent decades. Global burden of disease data analysis has reported >1 million premature deaths due to air pollution in 2015 in India. The Asia Pacific Association of Allergy, Asthma, and Clinical Immunology (APAAACI) white paper has highlighted the impact of air pollution (both outdoor and indoor) and global warming on aeroallergies. Global warming is associated with increase in CO_2

TABLE 1: Effects of climate change and pollutants on allergens and pollen-related allergenicity.

Pollutants	*Climate change*
Pollution amplifies allergenicity by acting as adjuvants	Extended duration of pollen seasons
Altered expression of allergens in pollen grains	Increased production of pollens
Increased allergen concentration in pollen grains	Increased allergen expression in pollen grains
Increased pollen protein expression with possibility of generating new allergens	Increased allergen content in pollen grains
Post translational modification of pollen allergens	Change in distribution of pollen producing agents
Increased antigen presentation	Releasing additional allergens due to stimulation of fungal sporulation.

Source: Adapted from Burks AW, Holgate ST, O'Hehir MD RE, Bacharier LB, et al. Middleton's Allergy principles and Practice., 9th edition. USA: Elsevier; 2020.

concentration, pollen production, allergen potency, and premature onset as well as extended pollen season. Larger wheals are induced in skin prick test by pollen from birch trees which are exposed to higher O_3 levels than by pollen exposed to lower O_3 levels, indicating that O_3 may increase the allergenicity of any pollen. About 23% of asthma ER visits in India were linked to O_3, 30% to PM2.5 (PM with a diameter of 2.5 μm or less), and 15% to NO_2. According to estimates, 57% of children nationwide suffer from asthma, which may be brought on by PM2.5. In vulnerable people, 85 PM2.5, O_3, NO_2, and SO_2 can worsen airway inflammation, leading to increased allergen permeability into mucous membranes and improved interaction with immune cells.

CONCLUSION

Climate change has emerged as a major amplifier of allergic diseases, acting through rising temperatures, worsening air quality, altered aeroallergen patterns, and disruption of epithelial barrier integrity. Heat waves, PM, wildfires, and changing pollen dynamics interact to enhance allergenicity, prolong pollen seasons, and increase susceptibility to asthma, AR, and AD. Evidence clearly shows that epithelial barrier dysfunction—both cutaneous and respiratory—forms a central link between environmental stressors and type 2 immune responses.

For India, the combined burden of rapid urbanization, escalating pollution levels, and emerging novel aeroallergens places children at particular risk. Strengthening environmental surveillance, improving air-quality mitigation strategies, and raising awareness about climate-related health hazards are essential public health priorities. As pediatricians and allergists, understanding these evolving environmental drivers allows timely recognition, early management, and appropriate preventive guidance for allergic disorders in the changing climate landscape.

KEY POINTS

- Climate change causes atopy in a number of ways, including heat waves, air pollution, sandstorms, and bushfires.
- In AR, elevated TRPV1 expression compromises the epithelial barrier.
- Because the skin barrier is compromised in AD patients, allergens and pollutants can enter the body and cause a type 2 immune response.
- Aeroallergens can rise in response to a variety of stimuli, including rising temperatures and pollutants, and are bioindicators of climate change.
- Pollution and change in climate can coexist, creating a domino effect that raises the incidence of atopy.
- Pollen production, allergen potency, pollen release, and pollen dispersion may all be improved by global warming linked to rising CO_2 concentrations.

SUGGESTED READING

1. Aghapour M, Ubags ND, Bruder D, Hiemstra PS, Sidhaye V, Rezaee F, et al. Role of air pollutants in airway epithelial barrier dysfunction in asthma and COPD. Eur Respir Rev. 2022;31:210112.
2. Goldizen FC, Sly PD, Knibbs LD. Respiratory effects of air pollution in children. Paediatric Pulmonol. 2016;51;94-108.
3. Kaushik MS, Chakraborty S, Veleri S, Kateriya S. Mucociliary respiratory epithelium integrity in molecular defense and susceptibility to pulmonary viral infections. Biology. 2021;10:95.
4. Pacheco SE, Guidos-Fogelbach G, Annesi-Maesano I, Pawankar R, D' Amato G, Latour-Staffeld P, et al. Climate change and global issues in allergy and immunology. J Allergy Clin Immunol. 2021;148(6):1366-77.
5. Shaheen S, Maqbool K, Beg OA, Gul F. Thermal analysis of airway mucus clearance by ciliary activity in the presence of inertial forces. SN Appl Sci. 2021;3:1-11.

6. Silverman HA, Chen A, Kravatz NL, Chavan SS, Chang EH. Involvement of neural transient receptor potential channels in peripheral inflammation. Front Immunol. 2020;11:590261.
7. Urrutia-Pereira M, Badellino H, Ansotegui IJ, Guidos G, Solé D. Climate change and allergic diseases in children and adolescents. Allergol Immunopathol (Madr). 2022;50(S Pt 1):7-16.
8. Wolf J, O' Neil NR, Rogers CA, Muilenberg ML, Ziska LH. Elevated Atmospheric Carbon dioxide concentrations amplify Alternaria alternata sporulation and total antigen production. Environ Health Perspect. 2010;118:1223-8.
9. World Health Organization. (2021). New WHO Global Air quality guidelines. News release.[Online] Available from https://www.who.int/news/item/22-09-2021-new-who-global-air-quality-guidelines-aim-to-save-millions-of-lives-from-air-pollution [Last accessed December, 2025].
10. Çelebi Sözener Z, Treffeisen ER, Özdel Öztürk B, Schneider LC. Global warming and implications for epithelial barrier disruption and respiratory and dermatologic allergic disease. J Allergy Clin Immunol. 2023;152(5):1033-46.

25 CHAPTER

Allergy and Infections: Intertwined Pathways and Clinical Implications

Nayan Mani Deka

INTRODUCTION

Allergic diseases and infectious illnesses have traditionally been perceived as distinct clinical entities. Allergy involves an exaggerated immune response to typically harmless environmental antigens, whereas infection results from pathogenic invasion by viruses, bacteria, fungi, or parasites. However, recent advancements in immunology and epidemiology reveal a complex interplay between these two domains. Increasing attention is being paid to how infections in early-life influence immune system maturation, and consequently, the development of allergic conditions such as asthma, atopic dermatitis, and allergic rhinitis. Over the last decades, the importance of microbes, especially the role of the early-life gut microbiota, in immune development and tolerance, including its role in allergy, has been extensively acknowledged.

The modern environment, characterized by urban living, improved sanitation, and widespread vaccination, has significantly reduced the infectious disease burden. Simultaneously, there has been a dramatic rise in allergic diseases, particularly in industrialized countries—a trend suggesting that reduced microbial exposure might contribute to allergy pathogenesis. The hygiene hypothesis and its extensions, including the microbial and "old friends" hypotheses, propose that a lack of exposure to diverse microorganisms during early-life results in immune dysregulation.

Three major concepts anchor this discussion—(1) the hygiene hypothesis, which explains the increase in allergies as a result of reduced microbial exposure; (2) the viral trigger theory, which implicates specific viruses in the initiation and exacerbation of allergic disease; and (3) the evolving understanding of infection-allergy balance, which emphasizes the timing, type, and context of infectious exposures in determining allergic outcomes.

EPIDEMIOLOGY

The global burden of allergic diseases has witnessed a dramatic rise over the past few decades, with asthma, allergic rhinitis, and atopic dermatitis now recognized as major public health concerns. According to the Global Asthma Report 2018, asthma affects over 339 million people worldwide. The prevalence of allergic rhinitis is estimated at 10–30% globally, and atopic dermatitis affects up to 20% of children in developed countries. The upward trajectory of allergic diseases parallels urbanization, westernization of lifestyles, reduced family sizes, antibiotic overuse, and diminished microbial exposures.

India reflects this global trend with regional variability. Data from the ISAAC Phase III study (2001–2003) showed a prevalence of current wheeze in children aged 6–7 years at 5.35%, with some cities like Bangalore reporting rates as high as 9.1%. Follow-up studies indicate continued rise in urban areas. A 2020 ICMR survey reported that nearly 10–15% of Indian school children show features of allergic rhinitis, while atopic dermatitis is being increasingly recognized in pediatric dermatology clinics.

Interestingly, in rural and semi-urban populations, where the burden of infections—particularly parasitic and bacterial—is higher, the prevalence of allergic conditions remains lower. This inverse correlation has been consistently observed in comparative studies and is one of the primary epidemiological pillars supporting the hygiene hypothesis. The diversity of microbial exposures, dietary habits, and lower antibiotic use in these regions appears to modulate immune responses in a way that is protective against allergic sensitization.

IMMUNOLOGICAL BASIS OF ALLERGY AND INFECTION

The development of allergic diseases is underpinned by a complex interplay between genetic susceptibility and environmental exposures. Individuals with a family history of atopy are at significantly higher risk of developing allergic diseases. However, genetics alone cannot account for the rapid rise in allergy prevalence over recent decades, underscoring the role of environmental and epigenetic factors. The immune system constantly navigates between tolerance and activation, a balance that determines whether an antigen will lead to immunity, infection clearance, or allergic sensitization.

The immunopathology of allergic diseases involves a skewed T-helper 2 (Th2) immune response, characterized by the production of interleukins such as interleukin 4 (IL-4), IL-5, and IL-13. These cytokines promote immunoglobulin E (IgE) production, eosinophil recruitment, and mast cell activation—all hallmark features of allergic inflammation. In contrast, viral infections tend to elicit Th1 or interferon-dominated responses aimed at antiviral defense. These include the production of interferon gamma (IFN-γ) and IL-12, as well as activation of cytotoxic T lymphocytes and natural killer (NK) cells. In some cases, chronic or severe infections may induce regulatory T cells (Tregs) that suppress both Th1 and Th2 responses to maintain immune homeostasis.

This balance between Th1 and Th2 responses is critical during the neonatal period, which is a window of immunological plasticity. Newborns are inherently biased toward Th2 responses, presumably to prevent maternal immune rejection. Exposure to microbial agents, including commensals and pathogens, drives the maturation of Th1 responses and promotes the development of Tregs. Tregs play a central role in maintaining immune homeostasis and tolerance to self and environmental antigens.

Disruption of this maturation process—due to excessive hygiene, cesarean delivery, lack of breastfeeding, or antibiotic exposure—can lead to persistence of a Th2-skewed profile, thereby predisposing to allergies. The emerging role of the microbiome in immune education adds another layer of complexity, with gut and airway dysbiosis increasingly linked to allergic sensitization. For instance, reduced colonization by Bifidobacteria and increased prevalence of *Clostridia* species in infancy have been associated with eczema and asthma.

The cross-regulation between Th1 and Th2 pathways formed the foundation of the original hygiene hypothesis—suggesting that reduced Th1 stimulation from infections may allow unchecked Th2 responses to allergens. However, this model has evolved to incorporate the role of Tregs, epithelial barrier integrity, and the microbiome, which more holistically influence immune development.

Thus, infection can both suppress or enhance allergic responses, depending on the context, making the interaction highly dynamic. The etiopathogenesis of allergy is best understood as a multifactorial process involving host genetics, immune programming, environmental exposures, and microbial interactions.

VIRAL TRIGGERS IN ALLERGY

Viral infections are now recognized not only as potential instigators of allergic sensitization but also as significant contributors to disease exacerbation in individuals with established allergies. Several key respiratory viruses have been implicated in these dual roles.

Respiratory syncytial virus (RSV) is one of the most thoroughly studied pathogens in this regard. Severe RSV bronchiolitis in infancy has been consistently linked to an increased risk of recurrent wheezing and childhood asthma. RSV induces profound damage to the respiratory epithelium and promotes the release of epithelial-derived cytokines such as IL-33, IL-25, and thymic stromal lymphopoietin (TSLP). These molecules activate innate lymphoid cells (ILC2) and skew adaptive immunity toward a Th2 phenotype, laying the groundwork for atopic airway disease.

Rhinoviruses, particularly RV-A and RV-C, are also strongly associated with asthma development and exacerbations. Studies have shown that infants with RV-induced wheezing episodes, especially in the context of atopic dermatitis or eosinophilia, have a higher likelihood of developing asthma. Rhinoviruses enhance airway inflammation, increase mucus production, and impair epithelial barrier function.

Other viruses such as influenza, parainfluenza, and coronaviruses [including severe acute respiratory syndrome coronavirus 2 (SARS-CoV-2)] have also been linked to transient worsening of allergic conditions. These viruses provoke intense immune responses, often with overlapping Th1 and Th2 features, and may disrupt epithelial integrity, increasing allergen sensitization risk.

Mechanisms of Viral-allergy Linkage

- Epithelial barrier disruption → increased allergen access.
- Dendritic cell activation → promotes IgE production.
- Type 2 ILC2s activated by epithelial cytokines (IL-25, IL-33, and TSLP).
- Delayed or deficient interferon response in some children predisposes to both severe viral infections and allergic inflammation.

Interestingly, Timing Matters

- Early viral infection during a window of immune immaturity may promote allergy.
- Later exposures may train the immune system and reduce risk.

Importantly, the host's response to viral infections is modulated by genetic factors, atopic status, and the existing microbiome. Children with allergic predispositions exhibit altered antiviral responses, including deficient production of interferons, which may lead to prolonged viral persistence and heightened inflammatory responses.

Controversy exists whether viral infections "cause" allergy or simply unmask it in genetically predisposed children. Nevertheless, managing viral respiratory infections is key in allergy prevention strategies.

These insights suggest that preventing or modifying early-life viral infections could represent a potential strategy for allergy prevention.

HYGIENE HYPOTHESIS AND BEYOND

Proposed by David Strachan in 1989, the hygiene hypothesis postulated that fewer childhood infections in smaller families led to increased allergy risk due to insufficient immune system education. This theory sparked an array of epidemiological and experimental studies.

Core Contents of the Hygiene Hypothesis

- Lack of microbial exposure leads to immune dysregulation.
- Rural environments, animal exposure, and larger family size are protective.
- Excessive hygiene, antibiotic overuse, and cesarean births reduce microbial diversity.

Over Time, this Concept Expanded

- *"Old Friends Hypothesis":* It is not just any infection, but exposure to ancient microbes (e.g., gut flora, helminths, and soil bacteria) that matter.
- *Microbiome hypothesis:* Gut and airway microbiota composition in early-life influences immune development.
- *Farm effect:* Children growing up on farms show lower allergy and asthma rates, partly due to exposure to diverse environmental microbes and unpasteurized milk.

Key Studies Supporting This

- *PASTURE study:* Farm exposure during pregnancy and early-life → reduced eczema and asthma.
- *GABRIELA study:* Confirmed protective effects of microbial-rich environments in European farming communities.
- *Amish versus Hutterite study (Stein MM et al., NEJM 2016):* Despite similar genetics, Amish children had lower asthma prevalence due to microbial exposures.

Still, the hygiene hypothesis does not explain all allergy patterns (e.g., rise in food allergy in less "hygienic" settings), and may oversimplify complex host-environment interactions.

Factors that negatively impact microbial diversity—such as cesarean section, formula feeding, early antibiotic use, and urban living—are now considered risk factors for allergy. Conversely, exposure to farm environments, pets, and siblings may confer protection by enhancing microbial diversity and immune tolerance.

Thus, the hygiene hypothesis has matured into a multifaceted framework that incorporates microbial diversity, immune education, and environmental context. This understanding opens avenues for preventive strategies such as microbial supplementation, natural childbirth promotion, and controlled environmental exposures.

Infection Allergy Balance

The balance between infections and allergic diseases is influenced by numerous factors, including the nature of the pathogen, timing of exposure, host immune status, and environmental background. While some infections may confer protection against allergic sensitization, others are capable of enhancing the risk and severity of allergic diseases.

Protective infections often include helminths and certain bacterial exposures that induce regulatory immune responses. For instance, chronic helminth infections stimulate the expansion of Tregs and the production of immunosuppressive cytokines such as IL-10 and transforming growth factor-beta (TGF-β). These immune changes dampen excessive inflammatory responses and may reduce the risk of allergy. Epidemiological studies in sub-Saharan Africa and South America have consistently shown lower rates of allergic diseases in regions with high parasitic burden.

Conversely, infections caused by respiratory viruses such as RSV and rhinoviruses are associated with increased risk of allergy and asthma, particularly when they occur early in life. These viruses damage the respiratory epithelium, enhance allergen penetration, and create a proinflammatory milieu conducive to allergic sensitization. Repeated infections can lead to airway remodeling, chronic inflammation, and bronchial hyper-responsiveness—hallmarks of asthma.

The timing of infection is also crucial. Early-life exposures, especially during infancy when the immune system is still maturing, have the greatest influence. Infections during this window can permanently shape immune trajectories. While some exposures may promote immune tolerance, others can trigger persistent Th2 dominance and allergic inflammation.

Additionally, the site of infection plays a role. Gut infections may influence systemic immunity via the gut-associated lymphoid tissue (GALT), while respiratory infections impact the mucosal immune system in the lungs. The interplay between different mucosal sites further complicates this relationship.

These findings underscore the complexity of the infection-allergy interface. They also suggest that any interventions—such as deworming programs or vaccination policies—should be carefully designed to maintain immune homeostasis. Thus, infections and microbial exposures play a context-dependent role—shaping whether the immune system becomes tolerant or hyper-responsive.

CLINICAL AND PREVENTIVE IMPLICATIONS

The intricate relationship between allergy and infections has important implications for the prevention, diagnosis, and treatment of allergic diseases. Effective management requires an integrated approach that takes into account the patient's infection history, immune profile, environmental exposures, and genetic predisposition.

Understanding the infection-allergy interplay has major implications for pediatric and public health strategies.

Prevention

- Avoid unnecessary antibiotic use and excessive hygiene in early life.
- Encourage breastfeeding, vaginal delivery where feasible.
- Promote microbial diversity via diet, probiotics, and natural environments.

Management of Viral-triggered Wheeze

- Recognize viral wheeze phenotypes distinct from classical atopic asthma.
- Use of montelukast, inhaled steroids, and in some cases biologics in prevention of viral-induced exacerbations.

Vaccination

Vaccinations against common respiratory pathogens such as influenza, pneumococcus, and SARS-CoV-2 are essential in individuals with asthma and other allergic conditions. These vaccines reduce the risk of severe respiratory infections that can exacerbate underlying allergic diseases. Importantly, vaccines do not increase allergy risk and are generally safe in atopic individuals.

Public Health and Environmental Measures

Policymakers and public health professionals must strike a balance between hygiene and microbial exposure. While clean water and sanitation are essential for infection control, over-sanitization may reduce beneficial microbial exposures. Recommendations include encouraging outdoor play, interaction with pets, and avoidance of excessive antimicrobial cleaning products.

Hence managing allergy in the context of infection requires a nuanced understanding of immunology, microbiology, and environmental health. Personalized approaches that consider individual risk factors and exposures are essential.

Future Directions

- Microbiome modulation (synbiotics, microbial transplants)
- Personalized prevention strategies based on immune and microbial profiling

CONCLUSION

The relationship between infection and allergy is both multifaceted and bidirectional. Viral infections, particularly in early life, can act as triggers for allergic sensitization and asthma, while other microbial exposures may provide protection by fostering immune tolerance.

The evolving understanding of the hygiene hypothesis, the role of the microbiome, and the timing and nature of infections points to a delicate balance in early immune development. There is no one-size-fits-all explanation—genetic, environmental, and microbial factors interact in complex ways.

In clinical practice, a deeper appreciation of the infection-allergy relationship can help pediatricians and allergists adopt holistic, evidence-based approaches to patient care. Ultimately, understanding and leveraging this relationship may unlock new pathways for preventing and treating allergic diseases in the 21st century.

KEY POINTS

- *Allergy and infection are deeply interconnected,* not separate entities—early microbial and viral exposures shape immune development and influence allergy risk throughout life.
- *Reduced microbial exposure in early life,* due to urban living, excessive hygiene, antibiotic use, and cesarean births, disrupts immune balance and promotes allergic diseases—supporting the evolved *hygiene and microbiome hypotheses.*
- *Viral infections,* especially *RSV and rhinovirus,* can act as triggers for allergic sensitization and asthma, particularly when occurring in infancy during immune immaturity.
- *Balanced microbial exposure*—through breastfeeding, natural birth, outdoor activity, and microbial diversity—is vital for developing immune tolerance and preventing allergy.
- *Future strategies* should focus on *microbiome modulation and personalized prevention,* integrating infection control with immune education to achieve long-term allergy prevention and health resilience.

SUGGESTED READING

1. Asher MI, Montefort S, Björkstén B, Lai CK, Strachan DP, Weiland SK, et al. Worldwide time trends in the prevalence of symptoms of asthma, allergic rhinoconjunctivitis, and eczema in childhood: ISAAC phases one and three repeat multicountry cross-sectional surveys. Lancet. 2006;368(9537):733-43.
2. Blanken MO, Rovers MM, Molenaar JM, Winkler-Seinstra PL, Meijer A, Kimpen JL, et al. Respiratory syncytial virus and recurrent wheeze in healthy preterm infants. N Engl J Med. 2013;368(19):1791-9.
3. Fujimura KE, Lynch SV. Microbiota in allergy and asthma and the emerging relationship with the gut microbiome. Cell Host Microbe. 2015;17(5):592-602.
4. Jackson DJ, Gangnon RE, Evans MD, Roberg KA, Anderson EL, Pappas TE, et al. Wheezing rhinovirus illnesses in early life predict asthma development in high-risk children. Am J Respir Crit Care Med. 2008;178(7):667-72.
5. Liccioli G, Pucci N, Azzari C, Novembre E. The hygiene hypothesis and its implications for allergy prevention strategies in children. Pediatr Allergy Immunol. 2020;31(Suppl 24):30-2.
6. Papadopoulos NG, Arakawa H, Carlsen KH, Custovic A, Gern J, Lemanske R, et al. Promoting health and preventing disease: The contribution of allergology to public health. Allergy. 2011;66(4):500-12.
7. Strachan DP. Hay fever, hygiene, and household size. BMJ. 1989;299(6710):1259-60.

26 CHAPTER Vaccination in Allergy

Tina N Goel

INTRODUCTION

Vaccination is vital for public health, but it poses special considerations in patients with allergic disorders. Misattribution of allergic reactions to vaccines is common; therefore, distinguishing true vaccine allergies from unrelated events is essential for safe immunization practices. This chapter presents a contemporary, practical approach for handling vaccination in individuals with suspected or confirmed allergies.

UNDERSTANDING VACCINE REACTIONS

Vaccines can provoke a spectrum of reactions, which may be:

- *Nonallergic reactions:* For example, localized pain, fever, or vasovagal events, usually self-limited and resolving within a week
- *Mild allergic reactions:* For example, urticaria, flushing, or minor facial/lip swelling, typically arising within 0–72 hours post vaccination
- *Severe allergic reactions (anaphylaxis):* Characterized by abrupt symptom onset (5 minutes to 2 hours), including skin rash, respiratory distress, hypotension, and gastrointestinal symptoms **(Table 1)**

TABLE 1: Typical timing and manifestations of vaccine-related reactions.

Reaction type	*Symptoms range*	*Onset after vaccination*
Nonallergic local	Rash, joint pain, swelling	1–7 days
Nonallergic systemic	Fever, headache, gastrointestinal upset	1–7 days
Vasovagal	Hypotension, bradycardia	Immediate
Mild allergic	Hives, flushing, lip/eye swelling	0–72 hours
Anaphylaxis	Hives, bronchospasm, hypotension	5 minutes to 2 hours

VACCINE ALLERGENS: COMPONENTS THAT MAY TRIGGER REACTIONS

A variety of vaccine constituents—not just the antigens—may act as allergens. Key culprits are given in the **Table 2**.

Diphtheria, Tetanus, and Pertussis Vaccine

Allergic Reaction Profile

Diphtheria, Tetanus, and Pertussis (DTaP) vaccines cause allergic reactions in approximately 2 per million doses administered. These reactions may occur during booster dose administration due to specific IgE antibodies against acellular pertussis components.

Primary allergen: Casein
The main allergenic concern with DTaP vaccines is casein, a milk protein used as a nutrient medium during vaccine production. Despite theoretical concerns, allergic

TABLE 2: Components of allergens that trigger reactions.

Allergen	*Common vaccines*	*Role in vaccine*
Ovalbumin (egg)	MMR, influenza, yellow fever	Medium/stabilizer
Dextran	MMR, rotavirus	Stabilizer
Gelatin	MMR, varicella	Stabilizer
Casein (milk)	DTaP	Medium nutrient
Neomycin	DTaP, HepA, influenza, MMR, varicella	Antimicrobial
Thiomersal	Influenza, HPV	Preservative
Aluminum	Meningococcal, pneumococcal, Tdap	Adjuvant
Yeast	Meningococcal, pneumococcal	Medium nutrient
Latex	Meningococcal, rotavirus, Tdap	Vial/syringe cap
Polyethylene glycol	COVID-19	mRNA surfactant

reactions to casein in DTaP vaccines are exceptionally rare, even among children with severe milk allergies and high IgE levels against milk proteins.

Clinical Considerations

Large swelling reactions (over 4 inches) can occur in approximately 5% of children receiving their 4th or 5th DTaP dose. However, these reactions are not allergic in nature and do not contraindicate future DTaP vaccinations. There is no evidence suggesting that DTaP vaccines contribute to the development of allergic diseases or that atopy represents a contraindication for vaccination.

Influenza Vaccine

Allergic Reaction Profile

Influenza vaccines have an anaphylaxis rate of approximately 1.35 per million doses, which is consistent with other routine vaccines. Historical concerns about egg allergies have been largely addressed through modern vaccine production methods.

Ovalbumin Content and Safety

Modern influenza vaccines contain very low levels of ovalbumin (typically less than 0.12 μg/mL). Multiple studies, including the SNIFFLE study, have found no significant systemic reactions even in patients with severe egg allergies. Current guidelines from the Advisory Committee on Immunization Practices (ACIP) recommend that influenza vaccines can be safely administered to patients with egg allergies, including those with severe reactions, under standard clinical supervision.

Clinical Evidence

A comprehensive study of 292 patients with confirmed egg allergies receiving influenza vaccination found no systemic reactions, regardless of skin test results, administration method, or ovalbumin content. Even vaccines containing up to 1.421 μg/mL ovalbumin were well tolerated, suggesting that the safety threshold may be higher than previously estimated.

Measles, Mumps, Rubella Vaccine

Allergic Reaction Profile

Measles, Mumps, Rubella (MMR) vaccines have an anaphylaxis rate of approximately 1.8 per million doses. However, gelatin-specific allergic reactions can occur at higher rates of 5.3 per 100,000 first doses in susceptible individuals.

Primary allergen: Gelatin
Gelatin, used as a stabilizer in MMR vaccines, is responsible for the majority of allergic reactions to this vaccine. Both bovine and porcine gelatin can trigger IgE-mediated reactions. The British Society of Allergy and Clinical Immunology has confirmed that MMR vaccines are safe for children with egg allergies, as reactions are typically due to gelatin rather than egg proteins.

Alpha-Gal Syndrome Considerations

Patients with alpha-gal syndrome (AGS), caused by tick bites and characterized by delayed allergic reactions to mammalian products, may experience reactions to gelatin-containing vaccines 2–6 hours post vaccination. This delayed presentation can complicate diagnosis and management.

Clinical Management

In the United Kingdom, the Priorix brand MMR vaccine does not contain gelatin and can be safely administered to gelatin-allergic individuals, while many MMR vaccines contain porcine gelatin and should be avoided in such patients. Prior to vaccination with gelatin-containing vaccines, confirmation through skin testing or serum-specific IgE antibody testing is advisable for patients with a history of immediate-type reactions to gelatin.

Hepatitis B Vaccine

Allergic Reaction Profile

Hepatitis B vaccines cause severe allergic reactions (anaphylaxis) at a rate of approximately 1 per 600,000 doses (1.67 per million doses). A comprehensive study of 43,618 persons receiving 101,360 doses found that most adverse reactions were coincidental rather than vaccine-related.

Yeast Proteins as Potential Allergens

Hepatitis B vaccines are produced using yeast cells, leading to theoretical concerns about yeast protein allergies. However, no confirmed cases of allergic reactions to yeast proteins in hepatitis B vaccines have been documented. The manufacturing process effectively removes most yeast proteins, making allergic reactions extremely unlikely.

Clinical Manifestations

When allergic reactions do occur, they typically present with symptoms including chest pain, difficulty breathing, fast heartbeat, hives, and swelling. Commonly, postvaccination reactions occur within 15 minutes of vaccination, emphasizing the importance of postvaccination observation.

Human Papillomavirus Vaccine

Allergic Reaction Profile

Human papillomavirus (HPV) vaccines elicit variable rates of anaphylaxis across different populations. An Australian school-based program reported 2.6 per 100,000 doses (26 per million doses), which is significantly higher than rates observed with other vaccines.

Potential Allergens

The specific allergens responsible for HPV vaccine reactions remain unclear. Polysorbate 80, present at 50 µg per dose, has been suggested as a potential cause of anaphylactoid reactions, though skin testing has not consistently supported this hypothesis. Yeast proteins from the production process represent another theoretical concern.

Clinical Characteristics

Most HPV vaccine allergic reactions occur within minutes of vaccination, with a median age of 16.5 years among affected individuals. Approximately 50% of patients experiencing reactions had a history of allergic conditions, though the significance of this association remains unclear. All documented anaphylactic reactions were successfully treated without serious sequelae.

Pneumococcal Vaccines

Allergic Reaction Profile

Pneumococcal vaccines (both PCV and PPSV) have low rates of allergic reactions, with anaphylaxis occurring rarely. More concerning are cellulitis-like inflammatory reactions that can occur, particularly with the PPSV23 vaccine.

Inflammatory versus Allergic Reactions

A case series of five adult patients receiving PPSV23 vaccine developed fever, leukocytosis, and large local inflammatory reactions that mimicked cellulitis. These reactions occurred within 24 hours of vaccination and did not respond to antibiotics, suggesting a noninfectious inflammatory response rather than true allergic reactions.

Clinical Management

Patients experiencing severe local reactions to pneumococcal vaccines should be evaluated for inflammatory responses rather than infectious complications. Treatment with oral anti-inflammatory medications and cold compression may be more appropriate than antibiotics for the reaction,

SAFE VACCINATION PROTOCOLS FOR ALLERGIC PATIENTS

Risk Assessment

Healthcare providers should screen for:

- Previous allergic reactions to vaccines
- Known allergies to vaccine components
- History of severe allergic reactions requiring emergency treatment
- Multiple drug allergies

However, general allergic history (food allergies, environmental allergies, asthma) does not significantly increase the risk of vaccine allergic reactions and should not delay vaccination.

Prevaccination Testing and Graded Dosing

- *Skin testing:* If an allergy to a specific vaccine is suspected, perform skin testing with the vaccine and its components.
    - *Negative result:* Proceed with standard vaccination.
    - *Positive result:* Employ *graded dosing* under close supervision.
- *Graded dosing protocol:* For a standard 0.5 mL vaccine dose:
    - Start with 0.05 mL of 1:10 dilution.
    - If tolerated, administer stepwise full-strength aliquots at 15-minute intervals: 0.05, 0.1, 0.15, and 0.2 mL
    - Observe the patient at each step. Ensure that resuscitation equipment and epinephrine are immediately available.
    - Conduct in a hospital or office setting depending on the severity of previous reactions and patient comorbidities.

Postvaccination Monitoring

- All cases should be monitored for 30 minutes after any vaccination.
- High-risk cases should be observed in emergency with cash cart readily available.

Special Cases and Contraindications

- *Pertussis vaccines:* Absolute contraindication if encephalopathy or severe neurological sequelae follow previous vaccination
- *Rubella vaccine:* May cause transient arthritis in women but is not a reason to avoid further MMR doses

PRACTICAL CONSIDERATIONS

- Ensure that vaccine administration in allergic patients is done where emergency care can be provided.
- Education is critical—clinicians, ancillary health staff, and families must understand the distinction between true vaccine allergies and unrelated events.
- Maintain updated protocols as vaccine formulations and recommendations evolve.

CONCLUSION

Most adverse events following vaccination are non-allergic, and true IgE-mediated vaccine allergies remain extremely rare. Misconceptions often lead to unnecessary vaccine avoidance, placing children at an increased risk of preventable infections. A clear understanding of vaccine components, typical reaction patterns, and appropriate evaluation strategies ensures safe and confident immunization practices in children with allergic disorders.

With systematic risk assessment, selective skin testing, and graded dosing protocols when required, nearly all children—including those with food allergies, atopy, or previous mild reactions—can be vaccinated safely. Only a small subset with confirmed severe vaccine or component-specific allergy require specialized precautions. Strengthening awareness among pediatricians, vaccinators, and caregivers is essential to avoid missed opportunities for immunization. Ultimately, informed decision-making and evidence-based protocols enable safe vaccination while preserving the critical benefits of immunization for every child.

KEY POINTS

- *Vaccination is safe for the vast majority of children with allergic diseases*, including asthma, atopic dermatitis, allergic rhinitis, and most food allergies.
- *True vaccine allergy is extremely rare*; most post-vaccination reactions are mild, non-IgE mediated, and self-limiting.
- *Children with egg allergy can safely receive MMR, influenza, and other routine vaccines*, with special precautions needed only for a small subset with previous anaphylaxis.
- *Preservatives and stabilizers (e.g., gelatin, latex, yeast, PEG)* may rarely cause reactions—careful history and allergist evaluation help identify the true culprit.
- *Immunization should not be delayed or avoided in allergic children*; risk–benefit strongly favors timely vaccination, and allergist-supervised graded dosing or desensitization is available when needed.

SUGGESTED READING

1. Barış HE, Boran P, Kıykım A, Barış S, Özen A, Aydıner EK. Immunization practices in children with a history of allergies. Turk Pediatri Ars. 2020;55(3):244-50.
2. Goel T. Immunisation in allergy. In: IAP case-based reviews in Pediatric allergy ed. Ramesh Kumar R, Krishna Mohan R, Gupta N, Ashok N (Eds). New Delhi: Jaypee Publication Brothers Medical Publishers; 2023. pp. 257-67.
3. Gupta N. Vaccination in an allergic patient. In: Comprehensive Textbook of Allergy: Striking the Right Balance. New Delhi: Jaypee Brothers Medical Publishers; 2024. pp. 757-61.
4. Kroger A, Bahta L, Long S, Sanchez P. General best practice guidelines for immunization. Best practices guidance of the advisory committee on immunization practices (ACIP). [online] Available from https://www.cdc.gov/vaccines/hcp/acip-recs/general-recs/downloads/general-recs.pdf [Last accessed December, 2025].
5. Radulovic S, Powell E. Managing a child with a possible vaccine allergy. Paediatr Child Health. 2025;35(3):88-95.
6. Tsai MH, Chiu CY. Allergic Reactions to Vaccines in Children: From Constituents to Specific Vaccines. Biomedicines. 2023;11(2):620.

6 SECTION Preventive and Holistic Care

Section Editors: Sinchana Bhat, Pavan Kalyan

27 CHAPTER Primary Prevention of Allergies

Sinchana Bhat

"Prevention is the action aimed at eradicating, eliminating, or minimizing the impact of disease and disability"

—John M Last

INTRODUCTION

The prevalence of allergic diseases has risen sharply in recent decades, with nearly 30–40% of the global population affected by at least one allergic condition. This rising burden highlights the importance of prevention as a critical strategy in reducing morbidity, progression of the allergic march, and healthcare costs. Primary prevention aims to prevent the onset of sensitization in genetically susceptible individuals, especially during the "window of opportunity" in early life. Preventive measures encompass optimizing maternal health and diet, reducing harmful exposures during pregnancy and childhood, encouraging breastfeeding, timely introduction of allergenic foods, and maintaining healthy environmental conditions. Advances in genetics, epigenetics, and microbiome science provide deeper insight into how prenatal and early-life exposures shape long-term allergic risk. Effective primary prevention therefore requires a multifaceted, evidence-based approach tailored to both individual and population needs. This chapter aims to give an overview of the existing evidence and future perspectives for primary prevention of allergies.

There are four levels of prevention described for any disease **(Flowchart 1)**:

1. Primordial prevention
2. Primary prevention
3. Secondary prevention
4. Tertiary prevention

Flowchart 1: Levels of prevention.

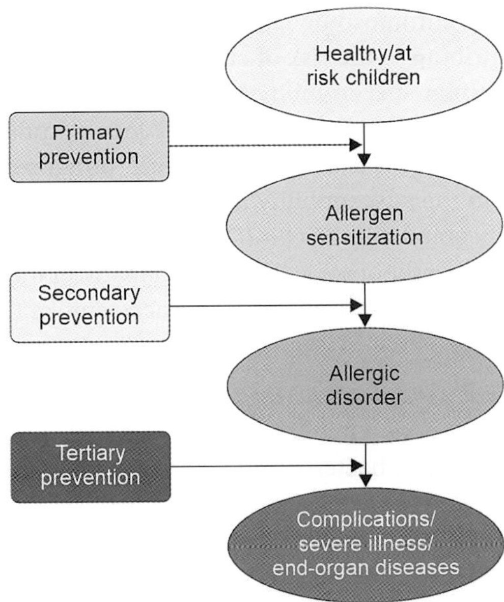

PRIMORDIAL PREVENTION

This concept is receiving special attention for prevention of chronic diseases. It is defined as prevention of emergence of risk factors in a population in which they have not yet appeared. It is the earliest preventive measure and gets promoted through laws and national policies. It mainly aims at individual and mass education regarding the adoption of healthy lifestyle. Promoting regular physical activity, implementing policies to discourage smoking, and encouraging good nutrition and healthy eating habits from early childhood are essential to prevent chronic illnesses, such as allergies. Strategies to reduce air pollution are the need of the hour to halt the epidemic of allergy.

PRIMARY PREVENTION

It is defined as the action taken prior to the onset of disease so as to reduce or remove the possibility of occurrence of the disease. It is a known fact that sensitization is the key step to the development of allergic diseases, and avoidance of sensitization in an individual is the main aim of primary prevention, especially during the window period of opportunity, i.e., the first 2 years of life. The target population is healthy individuals as well as high-risk and low-risk neonates, especially those with a genetic predisposition.

ROLE OF GENETICS IN PREVENTION OF ALLERGIES

A complex relationship exists between the genetic predisposition of an individual, environmental allergen exposure and disease manifestation. The genome-wide association analysis (GWAS) has been widely used to identify genetic variants that contribute to disease and influence asthma susceptibility. The first comprehensive GWAS of asthma reported by Moffatt et al. identified genetic variants at chromosome regulating *ORMDL3* expression and contribute to the risk of childhood asthma. The first novel asthma-susceptibility locus to be identified by a GWAS was on chromosome 17q12-21 locus. Studies have shown that several single-nucleotide polymorphisms (SNPs) on the susceptibility locus on this chromosome, which encompasses the *ORMDL3* and *GSDMB* genes, are confined to early-onset asthma, particularly in those who were exposed to environmental tobacco smoke (ETS) in early life.

Genes that modulate the response to environment: The *CD14/TLR4* gene encodes for the receptors needed to identify and clear bacterial endotoxins, which is important in innate immune response. SNPs of these receptors modify the effect of microbial exposure on immune system leading to early-life origins of allergic disease. Studies have shown interactions between a polymorphism of CD14 and exposure to farm environment, consumption of unpasteurized milk, and household dust endotoxin levels are involved in determining serum IgE levels, sensitization, and asthma. *GST* gene which encodes for glutathione-S transferase modulates the effect of environmental toxins such as tobacco smoke and air pollution. Children with *filaggrin (FLG)* gene mutations are more prone to eczema when they are exposed to cats. Defective epithelial barrier in children with this defect leads to early transcutaneous sensitization, thereby initiating the allergic march. Identifying the individuals with these genetic defects may help in early intervention by modification of environmental conditions. They may also serve as newer therapeutic targets in future.

EPIGENETICS

It describes mechanisms of (heritable) regulation of gene expression that occur without changes in DNA sequence. These mechanisms include DNA methylation, histone modification, and non-coding mRNA. Epigenetic processes can occur in response to the environment, aging, disease, and other factors. These changes can begin from in utero period and continue throughout lifetime. The fetal onset of adult disorders (FOAD) hypothesis proposes that during critical periods of early life, nutritional and environmental exposures can induce permanent long-term changes in metabolic and immune physiology of the host leading to susceptibility to allergies. Hence, the trajectory of allergic diseases begins from the in utero period itself. Prenatal smoking, stress, obesity, and asthma can cause DNA methylation resulting in asthma in the offspring.

STRATEGIES OF PREVENTION IN PERINATAL PERIOD

- *Tobacco smoking in pregnancy:* Both active and passive tobacco smoking by a pregnant woman have been postulated as a strong risk factor for allergies and asthma in the early childhood and eczema later in life. Therefore, exposure to tobacco smoke should be avoided by the pregnant woman.
- Consumption of a balanced diet with diverse food products is recommended during pregnancy. Diet high in sugar, sweetened beverages, and fast food should be avoided. Avoidance of potential allergens should not be followed in pregnancy or lactation.
- Excessive weight gain in pregnancy and high maternal prepregnancy body mass index (BMI) may affect the development of the immune system of the fetus, and increases the risk allergic diseases in childhood. It has been found as an independent risk factor for development of asthma. Hence, it is advisable for pregnant women mother to maintain normal BMI in pregnancy.
- *Vitamin D:* Vitamin D plays an important role in regulating the innate immune system and has anti-inflammatory properties. Vitamin D supplementation has not been shown to reduce the risk of eczema in offspring and has demonstrated only a modest reduction in the risk of allergic rhinitis, limited to evidence from observational studies. The long-term follow-up results of vitamin D Antenatal Asthma Reduction Trial (VDAART) concluded that vitamin D sufficiency in early and late pregnancy had a protective effect against active asthma in offspring at age 6 years. However, the doses recommended to achieve this effect are high, raising concerns of potential toxicity. The

doses of vitamin D supplementation recommended were at least 4,400 IU vitamin D_3 daily throughout their pregnancy, starting at the time of conception.

- *Probiotics supplementation:* Their potential role in allergy prevention is based on the hypothesis of modulation of the gut microbiota during the critical period of immune system development. Several RCTs and meta-analyses have evaluated their role in pregnancy, lactation, and early infancy. The most consistent evidence supports a modest benefit in the prevention of atopic dermatitis (AD) when they are supplemented to the mother during late pregnancy and the infant in the early life. However, there is no clear preventive effect on other allergies. The benefits depend on the strain used, the time of initiation, and duration and host factors.
- *Maternal stress:* Prenatal stress is associated with high cord blood IgE and allergies in childhood. Hence, all efforts should be made to reduce stress during pregnancy.
- *Delivery by vaginal route:* It increases the exposure to diverse microflora from the mother.

INFANCY AND CHILDHOOD

Exclusive Breastfeeding

Exclusive breastfeeding until 6 months of age is recommended as per the WHO and IAP Guidelines. Breastfeeding for 3–4 months is beneficial to reduce the incidence of AD in children below 2 years. Though its role in the prevention of all other allergies is still controversial, it confers overall health to the baby. There is no evidence that soy-based infant formulas and milk of other animals prevent allergies. In infants who cannot be exclusively breastfed for the first 4–6 months of life, hydrolyzed formula has no advantage over cow's milk formula (CMF) in prevention of allergic diseases. There has been a concern of the risk for cow's milk allergy (CMA) with early short-term exposure to CMF due to unavoidable circumstances, followed by exclusive breastfeeding. In such situations, research has proven that supplementation of small amounts of CMF (10 mL) daily until 2 months of age along with breastfeeding significantly reduces the risk of CMA associated with short-term supplementation.

Early Introduction of Major Allergenic Foods

This strategy is being promoted by most of the infant feeding guidelines around the world to prevent food allergy. The American and the Canadian guidelines recommend introducing well-cooked egg and peanut at around 6 months of age. Screening for sensitization is not necessary before introducing these foods; however, hesitant families can be offered testing. There is a lack of efficacy data regarding the frequency, quantity, and duration of allergen ingestion that supports ongoing tolerance. It has been suggested that regular exposure of the child to the allergen outweighs the dosing amount in supporting tolerance in the long term. The other common allergenic foods can be introduced gradually once these two foods are tolerated. Fish oil introduction at 4–6 months of age and fish intake later is protective against food allergy and asthma, respectively in children. Once the allergenic foods are introduced, infants should be fed a diverse diet rich in fruits and vegetables to prevent respiratory and food allergies.

Rapid Weight Gain in Infancy and Obesity in Childhood

The risk of asthma increased from 8 to 17% in overweight children whereas in obese children it increased from 26 to 38%. This could be possibly because of the common genetic background, changes in the lung function, changes in the physical activity and diet, and increased insulin resistance and systemic inflammation. It is one of the most important preventable risk factor and comorbidity associated with allergic diseases.

Hygiene Hypothesis

Early-life infections and exposure to diverse microbes help shape the immune system, promoting a balance between *Th1* and *Th2* responses. Lack of such exposures skews immunity toward *Th2 dominance,* which favors allergic inflammation. Reduced exposure to microorganisms in early childhood due to improved hygiene, smaller family sizes, urban living, and vaccination programs may lead to an understimulated TH1 immune system, increasing the risk of allergy. Growing up in a closed farm environment, consumption of raw farm milk, exposure to helminthic infections and day care, and older siblings in early childhood result in exposure to rich and diverse microflora thus protecting against allergies. Exposure of pregnant mother to such environment has been found to be more protective to the offspring. Keeping dogs as pets in the first 3 years of life has been found to help prevent future allergies and asthma, even in families with a history of allergies. However, early cat exposure may be associated with an increased risk of allergies, especially in susceptible children.

The microbiome hypothesis and the biodiversity hypothesis also postulate that the gut, skin, and airway microbiota play a crucial role in immune development. Disruption of microbiome may impair immune tolerance and promote allergies.

Antibiotics

Excessive use of antibiotics in the first 2 years of life has a moderate increased risk of asthma and higher risk of eczemas in later life. Meta-analytic studies have proven that five or more antibiotic courses, antibiotic exposure within 1 week of life leads to development asthma at 1–3 years of age Therefore, rational usage of antibiotics is advocated.

Exposure to Indoor Pollutants

Children can be exposed to this right from the in utero period and also in the early years of life due to confinement to indoors.

Environmental tobacco smoke—exposure, particularly in early life, is a major risk factor for asthma development and also leads to exacerbations of other airway conditions such as acute otitis media and upper and lower respiratory tract infections. A systematic review identified that exposure to maternal (prenatal and postnatal), paternal, and household sources of cigarette smoke was associated with an increased likelihood of children wheezing up to the age of 18 years. A meta-analysis done on the effect of passive smoking on children inferred that children exposed to passive smoking or second-hand smoke are twice likely to have severe asthma. Avoidance of exposure to tobacco smoke starting right from pregnancy and continuing as the child grows is beneficial.

Outdoor Air Pollutants

Exposure to outdoor air pollutants increases the risk of allergic disorders and is a significant risk factor for development of asthma and also triggering asthma exacerbations. Diesel exhaust particles (DEPs) are also known to increase IgE levels by 50-fold and also cause neosensitization. These pollutants increase systemic inflammation, oxidative stress, and bronchial hyperresponsiveness and decrease lung function. They can also bind with pollen and increase their allergenicity. Young children are particularly susceptible because of the growing lung and immature immune system. Atopy, stress, and obesity modify the susceptibility to air pollution.

General measures to reduce both indoor and outdoor pollution should be implemented to minimize exposure (explained in detail in the section on Pollution and Allergy).

CONCLUSION

Primary prevention of allergy requires a multifaceted approach targeting prenatal, perinatal, and early childhood periods. The emphasis is on promoting healthy maternal and infant practices, controlling environmental exposures, and supporting immune tolerance development. While some interventions are strongly evidence-based, others remain under investigation, and recommendations should be updated as new research emerges.

KEY POINTS

- *Allergy prevention starts early:* The trajectory of allergic diseases begins in utero; maternal health, smoking avoidance, balanced diet, and reduced stress are crucial in pregnancy.
- *Breastfeeding and early nutrition:* Exclusive breast-feeding for ~6 months, along with timely introduction of allergenic foods (egg, peanut, and fish), promotes immune tolerance and reduces food allergy risk.
- *Environmental factors matter:* Avoidance of tobacco smoke, air pollution, and unnecessary antibiotic use in early life are key modifiable risk factors.
- *Microbiome and immune development:* Early exposure to diverse microbes (farm environment, pets, and vaginal delivery) helps shape a balanced immune system and protect against allergies.
- *Prevention is multidimensional:* A combination of genetic insights, epigenetic influences, healthy lifestyle practices, and public health measures is essential to reduce the burden of allergic diseases.

SUGGESTED READING

1. Bawany F, Beck LA, Järvinen KM. Halting the March: Primary Prevention of Atopic Dermatitis and Food Allergies. J Allergy Clin Immunol Pract. 2020;8(3):860-75.
2. Bouzigon E, Corda E, Aschard H, Dizier MH, Boland A, Bousquet J, et al. Effect of 17q21 variants and smoking exposure in early-onset asthma. N Engl J Med. 2008;359: 1985-94.

3. Eder W, Klimecki W, von Mutius E, von Mutius E, Riedler J, Braun-Fahrländer C, et al. Opposite effects of CD 14/-260 on serum IgE levels in children raised in different environments. J Allergy Clin Immunol. 2005;116:601-7.
4. Fleischer DM, Chan ES, Venter C, Spergel JM, Abrams EM, Stukus D, et al. A Consensus Approach to the Primary Prevention of Food Allergy Through Nutrition: Guidance from the American Academy of Allergy, Asthma, and Immunology; American College of Allergy, Asthma, and Immunology; and the Canadian Society for Allergy and Clinical Immunology. J Allergy Clin Immunol Pract. 2021;9(1):22-43.e4.
5. Global Initiative for Asthma. (2020). Global strategy for asthma Management and Prevention. [online] Available from https://ginasthma.org/wp-content/uploads/2020/04/GINA-2020-full-report_-final-_wms.pdf [Last accessed December, 2025].
6. Kopp MV, Muche-Borowski C, Abou-Dakn M, Ahrens B, Beyer K, Blümchen K, et al. S3 guideline Allergy Prevention. Allergol Select. 2022;6:61-97.
7. Lang JE, Bunnell HT, Hossain MJ, Wysocki T, Lima JJ, Finkel TH, et al. Being Overweight or Obese and the Development of Asthma. Pediatrics. 2018;142(6):e20182119.
8. McWilliam V, Venter C, Greenhawt M, Perrett KP, Tang MLK, Koplin JJ, et al. A pragmatic approach to infant feeding for food allergy prevention. Pediatr Allergy Immunol. 2022;33(9):e13849.
9. Miller RL, Peden DB. Environmental effects on immune responses in patients with atopy and asthma. J Allergy Clin Immunol. 2014;134(5):1001-8.
10. Moffatt MF, Kabesch M, Liang L, Dixon AL, Strachan D, Heath S, et al. Genetic variants regulating ORMDL3 expression contribute to the risk of childhood asthma. Nature. 2007;448:470-3.
11. Ng PPC, Tham EH, Lee BW. Primary Prevention of Allergy - Is It Feasible? Allergy Asthma Immunol Res. 2023;15(4):419-36.
12. Osborn DA, Sinn JK, Jones LJ. Infant formulas containing hydrolysed protein for prevention of allergic disease. Cochrane Database Syst Rev. 2018;10(10):CD003664.
13. Thacher JD, Gruzieva O, Pershagen G, Neuman Å, Wickman M, Kull I, et al. Pre- and postnatal exposure to parental smoking and allergic disease through adolescence. Pediatrics. 2014;134(3):428-34.
14. Wang H, Li XB, Chu XJ, Cao NW, Wu H, Huang RG, et al. Ambient air pollutants increase the risk of immunoglobulin E-mediated allergic diseases: a systematic review and meta-analysis. Environ Sci Pollut Res Int. 2022;29(33):49534-52.
15. Weiss ST, Mirzakhani H, Carey VJ, O'Connor GT, Zeiger RS, Bacharier LB, et al. Prenatal vitamin D supplementation to prevent childhood asthma: 15-year results from the Vitamin D Antenatal Asthma Reduction Trial (VDAART). J Allergy Clin Immunol. 2024;153(2):378-88.
16. WHO. WHO Guidelines for Indoor Air Quality: Dampness and Mould. Geneva: WHO; 2009.
17. Yin Leung AS, Tham EH, Samuel M, Munblit D, Chu DK, Dahdah L, et al. Quality and consistency of clinical practice guidelines on the prevention of food allergy and atopic dermatitis: Systematic review protocol. World Allergy Organ J. 2022;15(9):100679.

28 CHAPTER

Secondary and Tertiary Prevention of Allergy

Sonia Bhatt, Nimmy Joseph

INTRODUCTION

Allergic diseases such as asthma, atopic dermatitis, allergic rhinitis, and food allergy are rising globally, often following the "atopic march," where early conditions like eczema progress to respiratory allergies. While primary prevention aims to block initial sensitization, secondary and tertiary prevention focus on children who are already sensitized or symptomatic. Secondary prevention seeks to halt progression before full-blown disease develops, while tertiary prevention targets established allergies to reduce morbidity, prevent complications, and improve long-term quality of life. Emerging evidence on early allergen introduction, microbiome modulation, environmental control, and allergen immunotherapy (AIT) has reshaped prevention strategies, shifting from strict avoidance to a more proactive, tolerance-inducing approach. Effective prevention requires timely identification of at-risk children, integration of multidisciplinary care, and individualized strategies that combine evidence-based medicine with practical, family-centered interventions.

Accordingly, allergy prevention strategies are categorized into three tiers:

1. *Primary prevention*—aimed at avoiding initial sensitization through environmental, nutritional, and microbial modulation.
2. *Secondary prevention*—which targets sensitized but asymptomatic individuals to halt progression.
3. *Tertiary prevention*—focused on managing established diseases to minimize long-term morbidity and improve quality of life.

Our aim is to focus on secondary and tertiary prevention, emphasizing clinically applicable interventions supported by current evidence.

SHIFTING PARADIGMS IN PEDIATRIC ALLERGY PREVENTION

Avoiding allergens, especially through dietary restrictions and environmental control, dominated preventive efforts for decades. This paradigm has, however, been drastically altered by research such as the LEAP (2015) and EAT (2016) trials, which show that introducing allergens such as peanuts and eggs under strict control early in infancy can greatly lower the risk of developing a clinical allergy. Global pediatric allergy guidelines were revised as a result of these findings, which reframed the idea of "exposure" as a preventive tactic rather than a provocative one in some situations.

New avenues for allergy modulation have also been made possible by growing research on the gut-skin-lung axis and the function of the infant microbiome. Immune dysregulation and an increased risk of allergies are increasingly associated with disruptions in early microbial colonization, which are made worse by caesarean delivery, breastfeeding cessation, and overuse of antibiotics. Probiotics, prebiotics, and synbiotics are examples of microbiome-targeted treatments that have demonstrated modest but encouraging results, especially for eczema and allergic rhinitis.

IMPORTANCE OF SECONDARY AND TERTIARY PREVENTION

Pediatricians must identify high-risk or already sensitized children in order to implement secondary and tertiary prevention strategies, which are clinically targeted, while primary prevention targets a larger population. Early risk stratification and the application of targeted interventions are made possible by the early detection of sensitization by skin prick testing (SPT), serum-specific immunoglobulin E (IgE), or component-resolved diagnostics. These consist of:

- Early introduction of allergens to nonreactive but sensitive infants.
- Environmental controls aimed at mold, pet dander, and house dust mites.
- Preventive medication for recurrent wheezing or subclinical asthma.
- Behavioral and educational interventions to guarantee adherence and symptom monitoring.

Tertiary prevention is crucial for children with known allergic diseases. AIT, long-term medication management, and thorough multidisciplinary care that addresses emergency preparedness, psychological health, and nutrition are all included in this. Research indicates that AIT can reduce new sensitizations, create long-term tolerance, and alleviate clinical symptoms.

Additionally, integrated care pathways are necessary for pediatric patients who have several comorbid allergic conditions. For instance, dietary restrictions and mental health issues such as anxiety or bullying frequently coexist for children who have both eczema and a food allergy. In order to prevent chronic distress and ensure normal growth and development, dietitians, psychologists, and school health professionals must be involved.

EARLY ALLERGEN INTRODUCTION, MICROBIOME MODIFICATION, AND DIET

It is becoming more widely acknowledged that a key component of secondary prevention in pediatric allergies is the interaction among diet, microbiome development, and allergic sensitization. The infant's gut microbiota rapidly colonizes during the first 1,000 days of life, which is crucial for immune education and tolerance induction.

Prebiotics and Probiotics

The immunomodulatory effects of probiotics, which are live microorganisms that offer health benefits, have been thoroughly investigated. It has been demonstrated that certain strains of *Bifidobacterium longum* and *Lactobacillus rhamnosus* GG suppress Th2-mediated inflammation and enhance regulatory T-cell responses.

According to a meta-analysis by Holt et al. (2018), probiotics given during pregnancy may cause high-risk infants' serum IgE levels to drop. The impact of probiotics on preventing asthma was inconclusive due to study of heterogeneity and strain specificity. Prebiotics, which are indigestible food ingredients that specifically promote good bacteria, have also drawn interest. Galactooligosaccharides (GOS) and fructooligosaccharides (FOS) supplements have been shown to positively modulate gut flora and reduce the incidence of eczema in infants, especially when paired with probiotics in synbiotic formulations.

International guidelines are still cautious despite growing interest. Although they acknowledged the potential benefit in certain populations, the European Academy of Allergy and Clinical Immunology (EAACI) recommended against routine probiotic supplementation for allergy prevention in 2023 due to limited consistency in results.

Early Introduction of Allergens

In recent years, there has been a significant shift in the paradigm surrounding the avoidance of allergens during infancy. According to the Learning Early About Peanut Allergy (LEAP) study, high-risk infants' incidence of peanut allergies was reduced by more than 80% when peanut-containing foods were introduced to them between the ages of 4 and 11 months. The Enquiring About Tolerance (EAT) study then expanded the findings to include other allergens, such as wheat, milk, and eggs.

International guidelines were revised as a result of these groundbreaking studies. The National Institute of Allergy and Infectious Diseases (NIAID), the American Academy of Paediatrics (AAP), and the EAACI now support the early, controlled introduction of allergens as a preventive measure, especially in infants with severe egg allergy or eczema.

This approach is further supported by recent cohort analyses, which show that higher rates of sensitization, particularly for peanuts and eggs, are correlated with delayed introduction beyond 12 months. Furthermore, the introduction of allergenic foods during active breastfeeding seems to strengthen oral tolerance, perhaps as a result of immunomodulatory factors in the mother.

In summary, a major development in the secondary prevention of childhood allergies is the combination of early allergen exposure and dietary modification. Although there is potential for microbiome-targeted interventions, their application needs to be guided by consensus guidelines, individual risk assessment, and new data.

Environmental Control: Aeroallergens and House Dust Mites

The most common causes of childhood allergic diseases, such as asthma, atopic dermatitis, and allergic rhinitis, are indoor environmental allergens, especially house dust mites (HDMs), pet dander, molds, and cockroach antigens. Because it can slow down the progression of the disease and reduce exacerbations, reducing exposure to these aeroallergens is essential to secondary and tertiary prevention strategies.

INTERVENTIONS BASED ON EVIDENCE

The Inner-City Asthma Study (ICAS) is among the most significant trials in this field. In the homes of children with moderate-to-severe asthma, this randomized controlled trial introduced a multicomponent environmental control intervention that included dust mite-impermeable bedding, high-efficiency particulate air (HEPA) air filters, integrated pest management, and professional cleaning. The research found a 20% reduction in the number of symptom days, a 13% decrease in urgent healthcare visits, and fewer missed school days.

These results, which show that integrated environmental strategies can significantly improve pediatric asthma outcomes, continue to be fundamental.

An updated 2022 meta-analysis examined studies on environmental changes in children with sensitization. In comparison to controls, multi-component interventions, including bedding encasements, humidity control, and HEPA filters, resulted in a 25–30% decrease in asthma exacerbations. The authors emphasized that better results were obtained by customizing interventions according to particular sensitizations (e.g., HDM-specific). Similarly, in 2023, the Global Allergy and Asthma European Network (GA2LEN) published guidelines supporting early environmental control in infants at high risk.

CLINICAL USE AND APPROACH

Regular environmental risk assessments should be conducted alongside diagnostic evaluations for pediatric allergists and clinicians, particularly for children who exhibit severe or persistent symptoms.

Key exposure sources can be found through a systematic household audit, which can direct interventions, such as:

- Installing HEPA air purifiers in the main living areas and bedrooms.
- Mattress and pillow encasings that are impermeable to dust mites.
- Cleaning bedding once a week at temperatures higher than 60°C.
- Removing soft toys and carpets from sleeping areas.
- Keeping the relative humidity inside the house below 50% (using dehumidifiers as necessary).
- Mold removal and safe pest control.
- Using natural, eco-friendly cleaners to lessen exposure to volatile organic compounds.

These policies provide viable, affordable choices for families from a range of socioeconomic backgrounds and have demonstrated efficacy in lowering morbidity and healthcare utilization.

ALLERGEN IMMUNOTHERAPY

The mainstay of tertiary prevention for pediatric allergic diseases, especially for allergic rhinitis, asthma, and venom hypersensitivity, is AIT. Through subcutaneous (SCIT) or sublingual (SLIT) exposure to particular allergens over time, it creates long-term immune tolerance. Data from >30 randomized controlled trials involving children aged 5–17 years were compiled in a systematic review. According to the analysis, AIT prevented monosensitized children from developing new sensitizations and decreased symptom scores and medication use by up to 40%. In order to achieve long-lasting immunological benefits, including increased allergen-specific IgG4 and suppression of Th2 responses, the review suggested a minimum treatment duration of 3 years.

The ability of AIT to modify disease is one of its main benefits. Compared to children receiving pharmacotherapy alone, children who finish entire courses of AIT have a lower chance of moving from rhinitis to asthma, according to longitudinal cohort studies. Crucially, when given in accordance with accepted practices, AIT is well tolerated in pediatric populations. Safety data show that there is still little chance of systemic reactions, with anaphylaxis happening about once every 2.5 million SCIT injections. AIT is a safe and efficient tertiary intervention that not only reduces present symptoms but also changes the long-term course of allergic disease in children, according to mounting data and better formulations.

HOME-BASED AND SUSTAINABLE APPROACHES

Home-based and sustainable methods are becoming more popular due to the rising prevalence of allergic diseases and the lack of access to specialized care in many places. These consist of:

- Using HEPA filters, humidity control, and indoor air purifiers to reduce allergens.
- Educating parents on asthma and anaphylaxis action plans.
- Using natural cleaning products, hypoallergenic bedding, and lowering volatile organic compounds (VOCs) in the house.
- Using smartphone apps for medication reminders and symptom tracking.

Additionally, through microbial diversity exposure, lifestyle interventions such as encouraging outdoor activities, exposing young children to green like encouraging outdoor activities, exposing young children to green spaces, and allowing them to interact with pets have demonstrated protective effects on immune tolerance. These ecoimmunological discoveries are currently influencing community-based allergy prevention models.

CONCLUSION

Beyond infancy, a continuum of preventive care is necessary for pediatric allergic disease. While tertiary strategies try to maximize control and reduce the disease burden in afflicted children, secondary prevention aims to stop the allergic cascade before clinical disease appears. Both strategies depend on accurate risk assessment, interdisciplinary teamwork, and the application of evidence-based, situation-specific interventions. Providing pediatricians and carers with useful, evidence-based resources for secondary and tertiary prevention is still crucial for public health, especially as allergy rates continue to rise worldwide. Improving outcomes for children with allergies or sensitivities requires secondary and tertiary prevention in pediatric allergy. The cornerstones are education, immunotherapy, early allergen introduction, and allergen avoidance. The sustainability and acceptability of interventions are increased when eco-friendly practices and home remedies are combined. The best course of action for pediatric allergists and carers is still a multidisciplinary, individualized strategy backed by continuing research.

KEY POINTS

- *Targeted prevention beyond infancy:* Secondary prevention aims at sensitized but asymptomatic children, while tertiary prevention addresses those with established allergic diseases to limit progression and complications.
- *Early allergen introduction:* Controlled introduction of allergenic foods (e.g., peanut, egg) in infancy has been shown to reduce the risk of food allergy development, marking a paradigm shift from prior avoidance strategies.
- *Environmental and lifestyle interventions:* Reducing exposure to aeroallergens, indoor pollutants, and tobacco smoke, along with optimizing home environments, can significantly reduce exacerbations and disease burden.
- *AIT:* AIT is the cornerstone of tertiary prevention, capable of inducing long-term immune tolerance, reducing new sensitizations, and altering the natural course of allergic rhinitis and asthma.
- *Multidisciplinary and holistic care:* Effective secondary and tertiary prevention requires integration of medical, nutritional, psychological, and educational support, ensuring improved outcomes and quality of life for children with allergies.

SUGGESTED READING

1. Bousquet J, Burney PG, Zuberbier T, Cauwenberge PV, Akdis CA, Bindslev-Jensen C, et al. GA2LEN (Global Allergy and Asthma European Network) addresses the allergy and asthma 'epidemic'. Allergy. 2009;64(7):969-77.
2. Calderón MA, et al. Allergen immunotherapy for allergic respiratory diseases: A review. Lancet. 2022; 400(10361):75-87.
3. Chan HY, Yuen YL, Leung DYM. Eco-friendly home cleaning and pediatric asthma outcomes: A six-month prospective cohort. Pediatr Pulmonol. 2021;56(7):2305-312.
4. Cronin A, et al. Pediatric allergy in the 21st century: Trends, mechanisms, and management. J Allergy Clin Immunol Pract. 2023;11(1):45-60.
5. Du Toit G, et al. Randomized trial of peanut consumption in infants at risk for peanut allergy. N Eng J Med. 2015;372(9): 803-13.
6. Haahtela T, Roberts G, Sayre PH, Bahnson HT, Radulovic S, Santos AF, et al. Biodiversity and immune tolerance. Allergy. 2022;77(3):833-47.
7. Holt PG, et al. Probiotic supplementation in infancy for prevention of allergic disease. J Allergy Clin Immunol. 2018;142(3):708-11.
8. Lack G, et al. Long-term outcomes of early allergen introduction: A 5-year follow-up. J Allergy Clin Immunol. 2023;151(1):45-54.
9. Morgan WJ, Crain EF, Gruchalla RS, et al. Results of a home-based environmental intervention among urban children with asthma. New Engl J Med. 2004;351(11):1068-80.
10. Murray CS, Simpson A, Custovic A. Environmental interventions for prevention and management of pediatric allergic diseases: A systematic review and meta-analysis. Thorax. 2022;77(4):370-9.
11. Perkin MR, Logan K, Tseng A, Raji B, Ayis S, Peacock J, et al. Randomized Trial of Introduction of Allergenic Foods in Breast-Fed Infants. N Engl J Med. 2016;374(18):1733-43.
12. Rancé F, Deschildre A, Bidat E, Just J, Couderc L, Wanin S, et al. [Secondary and tertiary prevention of allergic asthma in children]. Rev Mal Respir. 2010;27(10):1221-30.
13. Ren Z, Wang C, Xi L, Gao Y, Zhang Y, Zhang L. Long-term efficacy of house dust mite SCIT in children with allergic rhinitis. Allergy Asthma Clin Immunol. 2023;19:102.
14. Tang MLK, Proskin HM. Timing of food introduction and allergy development in children: A longitudinal analysis. Pediatr Allergy Immunol. 2022;33(2):189-97.
15. West CE, et al. Gut microbiota and pediatric allergy. Nat Rev Gastroenterol Hepatol. 2023;20(4):219-31.

7 SECTION Practical Considerations

Section Editors: *Naresh Grover, Surender Kagithapu*

29 CHAPTER

Setting Up an Allergy Clinic

Surender Kagithapu, Naresh Grover

INTRODUCTION

Allergic diseases are increasing worldwide, with a rising prevalence not only in high-income countries but also in low- and middle-income countries where infectious diseases continue to coexist. This growing burden of allergies adversely affects the quality of life of sufferers and represents a major public health challenge. Globally, nearly one-third of the population suffers from at least one form of allergic disease, making allergy one of the most pervasive chronic disorders.

The International Study of Asthma and Allergies in Childhood (ISAAC) Phase III reported prevalence rates in Indian children of 6–7 years and 13–14 years as follows: Wheezing in 7%, allergic rhinitis in 12.9% and 24.4%, respectively. In contrast, food allergy prevalence is estimated at 8% in the United States and Europe but remains very low in Indian children (0.11% in those aged 6–11 years). Allergy specialty services are highly developed in the Western world, but in developing countries such as India, allergy as a discipline is still in its infancy. Given the significant morbidity associated with allergic diseases and the increasing demand for care, it is both beneficial and timely to establish pediatric allergy services as an ancillary to routine pediatric practice. A dedicated and well-equipped pediatric allergy clinic; however, requires thorough background preparation and compliance with regulatory standards. This includes:

- Registration with local health authorities and compliance with the Clinical Establishments Act.
- Approval from the Pollution Control Board for biomedical waste disposal.
- Fire safety licenses and mandatory insurance (including professional indemnity coverage).

In addition, doctors managing children with allergies should undergo certified training in allergy practice. They must be familiar with the risks of procedures such as skin tests, provocation tests, and intentional allergen exposures, as well as emergency management of adverse reactions, particularly anaphylaxis.

The core objectives of an allergy clinic are accurate diagnosis, long-term management of allergic disorders, and safe handling of hypersensitivity conditions. Adverse reactions, while possible, can be minimized when care is delivered by trained specialists in a controlled environment.

An effective pediatric allergy service can substantially improve the quality of life for patients, reduce healthcare costs, and ensure safer, evidence-based practice in a field of growing importance worldwide.

SERVICES/SCOPE

History eliciting, testing/diagnostic allergy procedure, skin prick test (SPT)/intradermal test (IDST)/bronchial challenge, nasal allergen provocation test, nasal endoscopy/food challenge.

THERAPEUTIC ALLERGY PROCEDURE

Subcutaneous immunotherapy (SCIT)/sublingual immunotherapy (SLIT)/venom immunotherapy/drug desensitization/oral immunotherapy (OIT) for food allergy.

Treatment

Anti-immunoglobulin E (Anti-IgE)/other biological treatment with human plasma products. Nebulizer treatment.

MODEL CLINIC (FIG. 1)

Key Areas of a Pediatric Allergy Clinic

Reception Area

- Serves as the first point of contact for patients and attendants.
- Registration for outpatient consultations, procedures, and follow-ups should be streamlined.
- Display consultation timings, procedure schedules, and fee structures clearly.
- Organizes patient flow and reduces waiting time through effective scheduling.

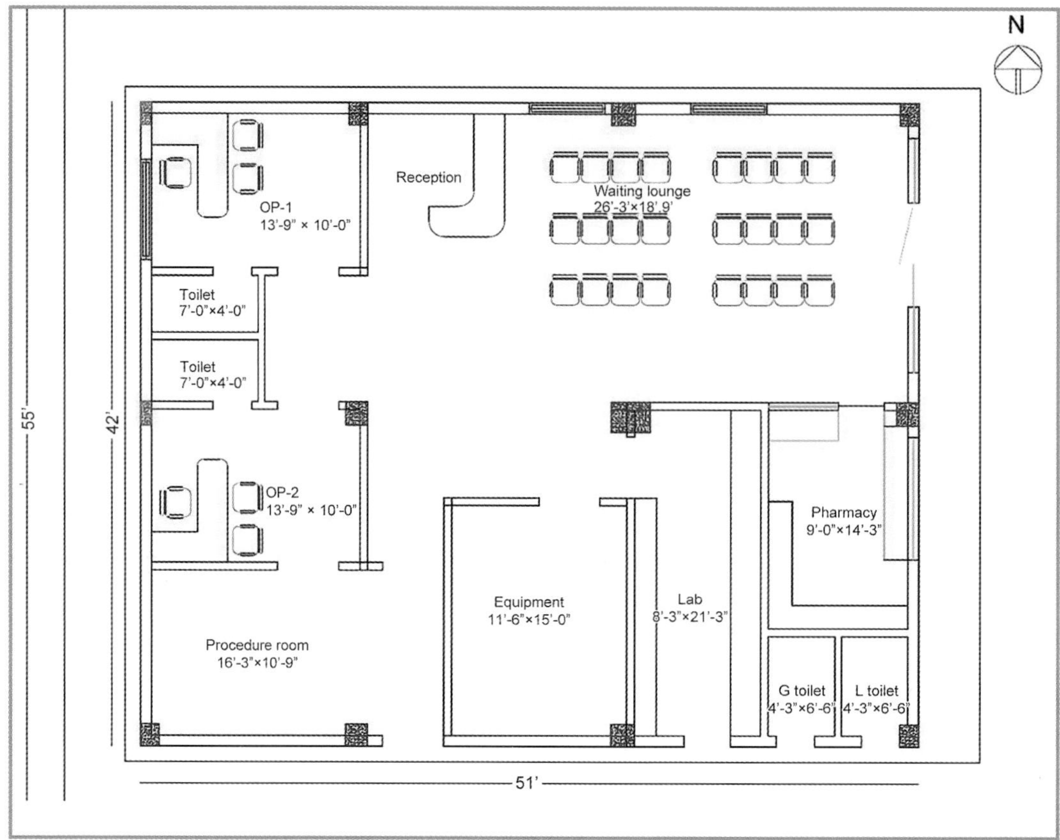

Fig. 1: Model clinic plan (300–400 ft^2).

Consultation Room

- Dedicated space for doctor–patient interaction.
- Activities include medical history taking, clinical examination, counseling regarding investigations and procedures, and obtaining informed consent.
- Treatment plans and follow-up schedules are discussed here.
- Comfortable, private, and adequately equipped for effective communication.

Procedure/Emergency Room

- Spacious enough to accommodate staff, patients, and family members.
- Patient chairs should be reclining to allow safe positioning in case of adverse events.
- Adequate access space for skin testing procedures.
- *Equipped with:*
  - Vitals monitoring equipment.
  - Emergency code cart for anaphylaxis and severe reactions.
  - Timer for accurate skin test reading intervals.
- *Essential storage:*
  - Dedicated refrigerator for allergens, vials, and medications (not for food or nonmedical specimens).
  - Temperature maintained at 2–8°C with alarms and daily logs to ensure potency and sterility.

Allergen Compounding Area

- Must comply with minimum standards for allergen immunotherapy mixing (as per USP recommendations).
- *There should be a dedicated Allergy Extract Compounding Area (AECA) with:*
  - Location at least 1 meter away from sinks and unsealed windows
  - No openings directly into kitchens, bathrooms, or high-traffic areas
  - Restricted access to authorized personnel only
  - Surfaces are disinfected after each session

    - Monthly disinfection of walls and doors, and scheduled ceiling cleaning
- If these criteria are met, compounded sterile preparations (CSPs) may be exempt from additional environmental monitoring requirements.

Waiting Area

Located close to the procedure room for postintervention observation.

- *Patients should remain for:*
    - *30 minutes* after injections or new vial administration to monitor for adverse events.
    - *15 minutes* following skin prick testing for reading results.
- Spacious enough to accommodate patients and attendants.
- Transparent glass panels allow monitoring by front desk staff for safety and quick response if needed.

Ancillary Staff

The physicians who should preferably have basic courses in allergy and immunotherapy. The physicians who have their own course in allergies are more efficient.

The Basic course training gives unique opportunities to interact with the faculty and to discuss critical issues and answer questions, as well as hands-on practice to demonstrate techniques.

Licensed practitioner nurses, registered nurses, can provide excellent patient education, and they strongly support the outpatient allergy practice.

Staff will perform both administrative and clinical tasks related to running an allergy practice. Administrative staff do not require any formal allergy technician certification course.

Allergy technicians are trained medical assistants who acquire the required knowledge in the allergy field by working and being trained under supervision in an allergy clinic.

All the staff should be trained in basic life support (BLS) and be able to recognize and respond to anaphylaxis.

All staff should participate in the ongoing observation process.

- *Allergy testing consumables:*
  For skin prick/intradermal testing:
    - Alcohol swabs, cotton swabs/gauze.
    - Adhesive tape or hypoallergenic micropore tape, sterile single-use skin prick lancets.
    - Intradermal syringes (1 mL, insulin-type).
    - Negative control solution (normal saline or glycerinated diluent).
    - Positive control solution (histamine dihydrochloride).
    - Allergen extracts (local and imported panels—pollen, dust mite, mold, animal dander, food allergens).
    - Adhesive labels; to mark test sites (optional), marker pens (skin-safe).
    - *Transparent millimeter ruler for wheal size measurement. For patch testing:*
        - Patch test chambers (aluminum or hypoallergenic plastic), hypoallergenic adhesive strips.
        - Preprepared allergen panels (e.g., cosmetics, metals, fragrances, and rubber chemicals).
- *Lung function and respiratory consumables:*
    - Nose clips
    - Mouthpieces (single-use) for spirometer/oscillometer, disposable peak flow meter mouthpieces.
    - Disposable bacterial/viral filters for spirometer
- *Immunotherapy consumables:*
    - Alcohol swabs, cotton/gauze pads.
    - Sterile single-use syringes (1 and 3 mL).
    - Needles (26–27 gauge).
    - Allergen immunotherapy vials (SCIT), sublingual allergen drops/tablets (SLIT), saline diluent for vial preparation (if needed), and vial cradles/sharps bins.
- *Emergency and first aid consumables:*
    - Adrenaline (ampoules or autoinjectors, epinephrine 1:1,000).
    - Antihistamine injections (e.g., chlorpheniramine).
    - Corticosteroid injections (e.g., hydrocortisone, methylprednisolone 125 mg vial).
    - IV stands
    - IV fluids (normal saline and Ringer's lactate).
    - IV cannulas (various sizes).
    - IV infusion sets.
    - Oxygen masks (adult and pediatric), Ambu bag, nasal canula, and face mask.
    - Nebulizer solution [salbutamol, ipratropium, and albuterol metered-dose inhaler (MDI)].
    - Disposable gloves (preferably, latex-free)
    - Suction machine and catheters
    - Oxygen cylinder
    - Glucagon 1 mg/mL

  - Heparin 10,000 units/mL
  - Atropine 0.5 mg/mL IV
  - Diphenhydramine 25–50 mg/mL
  - Ranitidine 25–50 mg/mL
- *General clinic consumables:*
  - Examination table roll/bed sheets (disposable or washable)
  - Disposable pillow covers.
  - Hand sanitizer bottles and refills.
  - Surgical masks and N95 masks.
  - Disposable aprons/gowns for staff.
  - Waste segregation bags (biohazard, general waste, and recyclable).
  - Sharps disposal containers.
  - Surface disinfectant wipes and sprays.
  - Paper towels/tissue boxes.
  - Drinking water cups for patients (preferably/biodegradable)
- *Office and patient education consumables:*
  - Appointment cards
  - File folders and stationery items
  - Patient consent forms (preprinted)
  - Test report forms and interpretation charts
  - Patient information leaflets (allergen avoidance, immunotherapy instructions)

DIAGNOSTIC PROCEDURES

Skin Prick Test

A typical diagnostic SPT kit consists of:
- Allergen extracts (liquid form, glycerinated, ready to use) with written expiry dates.
- Positive control (histamine dihydrochloride 10 mg/mL or 6 mg/mL).
- Negative control (diluent—saline with glycerin).
- Sterile single-use lancets (specialized for skin prick).
- Bottles with a dropper for each extract of allergen.
- Product insert with test panel specifics.
- World Allergy Organization (WAO) safety guidelines.

Setting: A hospital and outpatient clinic setting. Field (skin prick test only), e.g., epidemiology studies, may also be conducted by trained medical professionals.

Staff: Can be performed by a trained nurse/technician under the supervision of an experienced physician.

Emergency equipment availability: It must be accessible on site (mandatory).

Emergency staff (ICU) availability: Not necessary

Broncho Provocation Test or Nasal Provocation Test

- *Setting:* Ideally in a hospital. An outpatient clinic setting could be acceptable.
- *Staff:* The provocation test can be performed by a trained nurse/technician, but only under the supervision of a qualified clinician.

Emergency equipment availability: Should be available on site (mandatory).
- *Emergency staff (ICU) availability:* Should be available within 30 minutes.

Nasal Endoscopy

- *Setting:* Both hospital and outpatient clinics.
- *Staff:* Nasal endoscopic, either rigid or flexible, should be performed by a well-trained physician, either an otorhinolaryngologist or not (allergologist, pneumonologist, pediatrician, or even general practitioner).
- *Emergency equipment availability:* Not required.

THERAPEUTIC PROCEDURE

SCIT/SLIT/OIT:
- *Setting:* Treatment can be started and continued in an outpatient setting
- *Staff:* Only trained allergists are authorized to initiate and supervise SCIT/SLIT/OIT. The injections can be made by a nurse under a physician's supervision.
- *Emergency equipment availability:* Should be available on site (mandatory).
- *Emergency staff (ICU) availability:* Should be available on site (in <5 minutes) or within 30 minutes, depending on the risk assessment.

OPTIMAL PATIENT FLOW IN ALLERGY CLINICS: A COMPREHENSIVE ZONE-BASED APPROACH

This systematic patient flow model demonstrates evidence-based best practices for managing patients safely and efficiently through an allergy clinic. The five-zone approach ensures optimal care delivery while minimizing risks and maximizing patient satisfaction.

Zone 1: Entry and Registration (Reception/Waiting Area)

Initial contact and preparation:
- Patient check-in with reception staff for appointment confirmation and registration.

- *Infection control protocols:* Hand sanitizer dispensing and mask provision when indicated.
- *Previsit documentation:* Completion of comprehensive allergy history questionnaires and informed consent forms during waiting time.
- This zone establishes the foundation for safe care by ensuring proper documentation and infection prevention measures are in place before clinical interactions begin.

Zone 2: Consultation (Clinical Assessment Room)

Comprehensive clinical evaluation:
- *Vital signs assessment:* Blood pressure, temperature, pulse, and oxygen saturation monitoring.
- *Detailed medical history:* Current symptoms, previous reactions, medication usage, and family history review.
- *Past testing review:* Analysis of previous allergy test results and treatment responses.
- *Physical examination:* Focused skin, respiratory, and ear, nose, and throat (ENT) assessment.

Clinical Decision Making

- Determination of appropriate diagnostic procedures (SPT, patch testing, and spirometry).
- *Medication timing considerations:* Assessment of recent antihistamine use that may interfere with testing.
- Scheduling decisions based on patient readiness and clinical appropriateness.

Zone 3: Diagnostic Testing Area

- *Skin prick testing station:*
  - *Sterile setup:* Prearranged allergen extracts, lancets, and control solutions.
  - *Patient isolation:* One patient at a time to prevent cross-contamination and mixups.
  - *Immediate observation area:* Positioned for rapid response to adverse reactions.
  - *Spirometry station:*
    - *Separated from waiting areas:* Reduces cross-contamination risk.
    - *Single-use equipment:* Disposable mouthpieces and bacterial/viral filters.
    - *Immediate waste disposal:* Proper handling of contaminated materials.
- *Patch testing application:*
  - *Controlled environment:* Dedicated space for precise allergen applications.
  - *48-hour protocol:* Patient scheduling for return visits for reading results.

Zone 4: Waiting/Observation (Postprocedure Monitoring)

- *Critical safety monitoring:*
  - *Dedicated observation bay:* Separate area for postprocedure surveillance.
  - *Standardized monitoring periods:*
    - 15–20 minutes for skin prick tests.
    - 20–30 minutes for immunotherapy injections.
    - Extended periods for high-risk patients.
- *Emergency preparedness:* Immediate access to an emergency trolley with epinephrine, oxygen, and resuscitation equipment. The observation period is critical for patient safety, as most severe allergic reactions occur within 20–30 minutes of exposure.

Zone 5: Counseling and Exit (Results and Discharge)

- *Patient education and follow-up:*
  - *Results of interpretation:* Clear explanation of test findings with visual aids.
  - *Comprehensive care planning:*
    - Allergen avoidance strategies.
    - Dietary modifications and restrictions.
    - Prescription medications and emergency action plans.
- *Follow-up scheduling:* Organized appointment booking for continued care.

Optimized exit strategy:
- *Unidirectional flow:* Separate exit pathways to prevent congestion with incoming patients.
- *Final safety check:* Confirmation of patient stability before departure.

Key Design Principles for Optimal Flow

- *Safety-first approach:*
  - *Proximity planning:* Testing areas positioned near emergency equipment and oxygen supply.
  - *Emergency accessibility:* All zones equipped with immediate access to anaphylaxis treatment.
- *Staff training:* All personnel, including administrative staff, trained in BLS and anaphylaxis recognition.

- *Efficiency optimization:*
  - *Clear signage and navigation:* Directional arrows and zone labels (Reception → Consultation → Testing → Observation → Exit)
  - *Pediatric considerations:* Dedicated children's waiting areas with appropriate entertainment
  - *Privacy protection:* Enclosed consultation rooms for sensitive medical discussions.
- *Patient experience enhancement:*
  - *Transparent glass observation:* Front desk staff can monitor waiting patients through glass partitions.
  - *Comfort amenities:* Reading materials, television, and internet access during waiting periods.
  - *Family accommodation:* Space planning to include family members during procedures.

EVIDENCE-BASED IMPLEMENTATION BENEFITS

This structured flow system has been shown to:

- Reduce adverse events through systematic safety protocols.
- Improve patient satisfaction by minimizing wait times and providing clear expectations.
- Enhance staff efficiency through standardized workflows and defined responsibilities.
- Optimize resource utilization by preventing bottlenecks and reducing patient flow interruptions.

The zone-based approach ensures that every patient receives standardized, safe, and efficient care while maintaining the flexibility to accommodate individual patient needs and emergencies.

Materials Required

- *Reception/documentation table:*
  - *Purpose:* Patient registration, record-keeping, and billing.
  - *Type:* Standard office desk with storage.
  - *Key features:*
    - Space for computers, printers, and files.
    - Lockable drawers for prescription pads and reports.
    - Smooth, easy-to-clean surface.
- *Examination/consultation table:*
  - *Purpose:* Patient physical examination and basic procedures.
  - *Type:* Standard examination couch or semi-fowler couch with adjustable backrest.
  - *Key features:*
    - Padded, washable, non-allergenic vinyl cover
    - Sturdy frame (SS or powder-coated steel)
    - Paper roll holder (for disposable sheets)
    - *Height:* ~75–80 cm for ergonomic examination
    - *Why important in the Allergy Clinic:*
      - Needed for systemic examination before SPT or spirometry.
      - Comfortable position for anxious or pediatric patients.
- *Allergy testing procedure table:*
  - *Purpose:* Laying out allergen extracts, controls, lancets, and documentation during SPTs or patch tests.
  - *Type:* Instrument table or Mayo trolley with wheels.
  - *Key features:*
    - Stainless steel or laminated top (easy disinfection).
    - At least two shelves or trays.
    - Wheels with brakes for mobility.
    - Can be positioned close to the patient during testing.
    - *Why important:* Especially useful if doing SPT/patch tests on the back.
- *Immunotherapy and injection table:*
  - *Purpose:* Preparing SCIT doses and holding emergency drugs.
  - *Type:* Small dressing trolley or compact stainless steel procedure table.
  - *Key features:*
    - Two shelves
    - Nonreactive stainless-steel surface.
    - Drawer for syringes, needles, and swabs.
    - Upper for procedure, lower for emergency kit.
    - *Why important:* Enables quick shift from preparation to administration, especially in case of reactions.

FACILITY EQUIPMENT AND EMERGENCY SUPPLIES CHECKLIST

Refer **Table 1**.

CONCLUSION

The prevalence of allergic diseases are alarmingly increasing worldwide. Lower- and middle-income countries are also showing an upsurge in allergic diseases, adversely affecting quality of life. Allergy specialty is in the naïve phase in developing countries like India, hence incorporating allergy into pediatric practice, and bringing awareness

TABLE 1: Facility equipment and emergency supplies checklist.

Equipment checklist	*Yes*	*No*
Basic:		
☐ Examination couch and stool		
☐ Otoscope, dermatoscope		
☐ Peak flow meter, portable spirometer		
☐ BP apparatus, stethoscope		
Allergy-specific:		
☐ Skin prick test lancets		
☐ Allergen extracts (local + international panels)		
☐ Patch test kits		
☐ Digital camera (to document skin reactions)		
☐ Epinephrine autoinjectors or adrenaline vials		
Emergency readiness:		
☐ Oxygen cylinder/concentrator		
☐ Ambu bag		
☐ Nebulizer with masks		
☐ Suction machine		
☐ IV-line setup with fluids		

among the patients can not only improve the quality of life but also cost savings.

KEY POINTS

- A well-planned, dedicated space for allergy practice is essential for better patient management and to prevent unwanted adverse events during diagnostic procedures or treatment. Proper layout and specialized zones improve safety and efficiency.
- All staff, including administrative assistants in the clinic, must be trained in BLS and be able to recognize and respond to anaphylaxis promptly. This preparedness is critical to managing emergencies effectively and ensuring patient safety.

  These measures ensure quality care, minimize risks, and enhance overall allergy service effectiveness.

SUGGESTED READING

1. American Academy of Otolaryngic Allergy (AAOA). (2021). Starting an allergy practice. [Online]. Available from https://www.aaoallergy.org/starting-an-allergy-practice/ [Last accessed December, 2025].
2. Australasian Society of Clinical Immunology and Allergy (ASCIA). (2024). Skin prick testing guide. [Online] Available from https://www.allergy.org.au/hp/papers/skin-prick-testing [Last accessed December, 2025].
3. Indian Academy of Pediatrics (IAP). (2020). IAP-KPJ guidelines. [Online]. Available from https://iap-kpj.org [Last accessed December, 2025].
4. Kowalski ML, Ansotegui I, Aberer W, Al-Ahmad M, Akdis M, Ballmer-Weber BK, et al. Risk and safety requirements for diagnostic and therapeutic procedures in allergology: World Allergy Organization Statement. World Allergy Organ J. 2016;9(1):33.
5. Krishna MT, Mahesh PA, Vedanthan P, Motta S, Mehra V, Christopher DJ. An appraisal of allergic disorders in India and an urgent call for action. World Allergy Organ J. 2020;13(7):100446.
6. Scleisma LT, Reynoldol LA, Turner SE, Finlay BB. The hygiene hypothesis: current perspectives and future therapies. Immunol Ther. 2015;4:143-57.

30 CHAPTER

Patient Education and Advocacy in Pediatric Allergy

Vipul Sharma

INTRODUCTION

Across India, pediatric allergic disease has become both more visible and more burdensome. This is partly because we're getting better at recognizing and diagnosing these issues, which helps explain the increase in cases. However, other factors, including urbanization, air pollution, changes in diet, reduced ventilation in homes, and variations in early-life exposure to microbes, have also contributed to the issue. In this setting, the traditional approach of "diagnose, prescribe, review" is often not enough, especially when children face long commutes, indoor smoke, damp housing during the monsoon, and uncertain food quality at school. Medicines are most effective when used correctly and consistently; however, they are often ineffective when fear, myths, or logistical barriers prevent families from following through.

The practical answer is a dual commitment. First, clinicians must make precise, correct diagnoses and prescribe minimal effective therapy with planned reviews. Second, they must educate and advocate. They must teach children and caregivers to recognize patterns, use devices properly, reduce exposure without turning home life into a chore, and respond decisively to emergencies. This chapter focuses on how to accomplish this work in the Indian context. It links local disease patterns with practical clinic advice, school readiness, community involvement, and minor policy changes that can make safer habits more straightforward to follow.

EDUCATION IN PEDIATRIC ALLERGY

Why Patient Education Matters in Pediatric Allergy?

Patient education is not just about providing information; it is about helping families adopt and change their daily habits. In pediatric allergy, this involves ensuring that the child, parents, and other caregivers are capable of recognizing early symptoms, avoiding triggers, administering medications correctly, and taking appropriate action during emergencies. For example, parents who understand asthma as a variable, controllable airway condition are more likely to continue preventive medicines even when symptoms improve. Consider a caregiver who practices the spacer technique during a clinic visit; they are much more likely to manage a late-night asthma situation confidently when it matters most. Similarly, a teenager who knows how to read food labels and ask questions about how meals are prepared is more likely to avoid potentially dangerous situations that could send them to the emergency department. Education succeeds when it is concrete, repetitive, without being tedious, and tied to the child's daily life.

Objectives of Patient Education in Pediatric Allergy

It includes:

- *Enhance disease understanding* by clarifying the diagnosis, outlining the expected course, identifying potential complications, and addressing common misconceptions.
- *Teach the correct use* of inhalers, spacers, nasal sprays, emollients, and adrenaline autoinjectors.
- *Encourage adherence* by explaining the role and benefits of preventive treatment.
- *Prepare families* to recognize anaphylaxis early and give adrenaline without delay.
- *Develop self-management skills,* particularly for adolescents moving towards independent care.

Key Principles of Education in the Indian Context

- *Language appropriateness:* Use the local language alongside English in written and verbal communication.
- *Visual aids:* Pictures, diagrams, and videos enhance understanding, especially for families with low literacy.
- *Involving the extended family:* In many Indian households, grandparents or hired caregivers play significant roles in childcare and must be educated alongside parents.

- *Cultural sensitivity:* Respect traditional practices but clarify when they may be harmful or ineffective.
- *Practical demonstration:* "Show-do-teach back" ensures that the child and caregiver can perform the skill correctly.
- *Reinforcement:* Revisit key skills at every follow-up; skills like inhaler technique decay quickly without regular checks.

Methods and Tools for Patient Education

- *Verbal counselling:*
  - Schedule structured education for diagnosis, follow-up, and treatment changes.
  - Include both parents; where relevant, involve grandparents and older siblings.
- *Written material:*
  - Allergen avoidance lists
  - Asthma action plans
  - Emergency allergy plans with caregiver and doctor contacts.
- *Digital tools:*
  - Recommend credible apps for asthma tracking, medication reminders.
  - Share short, trustworthy YouTube videos on inhaler use in Hindi/regional languages.
- *Demonstration and hands-on learning:*
  - Inhaler/spacer use should be shown, practiced, and rechecked at every visit.
  - For food allergies, teach families to read ingredient lists and recognize hidden allergens.

ADVOCACY IN PEDIATRIC ALLERGY

Advocacy is the process of influencing policies, systems, and community practices to improve outcomes for children with allergies.

Advocacy Targets in India

- *Schools:* Implement allergy action plans, stock emergency medication, and train teachers.
- *Policy makers:* Include epinephrine auto-injectors in the National List of Essential Medicines; standardize school health policies.
- *Food regulation:* Ensure compliance with FSSAI allergen labeling; advocate for enforcement in unorganized sectors like street food vendors.
- *Public awareness:* Use media campaigns to debunk myths and promote early treatment.
- *Healthcare systems:* Train primary care providers in allergy recognition and management.

SCHOOL ADVOCACY

Why Schools Matter?

Children spend one-third of their waking hours in school. Exposure to triggers, risk of accidental allergen ingestion, and absence of immediate medical care make schools critical partners in allergy care.

School Advocacy: Turning Policy into Practice (Table 1)

The school day brings multiple opportunities for exposure and risk. Children eat, run, share, and react under the eyes of adults whose training is variable and who may fear "doing the wrong thing." Effective school advocacy is about embedding simple routines that staff understand and trust. Each child with allergies should have an individual plan on file, and a copy provided to their class

TABLE 1: School allergy management workflow.

Step	*Action*	*Responsible person(s)*
1	Identify students with diagnosed allergy/asthma and obtain medical forms and action plans	School nurse/class teacher/parent
2	Store emergency medications (e.g., epinephrine, a reliever inhaler) in a readily accessible location	School nurse/health lead teacher
3	Train staff annually on recognizing symptoms and administering emergency medications	Pediatric allergist/school nurse
4	Implement daily management strategies [e.g., avoiding allergens and monitoring Air Quality Index (AQI)]	Class teacher/student
5	Respond to symptoms according to the action plan, administer emergency medication as needed, and call emergency services if necessary	Any trained staff present
6	Document the incident and inform parents immediately	School nurse/principal
7	Review the incident and update action plans if necessary	School nurse/pediatric allergist/parent

teacher. The school should maintain an emergency kit in a designated, accessible location known to all staff, stocked with epinephrine in its preferred form, a reliever inhaler with a spacer, a nonsedating antihistamine, and a laminated algorithm with clear, stepwise prompts. At least twice a year, staff should conduct a brief drill to practice recognizing a problem, retrieving the kit, administering the correct medicine, and calling for help. Repeated practice makes the process faster and more assured.

Food safety changes culture more than budgets. Canteens can prevent cross-contamination by dedicating specific utensils for high-risk items, thoroughly cleaning surfaces, and clearly labeling common allergens in plain language. Younger classes tend to do well with a "no sharing food" rule framed as a kindness to protect friends. Birthday celebrations and festival days are predictable for high-risk periods; advanced planning with parents and teachers allows joy without danger. The best programs begin small and expand. If a school has not yet stocked autoinjectors, start by training staff, having plans on file, and establishing a clear route to the nearest hospital. Involve parent-teacher associations and utilize their influence to institutionalize what works.

Practical tip: Ask the principal to nominate a "health lead" teacher who attends your clinic's annual refresher session and acts as the in-school point person for allergy and asthma.

ADVOCACY BEYOND SCHOOLS: MULTI-LEVEL APPROACH IN INDIA (TABLE 2)

While schools remain a high-priority environment for pediatric allergy advocacy, Indian children interact with multiple systems that influence their health and safety. Pediatricians and allergists can extend advocacy to the levels discussed further.

Community-level Advocacy

- *At the doctor's clinic:* One-page pictorial guides for spacers, nasal sprays, and auto-injectors; pharmacies will display them; a hundred families will learn without ever stepping into your outpatient department (OPD).
- *Parent groups and support networks:* Promote local or online allergy parent groups for peer learning, stigma reduction, and joint action for better services.
- *Religious and cultural gatherings:* Engage temple committees, mosque boards, and gurudwara langar organizers to promote allergen-free zones during events and festivals. This can prevent flares without diluting tradition.
- *Health camps:* Partner with nongovernmental organizations (NGOs), Lions/Rotary clubs for community "Asthma–Allergy Camps" offering diagnosis, training, and free multilingual educational materials.

TABLE 2: Advocacy at different levels in pediatric allergy (India).

Level	*Key activities*	*Stakeholders*
Individual/family	Provide bilingual action plans, train in device use, counsel on trigger avoidance, and empower children to self-advocate	Pediatric allergist, parents, and extended family
School	Implement allergy-friendly policies, train staff, maintain emergency kits, and run awareness programs	School administration, teachers, the school nurse, and parents
Community	Conduct health camps, promote clean air initiatives, address cooking smoke exposure, and involve religious and cultural groups	Local health authorities, NGOs, and resident associations
Healthcare system	Standardize referral pathways, ensure access to essential medications, and integrate allergy modules in training programs	Hospitals, primary health centers, medical colleges, and professional bodies
Policy/government	Mandate allergen labeling, subsidize essential devices, include allergy care in school health programs, and fund research	Ministry of Health, FSSAI, education boards, policy makers

(FSSAI: Food Safety and Standards Authority of India; NGOs: nongovernmental organizations)

- *Community talks:* In resident associations about burning leaves or garbage. It can change the local air within weeks.

Primary Healthcare Advocacy

- *Accredited social health activist (ASHA) and anganwadi training:* A one-day module can train them to identify wheeze, eczema, allergic rhinitis, and anaphylaxis, with clear referral protocols.
- *Pharmacist engagement:* Pharmacists can act as local teachers at the point of sale, instructing local chemists on inhaler techniques and rational prescribing to reduce misuse and under-treatment.
- *Family physician sensitization:* Continuing medical education (CME) programs for general practitioners to standardize diagnosis and management according to national guidelines.

Workplace and Adolescent Advocacy

- *Workplace readiness:* For older teens entering internships or jobs, coordinate with occupational health teams to ensure allergen-safe environments and accessible emergency medication.
- *Sports and coaching staff:* Train coaches to recognize and manage asthma flares, adapt activities during poor air quality, and maintain quick-relief inhaler access.

Media and Public Awareness

- *Radio and TV:* Media and messaging shape what parents believe. A short, credible, local-language radio segment aired before pollen season, advising families to check their inhaler technique and keep action plans handy, spreads faster than any pamphlet.
- *Social media:* Infographics, reels, and myth-busting posts in Hindi, Tamil, Bengali, and other languages. WhatsApp is powerful when used judiciously; a school broadcast of your ninety-second video on autoinjector steps will be watched and remembered.
- *Newspaper health columns:* Regular contributions during peak allergy seasons to normalize public discussion and encourage early diagnosis. When misinformation about "addictive inhalers" or miracle allergy cures trends, pediatricians who respond calmly with fact-based, empathetic explanations help anchor public conversation in reality.

Policy and Regulatory Advocacy

- *Inclusion in national programs:* Push for allergy modules in the National Health Mission's school and adolescent health programs.
- *Cost reduction:* Advocate for GST reduction or a subsidy on epinephrine autoinjectors and pediatric inhalers. Insurance coverage for immunotherapy and recommended diagnostics makes long-term control possible for more families.
- *Food labeling:* Collaborate with the Food Safety and Standards Authority of India (FSSAI) to mandate allergen labeling on packaged foods and enforce standards in sweets and bakeries.
- *Securing availability and affordability:* Professional bodies of pediatrics, respiratory medicine, dermatology, and allergy can speak together to regulators and industry to secure availability and affordability.

Professional and Academic Advocacy

- *Specialist networks:* Create a national Pediatric Allergy Advocacy Forum to unify efforts and amplify messaging.
- *Data dissemination:* Publish open-access Indian epidemiology data for use by schools, NGOs, and public health planners.
- *Curriculum integration:* Advocate for pediatric allergy teaching in MBBS and MD Pediatrics programs, so new doctors are advocacy-ready.

FUTURE DIRECTIONS FOR INDIA

- National pediatric allergy surveillance and regional pollen/aeroallergen calendars to inform school advisories.
- Inclusion of pediatric allergy modules in MBBS/MD pediatrics curricula and school health teacher training.
- Insurance/State procurement to improve access to epinephrine auto-injectors and pediatric inhaler devices.
- Tele allergy follow-ups for underserved districts; creation of multilingual microlearning libraries (sub-2-minute videos).

Vignettes from Indian Practice

- *Syrup for wheeze:* A 6-year-old from a small town presents with "recurrent colds" treated repeatedly with syrups and antibiotics. On examination, he has an

audible wheeze. His mother is reluctant to try inhalers. In the clinic, you demonstrate spacer use, observe him practicing, and send a bilingual plan along with a school letter. Two months later, his symptoms are under control, and he is active with his classmates. The change came from education and technique rather than a new medicine.
- *Festivals and food:* An 8-year-old with an egg allergy has a reaction during a class birthday celebration. The school is unsure how to respond. You meet with the principal and teachers, file an action plan, set up a labeled emergency kit, train staff through a mock drill, and introduce a no-sharing rule in lower grades as a way to protect friends. Subsequent celebrations are safe, and the child participates fully without feeling excluded.
- *Monsoon rash:* A 10-year-old with flexural eczema has predictable flares each monsoon. The family alternates strong steroids with herbal remedies, and infections are common. You explain fingertip-unit dosing, advise using daily emollients after short, lukewarm baths, recommend wearing cotton clothing, and discuss simple ways to limit sweating. You replace perfumed oils with plain petroleum jelly. At follow-up, the skin is stable, sleep is uninterrupted, and school attendance has improved. Steady, uncomplicated care proved more effective than frequent changes in treatment.

CONCLUSION

Pediatric allergy in India is influenced by social and environmental factors as much as by biological factors. Children move between homes, schools, transport, outdoor spaces, and places of worship; each setting can either add risk or subtract it. When pediatricians and allergists pair accurate diagnosis and minimal effective pharmacotherapy with clear, repeated education and realistic advocacy, families respond more quickly, schools act with greater confidence, and communities adopt preventive habits. The benefits are seen in improved sleep, regular attendance, active play, and more stable disease control. Education and advocacy are core components of treatment, not add-ons.

KEY POINTS

- *Education is central to allergy care:* Empowering families with knowledge and skills transforms treatment outcomes more effectively than medicines alone.
- *Advocacy extends beyond the clinic:* Schools, communities, and policymakers must work together to create safe environments for allergic children.
- *Culturally sensitive, practical teaching:* Use local languages, visual aids, and hands-on demonstrations to build confidence and adherence.
- *School readiness saves lives:* Clear action plans, trained staff, and accessible emergency kits ensure a timely response to allergic emergencies.
- *Unified effort ensures long-term control:* Collaboration between families, healthcare providers, and public systems fosters awareness, affordability, and prevention.

SUGGESTED READING

1. Asthma & Bronchitis Association of India (ABAI). Programs for asthma/allergy education, awareness, and community support in Mumbai; includes camps, newsletters, and discounted inhalers. Mumbai: ABAI; 2025.
2. Deshpande C. (2025). IAP launches nationwide initiative on paediatric allergic disorders from Nagpur. [Online] Available from https://timesofindia.indiatimes.com/city/nagpur/iap-launches-nationwide-initiative-on-paediatric-allergic-disorders-from-nagpur/articleshow/122844149.cms [Last accessed December, 2025].
3. Indian Society of Allergy, Asthma and Sleep (ISAAS). Mission statement emphasizing education, research, and advocacy in India. ISAAS; 2025.
4. Kumar R, Behera D, Singh AB, Gaur SN, Agarwal MK, Prasad R, et al. Indian guidelines for the diagnosis of respiratory allergies. Indian J Allergy Asthma Immunol. 2023;37(Suppl 1):S1-98.
5. Vedanthan PK, Christopher DJ, Gupta N. Allergy training in India. Clin Exp Allergy. 2022;52(7):833-5.

8 SECTION Future Directions

Section Editors: *Mangayarkarshi Sinha, Nihar Ranjan Mishra*

31 CHAPTER Advances in Allergy Research

Shalini Tyagi

INTRODUCTION

Allergic disorders are a major and growing health concern, particularly in children. Over the past few decades, rapid urbanization, lifestyle transitions, and environmental exposures have contributed to a rising prevalence of asthma, allergic rhinitis, atopic dermatitis, and food allergies. Advances in research have uncovered novel insights into the role of the microbiome, epigenetics, and environmental triggers in allergy pathogenesis. Breakthroughs in diagnostics, including component-resolved testing and non-invasive biomarkers, along with therapeutic innovations, such as biologics, immunotherapy, and precision medicine, are reshaping pediatric allergy care. This chapter reviews these advances with emphasis on their clinical relevance to India.

EMERGING CONCEPTS IN ALLERGY PATHOGENESIS

Microbiome and Allergic Disease

Recent advances emphasize the role of the gut microbiome in shaping immune tolerance. A balanced and diverse microbiota in early life promotes healthy immune regulation, while dysbiosis—caused by caesarean delivery, formula feeding, antibiotic exposure, or urban living—predisposes children to asthma, atopic dermatitis, and food allergies. Though interventions such as probiotics, prebiotics, and maternal dietary supplementation have been studied, results remain inconsistent. Select strains, such as *Lactobacillus rhamnosus GG*, show potential in improving tolerance, but large-scale trials are still needed, especially in Indian children, where dietary and environmental factors differ significantly.

Epigenetics in Allergy

Epigenetic modifications, including deoxyribonucleic acid (DNA) methylation and histone acetylation, link environmental influences with allergic predisposition. Maternal nutrition, pollution exposure, and infections can alter gene expression without changing DNA sequence, thereby modifying immune responses. Population studies have identified methylation changes in genes regulating T-cell activity and antigen presentation in children with food allergies. These epigenetic signatures hold promise as biomarkers for early identification and may pave the way for personalized prevention strategies in high-risk populations.

Hygiene Hypothesis Revisited

The hygiene hypothesis, first introduced by Strachan in 1989, suggested that declining exposure to infectious agents was associated with rising allergy prevalence. Contemporary research refines this view, showing that reduced microbial diversity in early life disrupts immune maturation, promoting Th2-driven allergic responses. Indian studies comparing rural and urban children reveal lower rates of atopy in rural populations, supporting the protective role of environmental microbial exposures. This highlights the influence of lifestyle transitions on allergic risk in India.

DIAGNOSTIC ADVANCES

Traditional diagnostic methods, including skin prick and serum IgE testing, have limitations in specificity. Recent innovations provide greater accuracy:

- *Component-resolved diagnostics (CRD):* Identifies sensitization to individual allergen epitopes, improving diagnostic precision in nut and pollen-food allergies.
- *Noninvasive biomarkers:* Fractional exhaled nitric oxide (FeNO) is validated for eosinophilic asthma; periostin, eosinophil counts, and urinary leukotrienes are promising. Nasal fluid immunoglobulin E (IgE) profiling demonstrates high accuracy and may soon become clinically relevant.
- *Basophil activation test (BAT):* A functional in vitro assay that measures allergen-induced basophil activation, offering higher diagnostic relevance than sensitization tests alone.

THERAPEUTIC INNOVATIONS

Biologics

Biologic therapies have revolutionized the management of severe allergic diseases. Omalizumab (anti-IgE) is effective in asthma and chronic urticaria. Anti-IL-5 agents (mepolizumab and reslizumab) target eosinophilic asthma, while dupilumab [anti-interleukin-4 (anti-IL-4)/IL-13] benefits refractory atopic dermatitis and asthma and may enhance tolerance to allergen immunotherapy. Though highly effective, access and affordability remain challenges in India, underscoring the need for locally relevant cost-effectiveness studies.

Allergen Immunotherapy

Allergen immunotherapy (AIT), via subcutaneous immunotherapy (SCIT) or sublingual immunotherapy (SLIT) routes, remains the only disease-modifying intervention for allergic rhinitis and selected food allergies. Novel approaches include allergoids, epicutaneous patches, and intralymphatic immunotherapy. AIT is gaining interest in India, though accessibility and standardization remain as the main challenges.

Oral Immunotherapy for Food Allergies

Oral immunotherapy (OIT) is gaining traction for food allergies such as peanuts and milk, with advances in safety protocols. Experimental strategies, such as messenger ribonucleic acid (mRNA)-based vaccines, are under exploration. Indian children, due to distinct dietary practices, require region-specific OIT protocols due to dietary habits and cultural practices.

Novel Pharmacologic Agents

Beyond standard antihistamines and leukotriene receptor antagonists, new therapies are being developed for refractory allergic diseases.

- *Janus kinase (JAK) inhibitors and phosphodiesterase-4 (PDE4) inhibitors* offer targeted control in severe atopic dermatitis.
- *Topical calcineurin inhibitors* remain important in steroid-sparing regimens.
- Research is also focused on next-generation antihistamines with improved safety and efficacy profiles.

These agents expand therapeutic options, particularly for patients unresponsive to conventional treatments.

PRECISION MEDICINE IN ALLERGY

Personalized Risk Prediction

Advances in genomics, proteomics, and metabolomics are enabling individualized prediction of allergic risk. Candidate genes regulating cytokines, chemokines, and immune pathways have been linked to asthma and food allergies. Predictive models integrating genetic susceptibility, environmental exposures, and biomarker profiles hold promise for early intervention in high-risk children.

Digital Health and Artificial Intelligence

Mobile applications, teleconsultation platforms, and wearable devices allow real-time symptom monitoring and treatment of adherence tracking. Artificial intelligence (AI) is increasingly applied to predict exacerbations and optimize therapy. In India, these technologies may help bridge the urban–rural care gap and improve accessibility to pediatric allergy services.

THE CHALLENGES IN THE INDIAN CONTEXT

Population-specific Research in India

Allergen Mapping

Regional studies reveal significant variability in sensitizing allergens. For example, *Parthenium hysterophorus* pollen is common in North India, while fungal spores and food allergens vary by geography. Local mapping is essential for accurate diagnosis and targeted immunotherapy.

Urbanization and Pollution

Rising vehicular emissions and industrial pollutants, particularly fine particulate matter (PM2.5), are strongly associated with the increasing prevalence of asthma and allergic rhinitis in Indian children. Ongoing research aims to elucidate mechanisms and inform public health interventions.

Socioeconomic and Cultural Factors

Traditional dietary practices, regional food exposures, and variable healthcare access influence both risk and management of allergies. Socioeconomic disparities further affect diagnosis, affordability of biologics, and uptake of immunotherapy. Cultural dietary practices, traditional medicine use, and health literacy are important considerations in designing effective allergy prevention and management strategies for Indian pediatric populations.

FUTURE DIRECTIONS

The future of pediatric allergy research and management is rapidly evolving:

- *Universal allergen vaccines* under development may provide broad protection.
- *Microbiome-based interventions* such as designer probiotics and postbiotics could restore immune tolerance.
- *Gene editing and cell-based therapies* may offer solutions for severe refractory cases.
- *AI-driven tools* will enhance diagnostic accuracy and personalized care.
- *Policy-level integration* of allergy prevention and treatment into national child health programs is urgently needed in India.

CONCLUSION

Allergic diseases in children are increasing at an alarming pace, driven by complex interactions between genetics, environment, and lifestyle. Advances in microbiome science, epigenetics, diagnostics, biologics, and immunotherapy are reshaping management, moving closer to disease modification and precision care. In India, unique challenges of pollution, regional allergens, and socioeconomic disparities demand context-specific solutions. Collaborative research, policy support, and clinical innovation will be critical to improving outcomes for children with allergies in the years ahead.

KEY POINTS

- *Microbiome and epigenetics:* Early-life microbial diversity and epigenetic modifications are crucial in shaping immune tolerance; dysbiosis and pollution-related epigenetic changes increase allergic risk.
- *Novel diagnostics:* Component-resolved diagnostics, nasal fluid IgE assays, and BATs offer greater accuracy and non-invasive assessment compared to traditional tests.
- *Therapeutic innovations:* Biologics (e.g., omalizumab and dupilumab), allergen immunotherapy, and oral immunotherapy for food allergies represent disease-modifying treatments with increasing applicability in India.
- *Precision and digital medicine:* Genomics, AI-based prediction tools, and telemedicine are paving the way for individualized allergy risk assessment and care.
- *Indian context:* Regional allergen mapping, the impact of pollution, and socioeconomic disparities necessitate locally relevant strategies for diagnosis, management, and prevention.

SUGGESTED READING

1. Chun Y, Lee JH, Bunyavanich S. Epigenomic and epigenetic investigations of food allergy. Pediatr Allergy Immunol. 2024;35(1):14065.
2. Delgado Dolset MI, et al. Dupilumab prior tobefore AIT improves tolerance and induces metabolomic changes. EAACI Abstracts. 2025.
3. Møiniche M, Johansen KH, Parrón-Ballesteros J, Corneliussen JK, Eriksen HH, Kringelum JV, et al. mRNA-delivered consensus allergens induce a neutralizing IgG response against food and pollen allergensmRNA-delivered consensus allergens induce neutralizing IgG. [Online]. Available from https://www.biorxiv.org/content/10.1101/2024.02.26.582073v1EAACI Abstracts. 2025. [Last accessed December, 2025].
4. Strachan D. Family size, infection and atopy: the hygiene hypothesis. Thorax. 2000;55(Suppl 1):S2-10.
5. Tan-Lim CSC, Esteban-Ipac NAR. Probiotics as treatment for food allergies among pediatric patients: a 2024 update. Pediatr Allergy Immunol. 2025;36(1):e700284.
6. Toda M, Ono SJ. Genomics and proteomics of allergic disease. Immunology. 2002;106(1):1-10.

32 CHAPTER Personalized Medicine in Allergy

Mangayarkarshi Sinha

INTRODUCTION

Personalized medicine is a rapidly evolving approach that tailors therapy to an individual's genetic, environmental, and lifestyle profile. In allergy, this strategy is particularly valuable because conventional uniform treatments often fail to address the diverse clinical patterns, immune pathways, and environmental exposures unique to each patient.

India presents a distinctive landscape for personalized medicine in allergy. Rapid urbanization, air pollution, dietary transitions, and diverse genetic backgrounds shape allergic disease expression in ways that differ from Western populations. Recent national initiatives—including the *Genome India Project (2020), Phenome India CSIR Cohort (2023),* and the establishment of *precision medicine centers at AIIMS Jammu (2025) and IIT Delhi (2025)*—are creating the infrastructure for genomics, proteomics, and AI-driven allergy research. These programs aim to integrate Indian-specific data into clinical decision-making, making personalized allergy care more relevant and affordable for the local population.

Although personalized medicine in allergy is still in its early stages in India, growing access to biomarkers [e.g., skin prick testing, fractional exhaled nitric oxide (FeNO), immunoglobulin E (IgE), and cytokine panels], biologics, and microbiome research is bridging the gap between science and practice. With these advances, Indian pediatricians and allergists are well-positioned to implement precision-based strategies that improve outcomes while considering resource constraints and population diversity.

PHENOTYPES AND ENDOTYPES OF ALLERGIC DISEASES

Patients with allergic diseases present and respond to treatments differently, which can create a major dilemma in providing optimal management. This is due to underlying phenotype, endotype, -omic (genetic, genomic, epigenomic, metabolomic, etc.), immune, environmental, and microbiome differences among patients.

One of the first steps is to diagnose an allergic disease based on the clinical and diagnostic criteria of the disease. It is then subdivided into phenotype with the help of some observable disease trait. The next most important part is to determine the endotype. Disease endotypes differ according to specific molecular pathophysiologic mechanisms driving the disease in question. Endotypes are not necessarily limited to a single molecular marker, but rather represent the unique constellation of factors mechanistically responsible for the phenotype/trait. For example, patients with asthma with high sputum eosinophilia or glucocorticoid-dependence respond well to biologics directed against interleukin 5 (IL-5) compared with asthmatics without these features. Similarly, asthmatics with IgE sensitization respond to IgE-directed therapy of omalizumab by decreased exacerbation rates and decreased seasonal peaks of symptoms.

Understanding allergic diseases through both clinical manifestations (phenotypes) and underlying mechanisms (endotypes) provides pediatricians and allergists with a powerful framework to deliver personalized care **(Fig. 1)**.

The accuracy of these distinctions will allow for specific, targeted therapy and truly allow for personalized medicine. If a disease endotype can be further refined, then individual patients could receive more endotype-specific diagnoses and thus optimized endotype-specific treatments, increasing the overall effectiveness of therapy **(Fig. 2)**. In order for personalized medicine to realize its potential for allergic diseases, we will need a much greater understanding of the landscape of allergic endotypes.

A *phenotype* refers to the observable characteristics or clinical presentation of a disease.

An *endotype* is a subtype of the disease condition defined by distinct pathophysiologic mechanisms

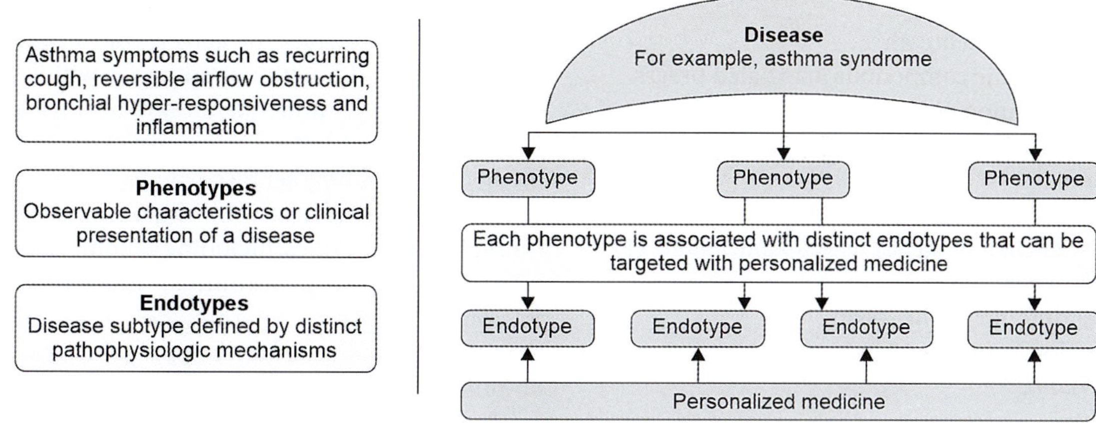

Fig. 1: Concept of phenotypes and endotypes of diseases.

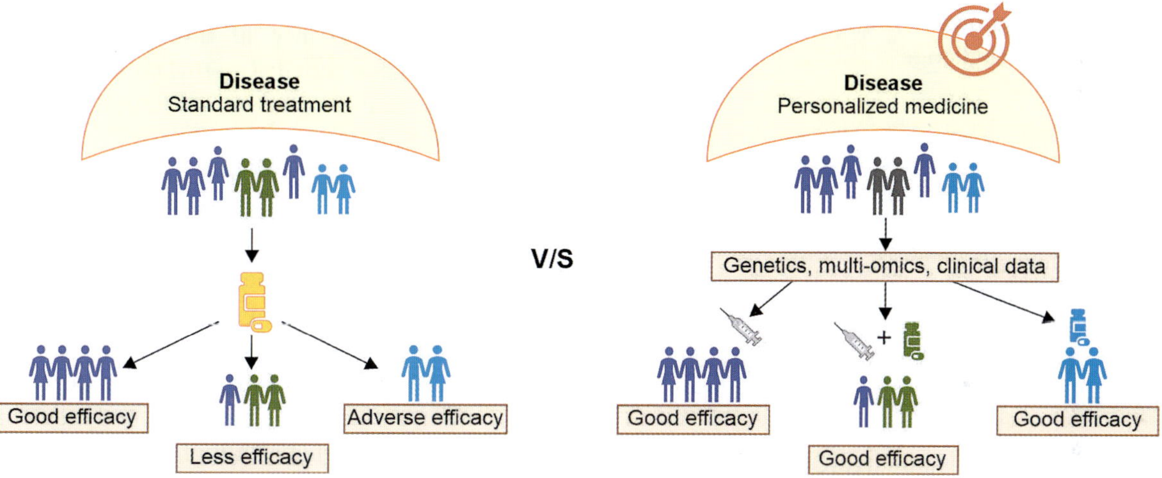

Fig. 2: Difference between traditional approach and personalized medicine in disease management.

ENDOTYPES AND BIOMARKERS IN ALLERGIC DISEASES

Endotypes are characterized by the immunological, inflammatory, metabolic, and remodeling pathways that explain the mechanisms underlying a clinical presentation (phenotype) of a disease. In allergic diseases, endotypes are an important tool for disease management. As part of determining endotypes, biologic markers or biomarkers are used to define different aspects of a disease such as severity or the likelihood of a response to a given treatment.

Biomarkers

Biomarkers or biological markers are measurable indicators used to examine any aspects of health or disease. Any type of analyses can be a biomarker and may provide information about the pathophysiology of an underlying disease, the course of an illness, and/or the response to treatment. In medicine, biomarkers play a crucial role in diagnosis, prognosis, and treatment monitoring. Biomarkers also help in determining endotypes of the disease.

Established and Emerging Biomarkers for Major Allergic Disorders

- *Asthma:*

  Biomarkers:
  - Serum IgE
  - Blood eosinophils
  - Serum periostin
  - Leukotriene E4 (LTE4) in urine

  - Metabolomic profile
  - FeNO in exhaled breath
  - Volatile organic compounds in exhaled breath
  - Sputum eosinophils
- *Atopic dermatitis:*
  Biomarkers:
  - Serum TARC/CCL17 (thymus- and activation-regulated chemokine/CC chemokine ligand 17)
  - Filaggrin genotype
  - Transcriptome profile—skin
  - Microbiome profile—skin
- *Allergic rhinitis:*
  Biomarkers:
  - Allergen sensitization—skin prick test
  - TARC/CCL17, endothelin-1—from nasal secretions
  - Eosinophils, IL-5, IL-6, and macrophage inflammatory protein from nasal lavage following nasal allergen challenge
- *Food allergy:*
  Biomarkers:
  - Allergen sensitization—skin prick test
  - Allergen-specific IgE levels
  - Basophil activation test
  - Mast cell activation
  - FOXP3 methylation in antigen-induced Treg cells
  - Eotaxins from tissue or serum

Sputum eosinophils, FeNO, and serum periostin show promising results as emerging biomarkers in type 2 allergic diseases.

In the Indian scenario, biomarkers like skin prick test, specific allergen sensitization, total IgE, blood eosinophils, and FeNO are easily available and can be used for assigning the endotype. Cytokine profiling leads to further subclassification of the diseases, helping us decide the biological to be used as treatment modality. For example, omalizumab (anti-IgE) and mepolizumab (anti-IL-5) opening up an entirely new era of personalized medicine.

Biomarkers are measurable indicators of biological processes, disease states, or responses to treatment.

Cytokine profiling involves measuring multiple cytokines simultaneously to understand underlying immune activity, particularly useful for identifying allergic endotypes (e.g., Th1 vs. Th2 responses).

ROLE OF OMICS IN PERSONALIZED MEDICINE

Omics Sciences is an emerging area of research that is advancing the use of personalized medicine in clinical practice. Omics sciences offer new perspectives on the complex interplay of genes, transcripts, proteins, metabolites, and functional pathways within organisms, providing a deeper understanding of health and disease.

Omics approaches are central to personalized medicine and biomarker discovery.

The term "omics" encompasses several high-throughput techniques, including genomics, epigenomics, transcriptomics, proteomics, metabolomics, and microbiomics and the interpretation of high-dimensional data through bioinformatics approaches, shedding light on unique biological processes, key functions, and their regulation.

The major types of omics data are:

- Genomics—study of the complete DNA sequence (genome)
- Epigenomics—study of chemical modifications regulating gene activity (methyl tags and histones)
- Transcriptomics—study of all RNA transcripts (gene expression)
- Proteomics—study of the entire protein complement
- Metabolomics—study of small-molecule metabolites (metabolites—amino acids, fatty acids, carbohydrates, vitamins, and nucleotides)
- Microbiomics—study of microbial communities (e.g., gut microbiota)
- Exposomics—study of exposures to allergens, toxins, pollution, diet, climate, radiation, and medicine

Omics technologies and high-dimensional analyses enable the generation of new data and the integration and reinterpretation of existing datasets. These innovative approaches offer unparalleled opportunities for endotyping diseases, discovering biomarkers, and developing drugs, thereby advancing personalized medicine.

Comprehensive integrative omics: Integrative omics (multi-omics) in allergy is the process of combining the information of multiple-omics layers. Although important insights into allergy and immunology have been gained by the study of single omic data types, the integration of multiple hierarchical levels of omic data has potential to provide the most complete biological insight into allergy pathobiology.

Furthermore, integrating omics with non-omics data (data obtained from clinical and demographic information, routine laboratory/diagnostic reports, environmental exposures, personal lifestyle data, etc.) will further increase our understanding of the disease, leading

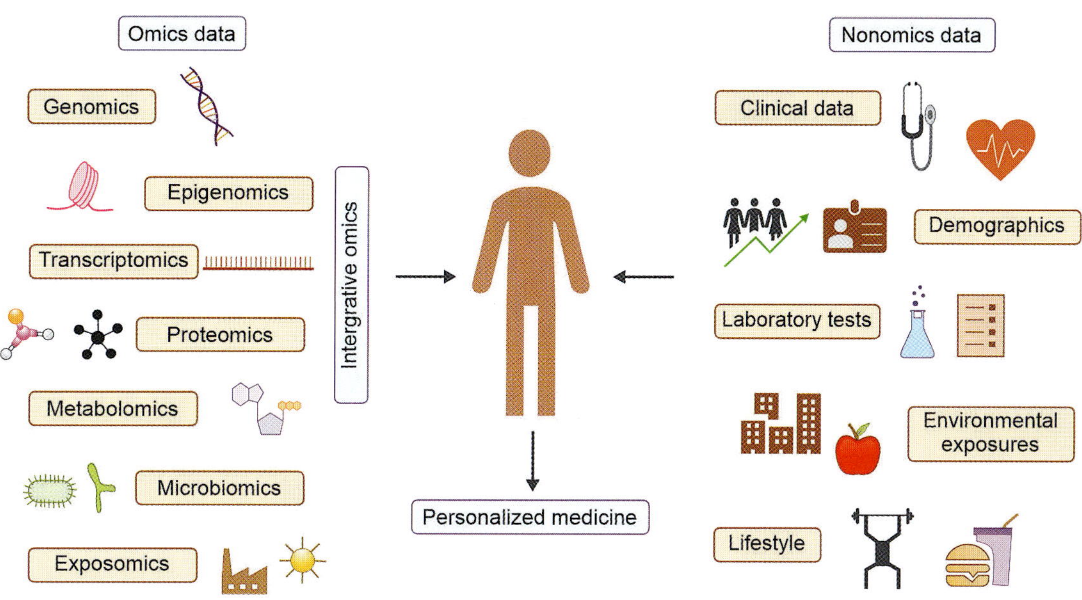

Fig. 3: The omics and non-omics data used for classification of disease endotypes.

to more meaningful classification of the disease endotypes and hence effective personized medicine for the patient **(Fig. 3)**.

In India, leveraging omics for allergy care is still in its early stages of development, but the foundation is being laid via established research institutions and government initiatives. Future efforts could include integrating multi-omics platforms into clinical trials, developing Indian pediatric omics cohorts, and validating biomarker-guided therapies for Indian population.

Omics = The large-scale, data-driven study of entire classes of biological molecules (genes, RNA, proteins, metabolites, and microbes), made possible by high-throughput technologies.

BIOLOGICS AND PERSONALIZED MEDICINE

Monoclonal antibodies (mAb) are the type of biologics that target various steps in the allergic inflammatory cascade. They refer to any type of medical therapy that is derived from living organisms such as humans, animals, or microorganisms. This contrasts with traditional nonbiologic pharmaceutical drugs **(Fig. 4)**.

Biologic therapies have been developed on the basis of a greater understanding of the immune system and disease pathogenesis. Biologics are designed to block specific immune molecules [e.g., IgE, thymic stromal lymphopoietin (TSLP), IL-5, and IL-4/13] implicated in the allergic pathway **(Table 1)**. Intervention at various stages of the allergic cascade offers the opportunity to prevent initiation and/or maintenance of the type 2 immune response and effectively provide therapeutic benefit to patients. Biologic therapies are therefore also called targeted therapies. This targeted approach allows therapies to be matched to individual disease drivers rather than applying a one-size-fits-all treatment. Thus, biologic therapies form part of evolving as well as established personalized treatment modality in allergy management. They represent an increasingly important means to use personalized medicine in allergic disorders.

A key area where personalized medicine could be useful in the rapidly developing landscape of biologic therapy for allergic diseases is to identify which patients would benefit most from a given biologic by using key patient biomarkers and other characteristics.

Thus, biologics are targeted therapies that interfere with specific immune mediators driving allergic inflammation, offering personalized treatment beyond conventional drugs. They have revolutionized the management of severe allergic diseases, particularly asthma and chronic urticaria. Careful attention to the clinical profile of the patient, targeted investigations of the phenotype and endotype of the individual, and a thorough knowledge of the available biologics should assist in decision-making as to the choice of biologic agent to be used.

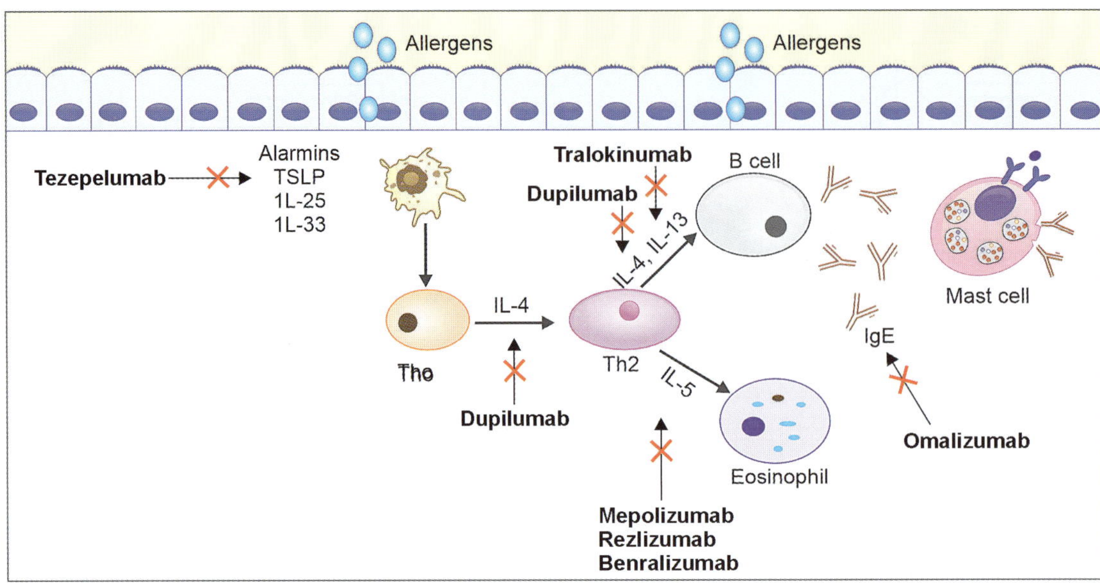

Fig. 4: Various sites of action of biologics.

TABLE 1: Biologics used in allergic diseases.

Sr. No.	*Biologic*	*Target*	*Primary mode of action*	*Allergic disease*
1.	Tezepelumab	TSLP (Alarmin)	Binds to TSLP, thus preventing receptor interaction and signaling, thereby reducing the production of IL-4, IL-5, and IL-13	• T2 Asthma (eosinophilic and allergic asthma) • Non T2 Asthma
2.	Dupilumab	IL-4Rα	Binds to the IL-4Rα receptor and inhibits signaling of both IL-4 and IL-13	• Asthma • Atopic dermatitis
3.	Tralokinumab	IL-13	Binds to the IL-13 receptor and inhibits signaling of IL-13	Atopic dermatitis
4.	Omalizumab	IgE	Binds to free circulating IgE and prevents IgE binding to the high affinity FcεRI on mast cells and basophils	• Allergic asthma • Chronic spontaneous urticaria (CSU) • Chronic rhinosinusitis with nasal polyposis (CRSwNP) • Food allergy • As adjunct in AIT
5.	Mepolizumab	IL-5	Binds to IL-5 that supports eosinophil maturation, activation, and survival and blocks eosinophil activity	• Asthma • Hypereosinophilic syndrome • Eosinophilic granulomatosis with polyangiitis (EGPA) • CRSwNP
6.	Reslizumab	IL-5	Binds to IL-5 cytokine	Asthma
7.	Benralizumab	IL-5Rα	Binds to IL-5Rα and that prevents eosinophil activation and survival and also induces apoptosis through antibody dependent cell-mediated cytotoxicity	• Asthma • EGPA

(AIT: allergen immunotherapy; IgE: immunoglobulin E; IL-4Rα: interleukin-4 receptor alpha; TSLP: thymic stromal lymphopoietin)

TABLE 2: JAK inhibitors used to block IL-4 pathway.

Sr. No.	*Molecule/drug*	*Target*	*Primary mode of action*	*Allergic disease*
1.	Upadacitinib (oral JAK inhibitor)	JAK-1	Inhibits downstream signaling of several cytokines	Atopic dermatitis
2.	Abrocitinib (oral JAK inhibitor)	JAK-1	Inhibits downstream signaling of several cytokines	Atopic dermatitis

(IL-4: interleukin 4; JAK: Janus kinase)

Biologics are therapeutic agents derived from living cells (such as mAbs or recombinant proteins) that specifically target immune pathways involved in allergic diseases.

Janus kinase (JAK) inhibitors are small molecule drugs that target Janus kinases, the signal transduction proteins. More than 50 cytokines signal via the JAK-signal transducer and activator of transcription (STAT) pathway. Thus, JAK inhibitors can block the IL-4 pathway **(Table 2)**.

MICROBIOME AND PERSONALIZED MEDICINE

The role of the microbiome in the molecular mechanisms underlying allergy has become highly relevant in recent years. The microbiome plays an essential role in developing a well-regulated immune system that does not respond to harmless allergens and self-antigens. Failure to establish a robust and diverse microbiome early in life can result in a dysfunctional immune system that lacks tolerance to innocuous environmental allergens, thereby increasing the risk of developing allergic conditions.

The microbiome develops primarily during infancy and early childhood. Initial exposure often occurs at birth, when infants born vaginally are exposed to beneficial commensal microbes in the maternal birth canal and gastrointestinal tract. Breastfeeding early in life can also shape infants' microbiomes, as breast milk has been shown to harbor these beneficial microbes. The composition of the human microbiota is dynamic and depends on host-associated factors such as diet, diseases, and lifestyle. The diversity of the microbiome is individual-dependent. This could make the microbiome a powerful tool in personalized medicine.

The microbiome influences the immune system through its effects on regulatory T cells (Tregs). Tregs are important for suppressing the allergic response. Both the Tregs, the thymic Tregs and the extrathymic Tregs, play a crucial role in regulating the activity of the immune system and maintaining tolerance to innocuous antigens, including both self and environmental antigens. In humans, certain commensal bacteria (such as Clostridia, *Bacteroides*, *Bifidobacterium*, *Faecalibacterium*, and *Enterobacter* species) have been found to induce Treg development, suggesting they may protect against the development of allergy. The microbiome affects Treg development through the generation of specific microbial metabolites. The commensal microbes in the gut break down dietary-derived components, such as fiber and tryptophan, as well as host-derived components, such as primary bile acids, to generate these metabolites. These metabolites, including short-chain fatty acids (SCFAs), indole, and secondary bile acids, cannot be produced by humans, and thus we rely entirely on commensal microbes for their generation. These metabolites promote gut barrier integrity and the generation of extrathymic Tregs directly or through the polarization of protolerogenic dendritic cells. The specific populations of Tregs that are generated in response to these metabolites induce tolerance to harmless antigens, especially those that can trigger food allergies. Commensals in the skin and lungs have been shown to be equally important in promoting the development of Tregs and reducing allergic responses at these sites.

Studies are increasingly suggesting that dysbiosis (reduced microbial diversity, loss of *Bifidobacterium* and *Lactobacillus*, and expansion of potentially pathogenic taxa) may result in local and systemic alteration of the immune response to specific allergens and can increase the risk of allergic diseases such as asthma, allergic rhinitis, atopic dermatitis, and food allergy.

Microbial composition and metabolites can act as biomarkers for allergic risk and therapeutic response. For instance, low gut microbial diversity in infancy predicts asthma development, while specific bacterial metabolites correlate with successful outgrowth of milk or peanut allergy. In atopic dermatitis, distinct skin microbiome patterns have been associated with disease severity and flare frequency. Integrating these biomarkers with clinical

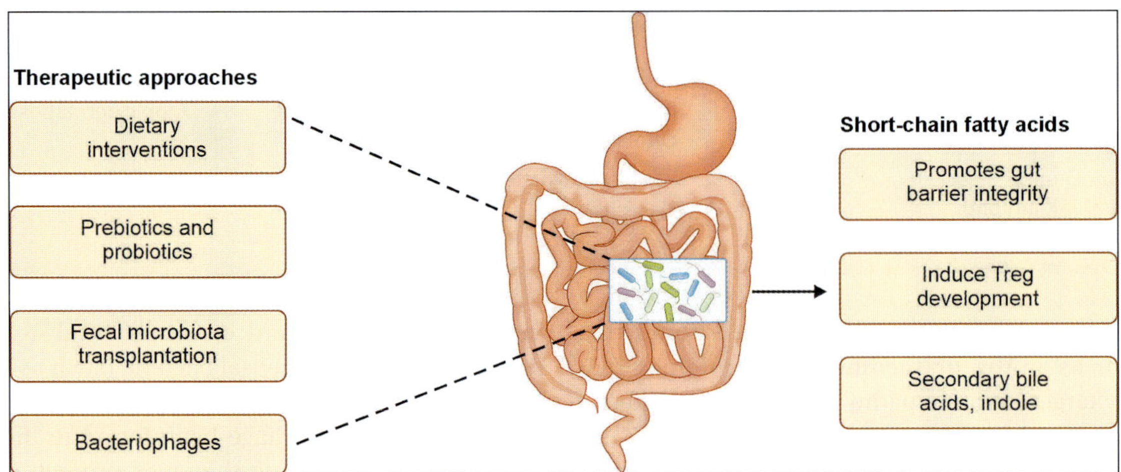

Fig. 5: Role of microbiome in health and therapy.

data allows stratification of patients into endotypes, guiding the choice of interventions.

Microbiota analysis techniques have advanced considerably in recent decades. Traditional culture-based methods, genomic studies (16S ribosomal *RNA* gene sequencing, shotgun metagenomics, and metatranscriptomics), and metabolomics are used to study the microbiome. Various therapeutic approaches such as probiotics and prebiotics supplementation, high fiber diet, and fecal microbiota transplantation (FMT) highlight the potential of microbiome-targeted interventions as personalized adjuncts to conventional allergy care.

Variability in microbiome composition across populations, lack of standardized assays, limited causal evidence in humans, and difficulties in translating findings into safe, effective therapies are the challenges in considering microbiomes for personalized medicine in allergy **(Fig. 5).**

Microbiota: The set of diverse microorganism communities (mainly bacteria, but also fungi, archaea, viruses, and parasites) that reside in our body.

Microbiome: The collection of microbiota along with their genomes and the environmental conditions in which they interact is known as Microbiome.

In summary, **Figure 6** clearly depicts the role of personalized medicine in allergy.

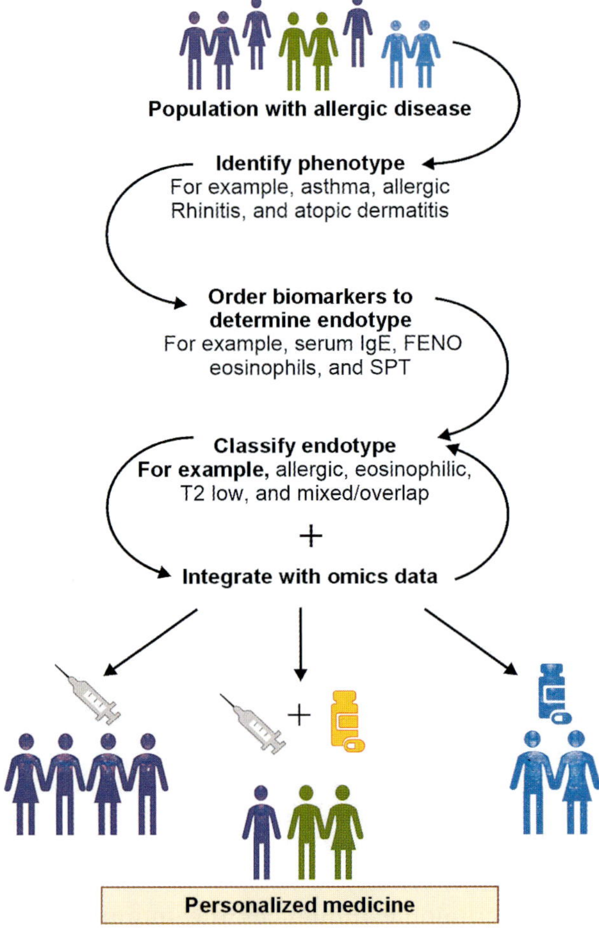

Fig. 6: Personalized medicine in allergy.

DID YOU KNOW?

- The term personalized medicine or precision medicine was first coined in 2008.
- This concept emerged in the late 2000s in the aftermath of the Human Genome Project and the advancement of next-generation sequencing along with other

technologies that rapidly increased the amount of genetic data available for the study of disease.

- *In 2011, the US National Research Council published a report called "Toward Precision Medicine:* Building a Knowledge Network for Biomedical Research and a New Taxonomy of Diseases", which further popularized the idea of precision medicine and a "Knowledge Network" of several data streams to drive further understanding of disease.
- In January 2015, President Obama launched the Precision Medicine Initiative (PMI).

PERSONALIZED MEDICINE IN INDIA

- The Genome India Project was initiated in 2020. Whole-genome sequencing of 10,000 individuals is already completed with a target to scale to 1 million sequenced genomes to enable precision interventions. This data is accessible through the Indian Biological Data Centre for research purposes.
- The Phenome India—CSIR Health Cohort Knowledgebase (PI-CHeCK) was officially launched on 7 December 2023 by the Council of Scientific and Industrial Research (CSIR). Phenome India is a longitudinal cohort study that focuses on Indian-specific risk factors for cardiometabolic diseases, facilitating personalized medicine research.
- Anusandhan (National Research Foundation) established under the Anusandhan National Research Foundation Act, 2023 is an autonomous body under the Department of Science and Technology (DST), Government of India to fund next-gen genomics and personalized medicine research. It supports genomics, proteomics, and AI-driven research, which are essential for personalized medicine in allergy and immunology and also promotes public-private collaboration to make biologics and personalized therapies more affordable in India.
- Centre for Advanced Genomics and Precision Medicine was inaugurated in AIIMS, Jammu on February 2, 2025 to integrate genomics with AI diagnostics, focusing on oncology, cardiovascular genomics, rare disorders, and affordable precision care via public health programs.
- CSIR-IGIB (Institute of Genomics and Integrative Biology) launched a central biobank in July 2025 to store biological samples tied to lifestyle, clinical, and genomic data.
- Centre of Excellence in Precision and Personalised Healthcare was established under Wadhwani Foundation at IIT Delhi's Research and Innovation Park on August 13, 2025 to fast-track AI-biotech innovations in diagnostics, personalized implants, wearables, and more.

  India is actively building the infrastructure and institutional framework necessary for personalized medicine, especially at the genomic and cohort levels. Major genomic sequencing efforts, new research centers, and policy-level recognition signal progress in this field in India.

CONCLUSION

Personalized medicine is reshaping the landscape of allergy care by shifting the focus from generalized treatment strategies to highly individualized approaches based on molecular, genetic, environmental, and clinical profiles. Advances in component-resolved diagnostics, biomarkers, genomic tools, and digital technologies now enable far more precise diagnosis and risk prediction. Integration of these tools allows clinicians to better differentiate true sensitization from cross-reactivity, anticipate disease severity, guide immunotherapy decisions, and monitor treatment response more accurately.

In pediatric allergy practice, personalized approaches hold particular promise in reducing diagnostic uncertainty, avoiding unnecessary dietary or environmental restrictions, and improving long-term clinical outcomes. As these tools become more accessible, their thoughtful incorporation into routine practice—along with clinician training and multidisciplinary support—will be essential. Personalized medicine ultimately paves the way for safer therapies, better disease control, and more efficient use of healthcare resources, laying the foundation for a new era of precision allergy care in India.

KEY POINTS

- *Diverse phenotypes and endotypes in India:* Allergic diseases in India are influenced by unique environmental exposures (air pollution, indoor biomass fuel, and climate variability) and genetic ancestry, making phenotype-endotype classification especially relevant.
- *Biomarkers in Indian practice:* Widely available tests—skin prick, total IgE, blood eosinophils, and FeNO—already allow basic endotyping. Cytokine and multi-omics profiling are emerging in select tertiary centers.
- *Omics and national initiatives:* Programs like the *Genome India Project* and *Phenome India* are

generating large-scale genomic and phenotypic data, which will guide biomarker discovery and endotype-specific management tailored to Indian populations.

- *Biologics access and affordability:* Biologics such as omalizumab and mepolizumab are available but costly. Government-supported research and *public-private collaborations* aim to reduce cost barriers and enable wider access to biologic therapy.
- *Microbiome and traditional practices:* India's dietary diversity (e.g., fiber-rich diets and fermented foods) and breastfeeding practices influence the microbiome, offering unique opportunities for microbiome-based personalized interventions alongside conventional allergy management.

SUGGESTED READING

1. Agache I, Akdis CA. Endotypes of allergic diseases and asthma: an important step in building blocks for the future of precision medicine. Allergol Int. 2016;65(3):243-52.
2. Atanasio A, Orengo JM, Sleeman MA, Stahl N. Biologics as novel therapeutics for the treatment of allergy: challenges and opportunities. Front Allergy. 2022;3:1019255.
3. Dhondalay GK, Rael E, Acharya S, Zhang W, Sampath V, Galli SJ, et al. Food allergy and omics. J Allergy Clin Immunol. 2018;141(1):20-9.
4. Donovan BM, Bastarache L, Turi KN, Zutter MM, Hartert TV. The current state of omics technologies in the clinical management of asthma and allergic diseases. Ann Allergy Asthma Immunol. 2019;123(6):550-7.
5. Fitzpatrick AM, Bacharier LB. One step forward, 2 steps back: the enigma of preschool wheeze. J Allergy Clin Immunol. 2019;143(5):1734-5.
6. Kumar V, Srivastava A. Mapping the future: personalized medicine and its impact on modern healthcare in integrative medicine. Int J Pharm Sci. 2025;3(5):425-33.
7. Long A, Bunning B, Borro M, Sampath V, Nadeau KC. The future of omics for clinical practice. Ann Allergy Asthma Immunol. 2019;123(6):535-6.
8. Matricardi PM, van Hage M, Custovic A, Korosec P, Santos AF, Valenta R. Molecular allergy diagnosis enabling personalized medicine. J Allergy Clin Immunol. 2025;156(3):485-502.
9. Precision medicine. In: O'Hehir RE, Holgate ST, Sheikh A, Khurana GK (Eds). Allergy Essentials, 2nd edition. Elsevier; 2022. pp. 25-39.
10. Proper SP, Azouz NP, Mersha TB. Achieving precision medicine in allergic disease: progress and challenges. Front Immunol. 2021;12:720746.
11. Tontini C, Radzikowska U, Aranda CJ, Tynecka M, Delgado Dolset MI, Eljaszewicz A, et al. The use of omics sciences in allergic diseases from bench to bedside: an EAACI position paper. Allergy. 2025;0:1-42.
12. Venkitakrishnan R, Augustine J, Ramachandran D, Cleetus M. Biological therapy for severe asthma – Indian perspectives and challenges. Lung India. 2023;40(3):253-9.
13. Virkud YV, Kelly RS, Wood C, Lasky-Su JA. The nuts and bolts of omics for the clinical allergist. Ann Allergy Asthma Immunol. 2019;123(6):558-63.
14. Zubeldia-Varela E, Barker-Tejeda TC, Obeso D, Villaseñor A, Barber D, Pérez-Gordo M. Microbiome and allergy: new insights and perspectives. J Investig Allergol Clin Immunol. 2022;32(5):327-44.

33 CHAPTER

Emerging Allergens and Global Trends

Nihar Ranjan Mishra, Vineeth Vijayan

INTRODUCTION

Within clinical immunology, food allergies are a complicated and developing topic with regional variations and new trends that go against conventional wisdom. Food allergies affect about 8% of children worldwide, and 10% of adults are diagnosed and treated for them. This is especially true in developed nations, where rates have dramatically climbed over the last three decades. Understanding both established and new triggers is necessary due to new allergens and shifting trends. The traditional "big eight"—fish, shellfish, peanuts, tree nuts, wheat, soy, milk, and eggs—remain the main contributors. However, recent concentration has been on allergens that are now identified by international authorities as priority allergens, such as sesame, lipid transfer protein (LTP) from lupin (a legume), and alpha-gal from tick bites.

The identification and treatment of food allergics are made more difficult by regional variations in allergen prevalence. Asians frequently respond to fish and shellfish, while Western cultures are primarily allergic to peanuts and tree nuts. The complicated development of food allergies is highlighted by the fact that these variances are caused by diet, genetics, and environment. Emerging allergens that impact perceptions of allergy onset and regional patterns, such as alpha-gal syndrome and nonspecific LTPs, provide challenges. Allergy patterns are altered by climate change, which also affects tick-borne sensitization and allergen exposure. Due to their environment and food, Indian populations have distinct sensitivity profiles. Targeted testing is necessary for allergens including chickpea, mustard, and eggplant, because Western techniques could overlook local sensitivity. Traditional ideas about allergies are also called into question by the awareness of delayed reactions.

With an emphasis on developments in diagnostics and their implications for management and treatment, this chapter explores the present difficulties in identifying new allergens. Along with fresh epidemiological data from India, the debate looks at global trends in allergen emergence and dissemination.

EPIDEMIOLOGY

Global trend: There are notable regional variations in emerging allergen patterns. In areas where endemic tick populations are present, alpha-gal syndrome is commonly observed. Alpha-gal syndrome may affect about 450,000 people in the United States, according to Centers for Disease Control and Prevention (CDC) estimates. This is a significant increase since the condition was initially discovered in 2009. In Europe, the prevalence ranges from 0.1 to 3% in areas with many ticks, with the highest rates among rural workers exposed to ticks.

Tick distribution patterns are linked to alpha-gal syndrome, mainly involving *Amblyomma americanum* in North America, *Ixodes ricinus* in Europe, and *Ixodes holocyclus* in Australia. Climate change alters tick habitats, causing a northward range expansion. Swedish research indicates up to 10% of the general population, and 35% of forestry workers, may be sensitized. The condition mostly affects middle-aged adults, with an average onset around age 50 years, unlike childhood food allergies.

Lipid transfer protein sensitization has been common in Mediterranean regions **(Table 1)** like Spain and Italy, where about 12% are sensitive to Pru p 3 (peach). Recent studies show expanding sensitization in Northern Europe, previously low-risk areas. Cross-reactivity suggests initial sensitization may also occur through exposure to *Cannabis sativa*, providing an alternative route outside the Mediterranean.

Sesame allergy has become a significant global concern, earning its status as a priority allergen by the CODEX Alimentarius Commission. Studies show prevalence rates of 0.1% in North American populations, with higher rates in Middle Eastern countries where sesame consumption is more common **(Table 1)**. The requirement to include sesame on mandatory labels in various regions reflects increased awareness of its clinical importance.

Indian trend: Unique food allergy patterns shaped by regional diets and environment. A study in Hyderabad of 1,622 patients identified chickpeas (28.8%), cabbage

TABLE 1: Global prevalence of emerging allergens by region.

Region	*Alpha-gal syndrome (%)*	*LTP sensitization (%)*	*Sesame sensitization (%)*	*Primary vector/source*
Southeastern USA	1.5–3.0	0.5	<0.1*	*Amblyomma americanum*
Mediterranean Europe	0.8–2.0	8–12	0.1–0.4*	*Ixodes ricinus*, Peach
Northern Europe	0.5–1.0	2–4	<0.1*	*Ixodes ricinus*, Cannabis
Australia	0.2–1.8	1–2	0.1–0.4*	*Ixodes holocyclus*

**Primary vector/source is Sesamum indicum.*
(LTP: lipid transfer protein)

(42.1%), and eggplant (24.6%) as common triggers. Western allergens like peanuts and sesame had low reports, reflecting population-specific sensitivities. Mustard is significant, with Sin a 3 as the main allergen. The prevalence of food allergies in India is low, with studies in Karnataka showing rates of 0.14% in children and 1.2% in adults.

Age-related prevalence patterns in Indian populations exhibit a peak in sensitization between the ages of 25 and 40 years. Chickpea, walnut, and cumin consistently trigger reactions across all age groups. Regional differences reflect local dietary habits; for instance, South Indian populations have higher sensitization rates to coconut and curry leaf compared to North Indian groups. Urban and rural areas have distinct patterns, with rural communities showing higher plant pollen cross-reactivity. India's low food allergy rate may be attributed to early exposure to antigens, traditional feeding practices, rural lifestyles, and genetic factors **(Table 2)**. Recent data indicate urban populations may be experiencing increased food allergies, especially cow's milk protein allergy in infants, possibly due to lifestyle changes. Hospital surveys from Indian cities like Hyderabad and Bangalore reveal that betel nut (29.3%) is the most common allergen, followed by regional staples. These findings underscore the importance of culturally specific allergen panels and the need for more epidemiological research beyond Karnataka.

ETIOPATHOGENESIS

Alpha-gal syndrome is a unique immune response caused by carbohydrate-specific IgE antibodies, leading to severe allergic reactions. Unlike typical allergies that target proteins, galactose-α-1,3-galactose is the first carbohydrate allergen known to cause anaphylaxis. Humans, apes, and Old-World monkeys lack the enzyme α-1,3-galactosyltransferase, making this epitope immunogenic upon exposure.

Tick saliva contains α-galactosyl glycoproteins that sensitize through the skin during feeding. Compounds like prostaglandin E2 in saliva enhance Th2 responses, thereby promoting IgE production. Multiple tick bites increase anti-α-gal IgE levels, which are more prevalent in middle-aged individuals, unlike childhood food allergies. Blood group B and AB individuals have protection due to the structural similarity between the α-gal epitope and the B antigen.

Nonspecific LTPs are small, cysteine-rich, heat- and digestion-resistant proteins that maintain allergenicity in processed foods. They bind lipid ligands, which may act as adjuvants, increasing allergenic potential. Peach Pru p 3, a key LTP allergen, shares IgE epitopes among Rosaceae fruits. Cross-reactivity occurs due to structural similarity within the LTP family, leading to multiple food sensitivities. Sensitization can come from oral, inhalational, or skin contact. *Cannabis sativa* (Can s 3) exposure through smoking, especially where legal, is an emerging sensitization route. Pollen from *Artemisia vulgaris* (Art v 3) or *Platanus acerifolia* (Pla a 3) can cause cross-reactivity. Climate change impacts allergies by altering pollen seasons, increasing allergen levels, expanding plant and tick habitats, and raising alpha-gal syndrome. Monitoring emerging sensitization patterns is essential.

Microbiome dysbiosis influences food allergies, with the early gut microbiota playing a crucial role in shaping immune development. Certain bacteria that produce short-chain fatty acids, like butyrate, protect against allergies. Disruptions from antibiotics, cesarean delivery, and low microbial diversity increase risk. Regulatory T cells (Tregs), particularly microbial-responsive RORγt+ Foxp3+ Tregs, play a crucial role in maintaining oral tolerance. Dysbiosis reduces the number of these cells, leading to a loss of tolerance and an increase in allergies.

TABLE 2: Other emerging allergens.

Allergen	*Mechanism*	*Predominant geographic area*	*Diagnostic modality*	*Treatment modality*
Lupin	Legume protein cross-reactive with peanut allergens	Europe, Australia	Skin prick test, specific IgE, and CRD for peanut/lupin cross-reactivity	Avoidance of lupin-containing foods, patient education on cross-reactivity
Chlorhexidine	Hapten-induced IgE-mediated anaphylaxis	Worldwide (healthcare settings)	Skin prick test, intradermal test, and basophil activation test	Strict avoidance, alternative antiseptics, and emergency management protocols
Insect proteins (cricket, mealworm)	Novel food proteins triggering IgE-mediated responses	Europe, Asia, and expanding globally	Skin prick test, specific IgE, and supervised challenge testing	Avoidance, improved food labeling regulations, and emergency epinephrine
mRNA vaccine excipients (polyethylene glycol)	IgE-mediated or complement activation-related hypersensitivity	Worldwide	Skin testing for PEG, basophil activation test, and clinical history	Avoidance in sensitized individuals, graded dosing protocols, and desensitization
Ambrosia artemisiifolia (Ragweed)	Pollen allergens induce seasonal allergic rhinitis/ asthma	North America, established in Europe since 1960s	Skin prick test, specific IgE, and nasal provocation test	Allergen avoidance, antihistamines, corticosteroids, and immunotherapy
Platanus (plane tree pollen)	Pollen protein allergens causing IgE-mediated respiratory allergy	Urban Europe and North America	Skin prick test, specific IgE, and CRD for cross-reactivity assessment	Allergen avoidance, pharmacotherapy, and specific immunotherapy
Biologics (Monoclonal antibodies, CAR-T)	Antidrug antibodies, cytokine release syndrome, and infusion reactions	Worldwide (healthcare/ biotech workers)	Serology for ADA, cytokine panels, and clinical monitoring	Premedication protocols, desensitization, and alternative therapies
Pea (Pisum sativum)	Vicilin, convicilin, and nsLTPs trigger IgE-mediated reactions	Global, increasing prevalence with plant-based products	Skin prick test, specific IgE testing, and component testing	Avoidance, improved food labeling, and emergency epinephrine
Hemp seed (Cannabis sativa)	Storage proteins (vicilins and edestins) cross-reactive with tree nuts	Regions with increasing hemp consumption	Specific IgE, immunoblots, ELISA, and component testing for cross-reactivity	Avoidance, patient education on cross-reactivity with tree nuts
Buckwheat proteins (Fag e 2)	2S albumin (Fag e 2) and other proteins cause IgE-mediated allergy	Increased exposure in gluten-free/ buckwheat-consuming areas	Skin prick test, specific IgE to Fag e 2, and supervised food challenge	Avoidance, specific IgE profiling for risk stratification
Invasive stinging insect venoms (Asian hornet)	Venom-induced IgE-mediated anaphylaxis	Europe (Asian hornet), expanding globally due to climate change	Venom skin tests, specific IgE, and detailed clinical history	Venom immunotherapy, avoidance strategies, and emergency epinephrine
Fire ants (Solenopsis invicta)	Venom allergens causing IgE-mediated systemic reactions	Southern US, expanding to northern regions	Venom skin test, specific IgE, and clinical assessment	Venom immunotherapy, environmental control, and emergency action plans
Oral mite anaphylaxis ("pancake syndrome")	Heat-resistant mite allergens (*Dermatophagoides* and *Blomia*) ingested in contaminated flour	Tropical/subtropical areas	Skin test to mite extracts, allergen detection in food samples	Proper grain storage, avoid mite-contaminated flour, and emergency epinephrine

(ADA: antidrug antibody; CRD: component-resolved diagnostic; ELISA: enzyme-linked immunosorbent assay; IgE: immunoglobulin E; PEG: polyethylene glycol)

CLINICAL FEATURES

Immediate-type reactions triggered by IgE antibodies occur within minutes to 2 hours after allergen exposure. Symptoms include skin issues such as urticaria, angioedema, and itching, affecting up to 80–90% of patients during acute episodes. Children often experience gastrointestinal problems such as nausea, vomiting, diarrhea, and cramps. Respiratory symptoms can range from rhinitis and asthma to severe laryngeal edema and bronchospasm. Anaphylaxis is the most severe form, involving rapid multisystem responses and possible cardiovascular collapse. It is the leading cause of food-related deaths in both children and adults, emphasizing its seriousness despite a low mortality rate.

Alpha-gal syndrome differs from typical food allergies because of its timing; symptoms usually start 2–6 hours after eating mammalian meat, making diagnosis difficult. Manifestations include gastrointestinal issues and anaphylaxis, with urticaria being most common, followed by GI symptoms, angioedema, and reactions like bronchospasm. Trigger foods include organ meats, especially kidney and liver, which are high in α-gal; some people tolerate lean meats. Dairy and gelatin can also cause delayed responses, requiring avoidance. LTP allergies have a more typical timing but vary clinically, with reactions ranging from mild to systemic, often influenced by cofactors like alcohol and exercise, and often still occur after cooking. Cross-reactivity is common among fruits, such as peach, apple, and cherry, as well as grains like wheat, with geographic differences in symptoms. Cofactors, such as exercise and medication, lower reaction thresholds, especially in LTP allergies; patient education is essential.

DIFFERENTIAL DIAGNOSIS

Differential diagnosis of emerging allergies requires systematic consideration of timing, trigger identification, and demographic factors. Alpha-gal syndrome's delayed presentation necessitates distinguishing it from *food poisoning, gastroenteritis,* or other conditions with delayed onset. The 2–6 hours delay sets it apart from immediate IgE-mediated reactions, while its specificity for mammalian meat differentiates it from broader food intolerances.

Chronic spontaneous urticaria should be considered as a key differential diagnosis, mainly because of the frequent urticarial symptoms seen in alpha-gal syndrome. Research indicates that approximately 31% of patients with chronic urticaria may have α-gal sensitization. Taking detailed dietary histories, particularly regarding mammalian meat consumption, is crucial for accurate diagnosis. Additionally, residing in tick-endemic regions can provide valuable diagnostic insight.

Nonspecific LTP allergies should be distinguished from *Bet v 1-related oral allergy syndrome and profilin cross-reactivity*. LTP reactions typically involve cooked foods and can cause systemic symptoms, whereas Bet v 1 cross-reactivity primarily causes oral symptoms. Using component-resolved diagnostics (CRDs) helps accurately differentiate these overlapping conditions. *Food-dependent exercise-induced anaphylaxis* should be considered in patients who experience exercise-related symptoms after consuming specific foods. LTP allergens, especially wheat Tri a 14, are common triggers. A detailed exercise and food history are vital for diagnosis. *Psychosomatic food reactions and eating disorders* can mimic food allergies through food avoidance behaviors. Careful psychological evaluation and objective testing are necessary to distinguish these from true allergic reactions.

DIAGNOSIS

Contemporary diagnostics for emerging allergens utilize molecular methods, such as CRD and cellular assays. Traditional extract-based tests are limited by cross-reactivity and new sensitization mechanisms. Molecular allergology accurately identifies allergenic components and differentiates proper sensitization from cross-reactive responses. Alpha-gal syndrome diagnosis mainly depends on serum-specific IgE testing against galactose-α-1,3-galactose **(Table 3)**.

Component-resolved diagnostics utilize purified allergens, such as Pru p 3, Art v 3, and Pla a 3, to identify cross-reactivity patterns, guide allergen avoidance strategies, and predict potential severity. Testing for *Cannabis sativa*, Can s 3, is especially valuable in regions

TABLE 3: Diagnostic modalities of alpha-gal syndrome.

Test	*Sensitivity (%)*	*Specificity*	*Cut off value*
Alpha-gal specific IgE	95.2	94.8	≥0.1 kUA/L
Bovine thyroglobulin IgE	100.0	92.3	≥0.35 kUA/L
Basophil activation test	88.5	96.2	≥15% CD63+

(IgE: immunoglobulin E)

TABLE 4: Diagnostic modalities of emerging allergens.

Test	*Sensitivity (%)*	*Specificity (%)*	*Clinical applications*
Skin prick test	85–95%	30–60%	Screening varies by allergen
Serum immunoglobulin E	80–95%	40–70%	Quantitative assessment
Component-resolved diagnosis	70–90%	80–95%	Risk stratification
Basophil activation test	75–90%	85–98%	Functional confirmation

where recreational cannabis use is prevalent. Multiplex platforms enable the simultaneous evaluation of multiple LTP components, thereby increasing testing efficiency. Basophil activation testing (BAT) measures cellular degranulation triggered by allergens, with flow cytometry detection of CD63 and CD203c showing greater correlation with clinical reactivity compared to serum IgE alone. BAT is particularly beneficial in diagnosing alpha-gal syndrome **(Table 4)**, which features delayed reactions that complicate food challenges. Standardized protocols incorporating glycolipids and glycoproteins enhance diagnostic accuracy. For emerging allergens, skin testing should prioritize fresh foods to improve sensitivity, as commercial extracts can be less reliable. Alpha-gal testing employs cetuximab or mammalian serum albumin; however, standardized extracts are limited. LTP skin testing correlates well with clinical reactions, especially when using fresh peach peel. Intradermal testing may increase sensitivity but requires careful monitoring due to the risk of severe reactions. *Oral food challenges remain the gold standard, but they require specialized facilities and experienced personnel.* Alpha-gal challenges involve mammalian meat preparations with extended observation periods of more than 6 hours. LTP challenges utilize graded dosing, considering cofactors. In India, personalized protocols using local foods, such as chickpeas and mustard, may be necessary.

Diagnostic Challenges with Emerging Allergens

Alpha-gal syndrome poses diagnostic challenges due to its delayed reactions and cross-reactivity. Diagnosis requires elevated alpha-gal-specific IgE levels, a clinical history, and a history of tick exposure. The BAT can verify clinical reactivity. Sesame allergy diagnosis benefits from component-resolved methods, although the best approach is still under development. Combining clinical history, traditional tests, and functional assays, such as BAT, offers the most accurate diagnosis.

MANAGEMENT

The European Academy of Allergy and Clinical Immunology (EAACI) guidelines, based on the GRADE methodology, emphasize a systematic approach to manage food allergies. After diagnosis, they recommend allergen avoidance education with a dietitian, written emergency plans, patient education on symptoms, and emergency medications like adrenaline autoinjectors.

Managing allergies involves patient education, avoidance, and emergency plans. Indian guidelines recommend culturally suitable diets and balanced nutrition. The Indian Council of Medical Research emphasizes allergen avoidance with monitoring and family education. Alpha-gal syndrome requires avoiding mammalian meat and products, which is hard in Indian diets due to dairy and ghee's importance. Highly sensitive individuals may need to avoid milk and hidden mammalian ingredients. Gelatin in medications and vaccines might require alternatives or premedication. Recent regulatory changes mandate allergen labeling for sesame, aiding management, but cross-contamination and extensive sesame use still pose challenges.

Pharmacological management follows established anaphylaxis protocols with modifications for delayed presentations. Epinephrine autoinjectors are the primary emergency treatment, with patient education on proper use. Indian guidelines recommend dual autoinjector prescriptions for high-risk patients, though access may be limited by availability and cost. Antihistamines have limited effectiveness but may lessen mild reaction severity. Allergen-specific immunotherapy research is still in early stages for new allergens **(Table 5)**. Sublingual immunotherapy shows promise for LTP allergies in European studies, but standardized extracts are unavailable in India. Epicutaneous patch therapy is an alternative under investigation. Oral immunotherapy requires caution due to potential severe reactions.

TABLE 5: Management modalities of emerging allergens.

Modalities	*Efficacy*	*Safety*	*Regulatory status*
Oral immunotherapy	60–80%	Moderate adverse events	Approved (peanut)
Omalizumab	65–75%	Good safety profile	Approved adjuvant
Epicutaneous immunotherapy	35–50%	Excellent safety	Investigational

Long-term management involves follow-up with IgE monitoring and clinical assessments. Alpha-gal IgE levels usually decrease without tick exposure, allowing some patients to develop tolerance. Preventing tick bites—through clothing, repellents, and environmental modifications—is the key, especially for Indian forest workers and rural populations. Adequate protein and vitamin consumption is ensured by nutritional advice; vegetarians may find it simpler to give up mammalian meat, but dairy patterns require modification. Meal planning is aided by discussing with dietitians, who may take into account a person's tolerance for different proteins such as fish, chicken, and legumes.

INDIAN CONTEXT

There are not many rules for handling food allergies in India, thus worldwide suggestions must be modified. When creating World Health Organization (WHO) guidelines, the Indian College of Allergy and Applied Immunology takes regional considerations into account. Opportunities and challenges are presented by the low prevalence of food allergies, while it lessens the burden, it may also limit access to specialized care and awareness. Even with low allergy rates, the possibility of severe reactions makes emergency management training essential.

FUTURE DIRECTIONS

Targeted immunomodulatory drugs, probiotics with modified components, and delivery methods based on nanoparticles are the examples of novel treatment techniques under investigation. Customized therapy choices can be developed with the aid of personalized medicine techniques that incorporate microbiome profiles, genetic variables, and biomarkers. One new area in the management of food allergies is the application of AI and machine learning to algorithms for diagnosis and treatment.

CONCLUSION

Emerging allergens highlight the dynamic and evolving nature of allergic diseases across the world. Shifts in environment, climate, dietary patterns, microbiome composition, and lifestyle are collectively shaping new sensitization trends, some of which differ markedly from traditional "big-eight" allergens. Conditions such as alpha-gal syndrome, LTP allergy, sesame allergy, lupin allergy, and reactions to novel proteins or biological agents reflect this changing landscape. These allergens often involve unique mechanisms, delayed reactions, complex cross-reactivity profiles, and distinct geographic associations, creating diagnostic and management challenges.

Modern tools such as CRDs and BAT are crucial for accurate identification and risk assessment. Management requires a combination of avoidance strategies, patient education, emergency preparedness, and—in select allergens—emerging immunotherapeutic or biologic options. For India, where sensitization patterns differ from Western countries, locally relevant epidemiology and context-specific diagnostic panels are essential. Continued research, improved surveillance, and clinician awareness will be key to recognize these allergens early and delivering patient-centered, evidence-based care in an increasingly globalized and changing world.

KEY POINTS

- Global variation in the prevalence of emerging allergens, due to the influence of environmental factors, lifestyle choices, and microbiome diversity on disease development
- Globally prevalent emerging allergens are alpha-gal syndrome, LTP allergies, and sesame allergy
- *Other emerging allergens:* Lupin, chlorhexidine, mRNA vaccines, biologics, cannabis, fire ants, chickpea, mustard, and eggplant
- Component-resolved diagnostics and BAT are revolutionizing diagnosis by offering greater specificity
- Newer treatment methods such as nanoparticle-based delivery systems, tailored probiotics, and targeted immunomodulatory drugs, in addition to oral/epicutaneous immunotherapy and omalizumab

SUGGESTED READING

1. Barber D, Diaz-Perales A, Escribese MM, Kleine-Tebbe J, Matricardi PM, Ollert M, et al. Molecular allergology and its impact in specific allergy diagnosis and therapy. Allergy. 2021;76(12):3574-94.
2. Commins SP. Diagnosis & management of alpha-gal syndrome: lessons from 2,500 patients. Expert Rev Clin Immunol. 2020;16(7):667-77.
3. Dadha P, Nimmagadda S, Venter C, Gupta R, Kumar PU, Warren CM. Reported food-related symptoms and food allergen sensitization in a selected adult population in Hyderabad, India: A hospital-based survey. J Allergy Clin Immunol Glob. 2025;4(1):100295.
4. Krishna MT, Mahesh PA, Vedanthan P, Moitra S, Mehta V, Christopher DJ. An appraisal of allergic disorders in India and an urgent call for action. World Allergy Organ J. 2020;13(7):100446.
5. Leung ASY, Xing Y, Fernández-Rivas M, Wong GWK. The relationship between dietary patterns and the epidemiology of food allergy. Allergy. 2025;80(2):345-59.
6. Platts-Mills TAE, Li RC, Keshavarz B, Smith AR, Wilson JM. Diagnosis and Management of Patients with the α-Gal Syndrome. J Allergy Clin Immunol Pract. 2020;8(1):15-23.e1.
7. Popescu FD, Preda M, Antolín-Amérigo D, Rodríguez-Otero N, Ramírez-Mateo E, Smolinska S. Biomarkers for the Molecular Diagnosis of IgE-Mediated Hymenoptera Venom Allergy in Clinical Practice. Int J Mol Sci. 2024;26(1):270.
8. Santos AF, Riggioni C, Agache I, Akdis CA, Akdis M, Alvarez-Perea A, et al. EAACI guidelines on the management of IgE-mediated food allergy. Allergy. 2025;80(1):14-36.
9. Sellaturay P, Nasser S, Ewan P. Polyethylene Glycol-Induced Systemic Allergic Reactions (Anaphylaxis). J Allergy Clin Immunol Pract. 2021;9(2):670-5.
10. Skypala IJ, Asero R, Barber D, Cecchi L, Diaz Perales A, Hoffmann-Sommergruber K, et al.; European Academy of Allergy and Clinical Immunology (EAACI) Task Force: Non-specific Lipid Transfer Protein Allergy Across Europe. Non-specific lipid-transfer proteins: Allergen structure and function, cross-reactivity, sensitization, and epidemiology. Clin Transl Allergy. 2021;11(3):e12010.
11. Skypala IJ, Jeimy S, Brucker H, Nayak AP, Decuyper II, Bernstein JA, et al. Cannabis-related allergies: An international overview and consensus recommendations. Allergy. 2022;77(7):2038-52.
12. Thompson JM, Carpenter A, Kersh GJ, Wachs T, Commins SP, Salzer JS. Geographic Distribution of Suspected Alpha-gal Syndrome Cases—United States, January 2017–December 2022. MMWR Morb Mortal Wkly Rep. 2023;72:815-20.
13. Zheng J, Jin Y, Wang C, Feng C, Lai X, Hua S, et al. Global, regional, and national epidemiology of allergic diseases in children from 1990 to 2021: findings from the Global Burden of Disease Study 2021. BMC Pulm Med. 2025;25:37.

Appendices

1 APPENDIX

Pediatric Allergy—Case Scenarios

Uppin Narayan Reddy, Pawankalyan Pinnamaneni

ALLERGIC RHINITIS

Ravi, a 9-year-old presented with persistent sneezing, nasal blockage, and watery rhinorrhea for 8 months, worse in winter mornings. His mother reported itchy, watery eyes, and poor concentration in school. Family history revealed that his father had asthma. On examination, Ravi had pale, boggy nasal mucosa **(Fig. 1)** watery discharge, and an allergic salute crease on the nose.

Diagnostic Reasoning

Chronic symptoms, morning worsening, ocular involvement, and family history suggest perennial allergic rhinitis, likely due to indoor allergens.

Investigations

- *Skin prick test:* Strongly positive for dust mites.
- *Complete blood count (CBC):* Mild eosinophilia (600 cells/μL).

Management Plan

Dust-mite avoidance measures, intranasal corticosteroid spray daily, oral second-generation antihistamines at night, and saline nasal irrigation twice daily.

Follow-up and Outcome

After 6 weeks, symptoms reduced significantly, and school attendance improved.

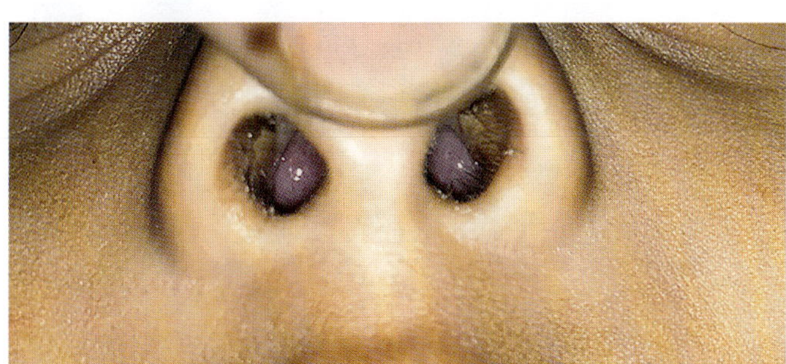

Fig. 1: Pale boggy nasal mucosa.

Teaching Points

- Indoor allergens like dust mites are major triggers in Indian children.
- Nasal steroids are first-line for persistent symptoms.
- Early treatment can prevent asthma progression.

ASTHMA AND ALLERGY

Meera, a 7-year-old, had recurrent episodes of cough, wheezing, and breathlessness for the past year, often after outdoor play. She also had a history of eczema in infancy. During one episode, she was brought to the emergency room (ER) with audible wheeze and difficulty speaking. She improved after nebulized salbutamol with oxygen.

Diagnostic Reasoning

History of atopy, recurrent wheeze triggered by outdoor allergens, and response to bronchodilators suggest allergic asthma.

Investigations

- *Spirometry:* Obstructive pattern reversible with bronchodilator **(Fig. 2)**.
- *Skin prick test:* Positive for grass pollen.

Management Plan

Low-dose inhaled budesonide twice daily, salbutamol inhaler for relief, and a written asthma action plan given to parents [according to Global Initiative for Asthma (GINA)].

Follow-up and Outcome

Marked improvement in symptoms and no ER visits over the next 6 months.

Teaching Points

- Allergy is a major risk factor for persistent asthma in children.
- Early introduction of inhaled corticosteroids (ICSs) improves control.
- Asthma action plans reduce emergency visits.

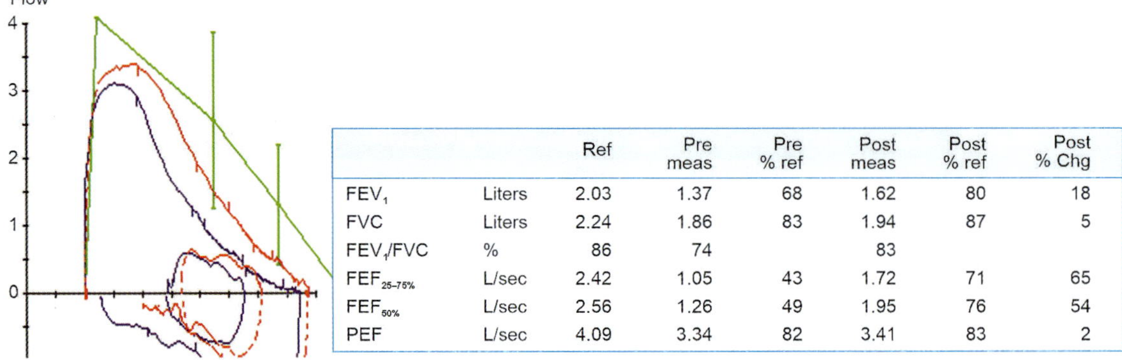

		Ref	Pre meas	Pre % ref	Post meas	Post % ref	Post % Chg
FEV_1	Liters	2.03	1.37	68	1.62	80	18
FVC	Liters	2.24	1.86	83	1.94	87	5
FEV_1/FVC	%	86	74		83		
$FEF_{25-75\%}$	L/sec	2.42	1.05	43	1.72	71	65
$FEF_{50\%}$	L/sec	2.56	1.26	49	1.95	76	54
PEF	L/sec	4.09	3.34	82	3.41	83	2

Fig. 2: Spirometry with obstructive pattern with bronchodilator reversibility.

EOSINOPHILIC LUNG DISEASES

Arjun, a quiet and soft-spoken 12-year-old boy, was brought in by his parents for a persistent cough and breathlessness that had been troubling him for nearly a year. His mother recalled that the symptoms began as occasional night-time coughing but gradually worsened, often leaving him breathless after minimal exertion. There was no history of fever or chest pain, but his parents noted that the symptoms were more pronounced after outdoor cricket practice.

On examination, Arjun had a mild increase in respiratory rate and occasional expiratory wheeze. Auscultation revealed scattered crackles over both lung fields. There was no clubbing or cyanosis.

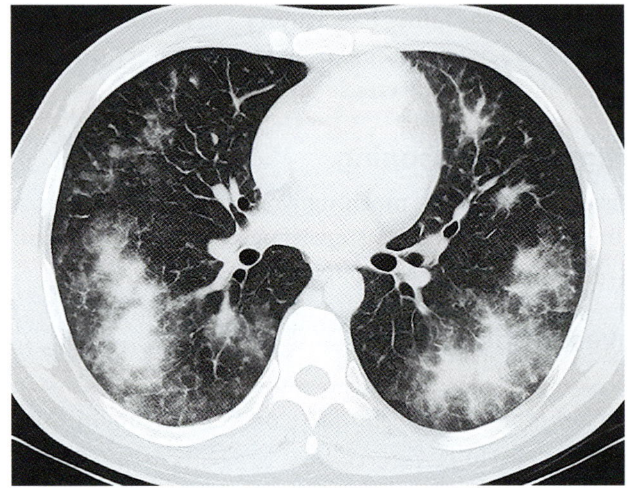

Fig. 3: High-resolution CT (HRCT) of chest revealed peripheral consolidations and ground-glass changes.

Diagnostic Reasoning

Given the chronicity and the presence of both wheezing and crackles, the initial differential diagnoses included asthma, bronchiectasis, allergic bronchopulmonary aspergillosis (ABPA), and eosinophilic pneumonia.

Investigations

Complete blood count showed marked eosinophilia (2,000 cells/μL). Chest X-ray demonstrated patchy, ill-defined opacities, and high-resolution CT (HRCT) revealed peripheral consolidations and ground-glass changes **(Fig. 3)**. Sputum cytology was negative for acid-fast bacilli but showed numerous eosinophils. Bronchoalveolar lavage confirmed elevated eosinophils (>25%) **(Fig. 4)**. These findings pointed strongly toward *chronic eosinophilic pneumonia.*

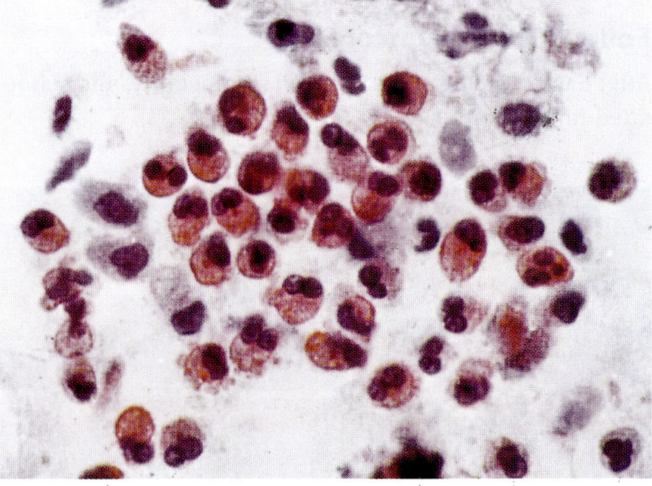

Fig. 4: Elevated eosinophils yield in bronchoalveolar lavage.

Management Plan

Arjun was started on oral prednisolone (1 mg/kg/day) with a gradual taper over 6 weeks. He and his parents were counseled on possible triggers, including environmental allergens. Follow-up at 2 weeks showed significant improvement in symptoms and exercise tolerance.

Follow-up and Outcome

Marked clinical and radiological improvement over 6 months.

Teaching Points

- Consider eosinophilic lung diseases in chronic cough with eosinophilia.
- Steroids are the mainstay of treatment.
- Relapses require careful follow-up.

HYPERSENSITIVITY PNEUMONITIS

Sana, a 14-year-old from a farming family, presented with dry cough, fever, and breathlessness that worsened after spending time in her family's paddy field storage area. Symptoms improved when she stayed away from the farm. On examination, Sana's oxygen saturation was 93% on room air, and auscultation revealed fine inspiratory crackles over both lung bases.

Diagnostic Reasoning

Exposure-related symptom pattern points to hypersensitivity pneumonitis (HP) from inhaled organic antigens.

Investigations

- *CBC:* Mild leukocytosis
- *HRCT chest:* Diffuse ground-glass opacities **(Fig. 5)**
- *Precipitin test:* Positive for mold antigens

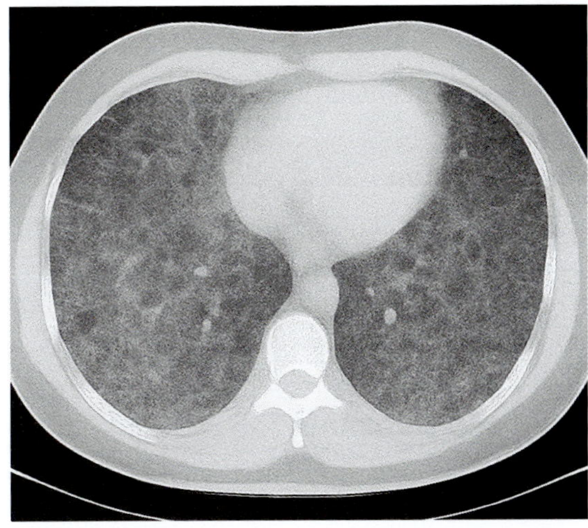

Fig. 5: High-resolution CT (HRCT) chest showing diffuse ground-glass opacities.

Management Plan

Complete avoidance of paddy field storage area, oral prednisolone for 4 weeks with taper, and education on protective masks.

Follow-up and Outcome

Full recovery after 2 months; no recurrence with continued avoidance.

Teaching Points

- HP is caused by repeated inhalation of organic antigens.
- Avoidance of antigen exposure is the cornerstone.
- Delayed diagnosis can lead to irreversible fibrosis.

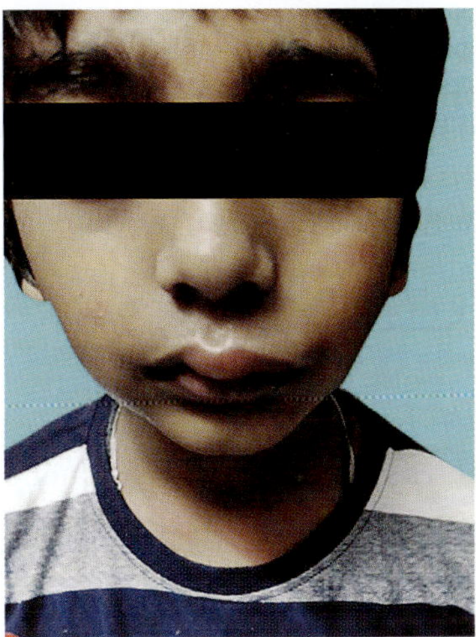

Fig. 6: Angioedema of lips.

FOOD ALLERGY—PEANUT

Rana, a 6-year-old redness, swelling of lips **(Fig. 6)**, and vomiting within minutes of eating peanut chikki at a wedding. He collapsed en route to the hospital. On arrival, she was hypotensive with urticaria over her body. He received immediate intramuscular (IM) adrenaline and intravenous (IV) fluids.

Diagnostic Reasoning

Acute onset of multisystem involvement after peanut ingestion confirms peanut-induced anaphylaxis.

Investigations

- No emergency laboratories are needed.

- *Acute tryptase levels (drawn within 2 hours):* Elevated
- Skin prick test later confirmed peanut sensitivity.

Management Plan

Strict avoidance of peanuts, prescription of epinephrine-loaded injection (0.01 mg/kg of 1:1,000 solution) kept in a spectacle box or imported autoinjector, and parental education on emergency management.

Follow-up and Outcome

No recurrence over 1 year with strict avoidance and school awareness.

Teaching Points

- Peanut is a common cause of severe food allergy in India.
- *Adrenaline is the first-line treatment for anaphylaxis* (0.01 mg/kg of 1:1,000 solution).
- School education is critical for prevention.

OCULAR ALLERGY

Vishal, a 10-year-old, presented with intense eye itching, redness **(Fig. 7)**, and tearing every March to May during cricket season. His mother noted frequent rubbing of eyes and sensitivity to sunlight. On examination, there was conjunctival redness, cobblestone papillae on the upper tarsal conjunctiva, and mild corneal punctate staining.

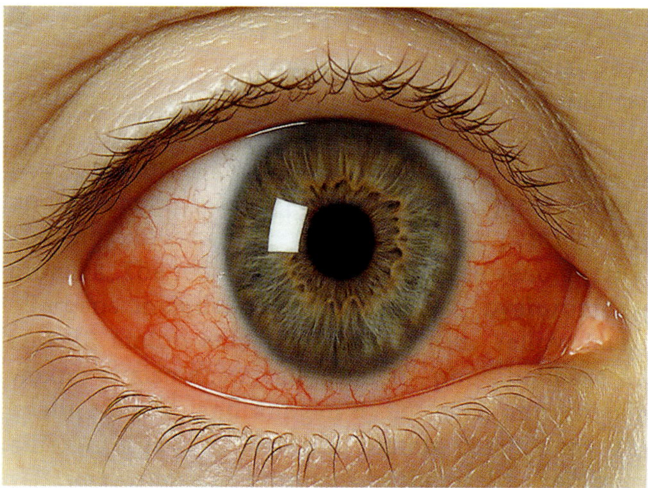

Fig. 7: Eye congestion and tearing.

Diagnostic Reasoning

Seasonal symptoms, signs of conjunctival inflammation, and papillary hypertrophy indicate vernal keratoconjunctivitis (VKC).

Investigations

No laboratories are required; slit-lamp examination confirmed diagnosis.

Management Plan

Topical antihistamine–mast cell stabilizer drops twice daily, lubricants, and sunglasses for outdoor play. Short course of topical steroids during flares.

Follow-up and Outcome

Marked reduction in symptoms over two seasons with maintenance therapy.

Teaching Points

- VKC is common in school-aged boys in India.
- Sunlight exposure is a trigger.
- Early treatment prevents corneal complications.

ATOPIC DERMATITIS AND CONTACT DERMATITIS

Mehul, an 8-year-old, had chronic itchy rashes in the elbow and knee folds since infancy, worsening after wearing a new synthetic sweater during winter. His mother observed redness and oozing in areas in contact with the sweater. Examination showed lichenified flexural eczema **(Fig. 8)** and acute erythematous patches over the neck.

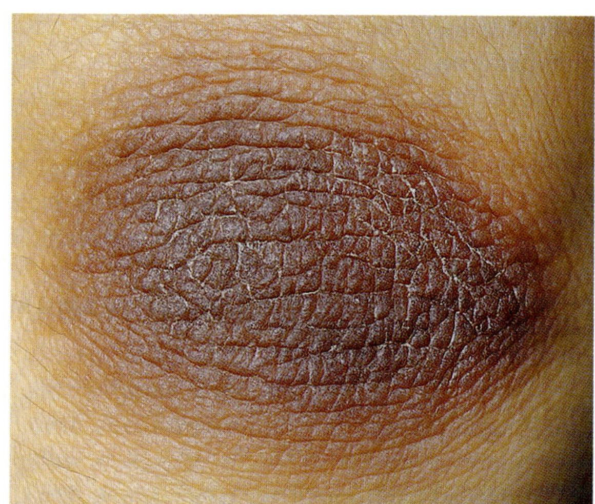

Fig. 8: Lichenification of flexural eczema.

Diagnostic Reasoning

History of chronic eczema with acute flare after contact suggests coexistence of atopic dermatitis and allergic contact dermatitis.

Investigations

Patch testing revealed sensitivity to textile dyes.

Management Plan

Emollients twice daily, topical corticosteroids for acute lesions, and avoidance of synthetic clothing.

Follow-up and Outcome

Significant improvement within 3 weeks; no recurrence with cotton clothing.

Teaching Points

- Atopic dermatitis is common in urban Indian children.
- Contact dermatitis can worsen atopic eczema.
- Patch testing helps identify triggers.

URTICARIA AND ANGIOEDEMA

Krishna, a 10-year-old, developed widespread itchy hives **(Fig. 9)** and swelling of lips within 30 minutes of taking ibuprofen for fever. He experienced mild throat tightness but no breathing difficulty. Examination confirmed urticaria and mild angioedema.

Diagnostic Reasoning

Temporal relation with nonsteroidal anti-inflammatory drug (NSAID) intake suggests NSAID-induced urticaria/angioedema.

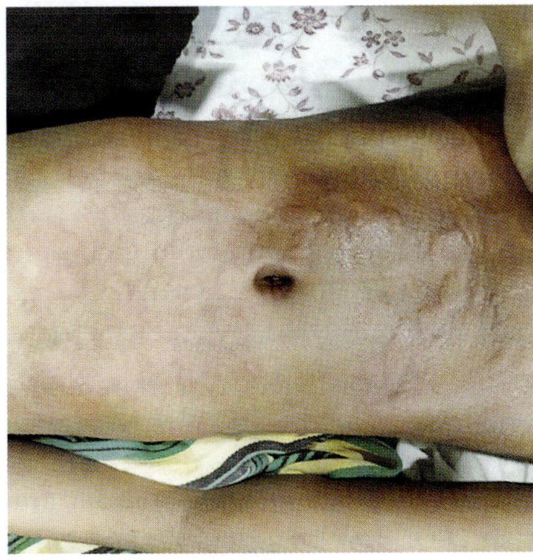

Fig. 9: Hives.

Investigations

No laboratories are needed for acute diagnosis.

Management Plan

Immediate oral second-generation antihistamines, avoidance of NSAIDs, and prescription of adrenaline autoinjector (imported) for potential severe reactions in future.

Follow-up and Outcome

No recurrence in 6 months after avoiding all NSAIDs.

Teaching Points

- NSAIDs are common drug triggers for urticaria in India.
- Airway involvement must be assessed urgently.
- Antihistamines are first-line for urticaria.

DRUG ALLERGY

Imran, an 11-year-old, developed widespread itchy maculopapular rash **(Fig. 10)** on day 4 of amoxicillin for throat infection. He had no breathing difficulty or systemic symptoms. Examination revealed blanchable erythematous maculopapular lesions over trunk and limbs.

Diagnostic Reasoning

Delayed-onset rash without systemic involvement suggests nonimmediate amoxicillin allergy.

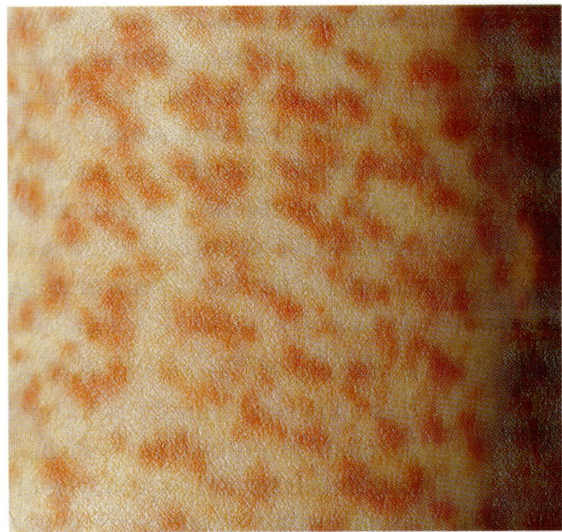

Fig. 10: Maculopapular rash after taking amoxicillin.

Investigations

No acute laboratories are required; drug provocation test considered after recovery.

Management Plan

Stopped amoxicillin, gave oral antihistamines for itch, and advised avoidance of penicillins until further evaluation.

Follow-up and Outcome

Rash resolved completely in 5 days.

Teaching Points

- Drug allergy diagnosis requires good history taking.
- Nonimmediate reactions are usually self-limiting.
- Avoid re-exposure to suspected drug until evaluated.

INSECT ALLERGY

Asha, a 15-year-old, developed rapid-onset dizziness, generalized hives **(Fig. 11)**, and breathing difficulty within 5 minutes of a bee sting while tending to her home garden. On arrival at the health center, she was hypotensive and wheezing.

Diagnostic Reasoning

Acute multisystem involvement after insect sting indicates systemic anaphylaxis.

Investigations

No emergency laboratories; venom-specific immunoglobulin E (IgE) testing later confirmed bee venom allergy.

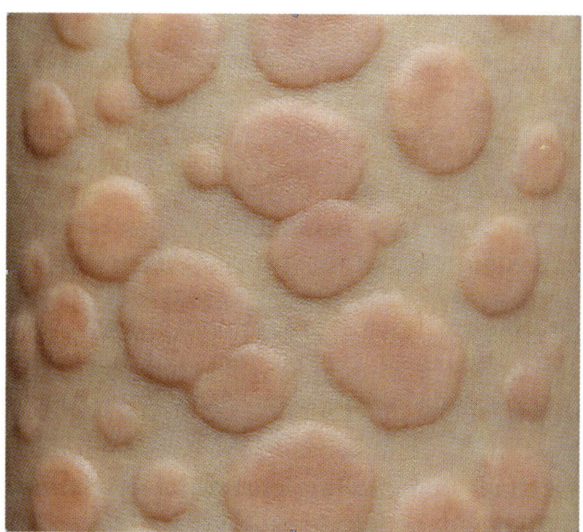

Fig. 11: Acute urticaria after a bee sting.

Management Plan

Acute management at presentation:

- *Immediate IM adrenaline*—0.01 mg/kg (max 0.5 mg) of 1:1,000 solution into mid-anterolateral thigh, repeated every 5–15 minutes if symptoms persist.
- *High-flow oxygen* administration.
- *Positioning*—supine with legs elevated, unless respiratory distress requires sitting position.
- *Rapid IV access*—isotonic crystalloid bolus 20 mL/kg for hypotension, repeat if needed.
- *Nebulized salbutamol* for bronchospasm/wheezing.
- *Observation*—minimum 6–8 hours in health facility (up to 24 hours in severe cases) to monitor for biphasic reactions.

Long-term prevention:

- Prescribed *adrenaline autoinjector* (0.3 mg) and demonstrated use to patient and family.
- Counseled on sting avoidance measures (protective clothing and avoiding flowering plants during peak bee activity).
- Referred to allergy specialist for consideration of *venom immunotherapy* (highly effective, where available).

Follow-up and Outcome

No recurrence in 1 year with preventive measures.

Teaching Points

- Adrenaline is the first-line, life-saving drug in anaphylaxis—do not delay for IV access or adjunct therapy.
- Venom immunotherapy offers long-term protection in insect sting allergy.
- Public education on early recognition and first aid for anaphylaxis can reduce mortality in rural India.

POLLUTION AND ALLERGY

Rahul, a 12-year-old with mild asthma, experienced worsening cough and wheeze every winter, particularly during post-Diwali smog episodes. He missed multiple school days and often required multiple hospital visits for the same. On examination: During a flare, he had expiratory wheeze and mild respiratory distress. Peak expiratory flow was 60% of predicted.

Diagnostic Reasoning

Seasonal exacerbations coinciding with hazardous Air Quality Index (AQI) levels suggested pollution-induced allergic asthma flare.

Investigations

- *AQI readings during symptom days:* >400 [severe-hazardous as per the Central Pollution Control Board (CPCB) classification].
- No new allergen sensitizations on skin-prick testing.

Management Plan

- Temporarily stepped-up ICS dose during high-pollution periods.
- Advised use of N95 mask when outdoors.
- Recommended staying indoors during early morning/evening peak smog hours.
- Coordinated with school for indoor activities on severe AQI days.
- Counseled family on monitoring AQI via CPCB/Safar India apps.

Follow-up and Outcome

The next winter, with preventive strategies and AQI-based ICS adjustments, his asthma remained well-controlled.

Teaching Points

- Air pollution significantly worsens allergic airway diseases in Indian metros.
- Preventive exposure reduction + medication optimization improves outcomes.
- Public health interventions such as clean fuel and crop residue management are essential long-term measures.

CLIMATE CHANGE AND ALLERGY

Neha, a 14-year-old, had seasonal allergic rhinitis and asthma since age 8 years. In the last 3 years, her pollen-related symptoms began earlier (late January) and persisted till September, compared to the earlier March–July season. On examination: Stable between seasons; more frequent use of maintenance and reliever inhaler reported during prolonged pollen months.

DIAGNOSTIC REASONING

Earlier onset and prolonged duration of pollen season—confirmed by meteorological data—pointed to climate change-related extension of allergen exposure.

Investigations

- Local meteorological reports showed increased pollen counts and extended flowering seasons.
- No new allergen sensitizations on repeat testing.

Management Plan

- Initiated prophylactic oral antihistamines 2–3 weeks before expected pollen season.
- Maintained optimized ICS/long-acting beta-agonist (LABA) [maintenance and reliever therapy (MART)] regimen for asthma.
- Educated family to monitor Indian Meteorological Department pollen bulletins.
- Advised keeping windows closed during high-pollen days and using indoor air filters.

Follow-up and Outcome

Neha's seasonal symptom burden reduced significantly with anticipatory therapy.

Teaching Points

- Climate change is shifting pollen seasons in India, increasing allergy duration.
- Anticipatory and preemptive treatment improves control.
- Regional pollen calendars are valuable tools in preventive allergy care.

ALLERGY AND INFECTIONS

Suresh, a 7-year-old with asthma, experienced frequent exacerbations during viral respiratory infection peaks in the monsoon and winter. Even mild colds triggered wheezing, requiring inhalational therapy. On examination: Normal respiratory findings between episodes and poor asthma control score noted.

Diagnostic Reasoning

Pattern suggested viral-triggered asthma exacerbations in an atopic child.

Investigations

- No evidence of bacterial infection during episodes.
- Influenza vaccination incomplete.

Management Plan

- Completed annual influenza vaccination before winter onset.
- Reinforced hand hygiene, mask use in crowded indoor spaces, and avoidance of sick contacts during viral peaks.

- Updated written asthma action plan, including early short-acting beta-agonist (SABA) and ICS use at first sign of cold symptoms.
- Educated parents on when to escalate care.

Follow-up and Outcome

Marked reduction in exacerbations over the next year after vaccination and preventive strategies.

Teaching Points

- Viral respiratory infections are a major asthma trigger in Indian children.
- Vaccination, hygiene, and early symptom action plans reduce morbidity.
- Preventive care is critical in atopic children with poor baseline control.

IMMUNIZATION AND ALLERGY

Tanya, a 6-year-old with a history of mild egg allergy (urticaria after egg ingestion), was due for her annual influenza vaccination. Her parents were concerned after reading online that vaccines were unsafe for egg-allergic children. *On examination:* No acute symptoms; stable vitals; and no active skin rash or respiratory distress.

Diagnostic Reasoning

Mild egg allergy without anaphylaxis is *not a contraindication* to influenza vaccination. Modern inactivated influenza vaccines available in India contain negligible egg protein (≤1 μg/dose) and are safe for most egg-allergic children.

Investigations

No allergy testing required before vaccination in cases of mild egg allergy [as per Indian Academy of Pediatrics (IAP) and World Health Organization (WHO) recommendations].

Management Plan

- Administered quadrivalent inactivated influenza vaccine in a hospital setting.
- Observed for 30 minutes postvaccination for any immediate reaction.
- Counseled parents on safety of routine vaccines in mild food allergy and dispelled common myths.

TABLE 1: Common pediatric allergic disorders—hallmark features.

Disorder	*Hallmark symptom/sign*	*Key trigger*
Allergic rhinitis	Sneezing, nasal blockage, and allergic crease	Dust mites and pollen
Asthma	Recurrent wheeze, cough, and exercise intolerance	Allergens and viral infections
Food allergy	Rapid urticaria, angioedema, and anaphylaxis	Peanut, milk, and egg
Atopic dermatitis	Chronic itchy eczema in flexures	Clothing and detergents
Ocular allergy (VKC)	Intense itching, photophobia, and cobblestone papillae	Sunlight and pollen
Drug allergy	Maculopapular rash and urticaria	Antibiotics and NSAIDs
Insect allergy	Sting → rapid anaphylaxis	Bee and wasp

(NSAIDs: nonsteroidal anti-inflammatory drugs; VKC: vernal keratoconjunctivitis)

- Scheduled follow-up for completion of other pending vaccines as per the National Immunization Schedule (NIS).

Follow-up and Outcome

Tanya tolerated the vaccine without any adverse events. She completed all other due vaccines in the subsequent months without issue.

Teaching Points

- Mild egg allergy is *not* a contraindication to influenza vaccination.
- Postvaccination observation is prudent but serious reactions are rare.
- Educating parents helps overcome vaccine hesitancy and prevents missed immunizations.

KEY POINTS

- Pediatric allergic diseases present with *diverse organ involvement,* but share common underlying immune mechanisms and hallmark symptoms/signs as highlighted in **Table 1**.

- *Detailed history and exposure correlation* are critical for accurate diagnosis.
- *Allergen avoidance and patient education* form the cornerstone of long-term management.
- *Intranasal corticosteroids, ICSs, and dual-action eye drops* are safe and effective first-line therapies for common allergic disorders.
- *Adrenaline is life-saving* in anaphylaxis and must be promptly administered without delay.
- Climate change, pollution, and infections are *emerging modifiers* of allergic disease severity in Indian children.
- Vaccinations are *safe in most allergic children,* including those with mild egg allergy.

2 APPENDIX

Drug Compendium

Reyaz A Malik

ORAL ANTIHISTAMINES

H_1 receptor antagonists block histamine competitively at its receptor sites. They were first developed in the late 1930s and are effective in countering histamine-induced effects such as bronchoconstriction, wheal, flare, and itching. These agents are particularly useful in type I hypersensitivity, where they provide relief from urticaria, itching, and angioedema, although they cannot fully prevent the severe fall in blood pressure that occurs in anaphylaxis.

First-generation H_1 blockers often cause drowsiness, the degree of which depends on the drug's ability to cross the blood–brain barrier and its binding strength to central H_1 receptors. Individual response varies widely, so some people experience significant sedation while others are only mildly affected.

Conventional H_1 antihistamines are well absorbed after oral or parenteral administration, metabolized in the liver, and eliminated through urine. They are widely distributed, including in the brain, which explains their sedating effect. Newer agents enter the brain poorly and therefore cause little or no sedation.

The action of most H_1 blockers lasts about 4–6 hours. However, certain drugs such as chlorpheniramine, mizolastine, loratadine, cetirizine, and fexofenadine—remain active for 12–24 hours or longer. Oral administration is the usual route, though some formulations are also available for intravenous (IV) or intramuscular (IM) use.

First-generation H_1 Antagonists

Chlorpheniramine

Allergic rhinitis:

- *6–12 years:* 2 mg orally every 4–6 hours; not to exceed 12 mg/day
- *>12 years:* 4 mg PO q4–6h; not to exceed 24 mg/day

Adverse drug reactions (ADRs): Central nervous system (CNS) depression, drowsiness, sedation ranging from mild drowsiness to deep sleep (most frequent), dizziness, lassitude, disturbed coordination, muscular weakness, restlessness, insomnia, tremors, euphoria, nervousness, delirium, palpitation, seizures (less common), epigastric distress, anorexia, nausea, vomiting, diarrhea, constipation, cholestasis, hepatitis, tachycardia, electrocardiogram (ECG) changes (e.g., widened QRS), arrhythmias (e.g., extrasystole and heart block), hypotension, hypertension, dryness of mouth, nose, and throat, dysuria, urinary retention, impotence, vertigo, visual disturbances, blurred vision, diplopia, tinnitus, acute labyrinthitis, insomnia, tremors, nervousness, irritability, facial dyskinesia, tightness of the chest, thickening of bronchial secretions, wheezing, nasal stuffiness, sweating, chills, early menses, toxic psychosis, headache, faintness, paresthesia, agranulocytosis, hemolytic anemia, leukopenia, thrombocytopenia, and pancytopenia.

Diphenhydramine

Allergic reaction:

- *2–6 years:* 6.25 mg every 4–6 hours; not to exceed 37.5 mg/day
- *6–12 years:* 12.5–25 mg every 4–6 hours; not to exceed 150 mg/day
- *>12 years:* 25–50 mg every 4–6 hours; not to exceed 300 mg/day

Cough: >12 years: 25–50 mg PO q4–6h; not to exceed 300 mg/day

ADRs: Sedation, confusion, anticholinergic effects, may decrease cognitive function in geriatric patients, xerostomia, dry nasal mucosa, pharyngeal dryness, thick bronchial sputum, agranulocytosis, hemolytic anemia, thrombocytopenia, convulsions, tachycardia, hypotension, nervousness, restlessness, blurred vision, palpitations, constipation, vertigo, menstrual irregularities, euphoria, anorexia, urinary retention, neuritis, diplopia, and tinnitus.

Hydroxyzine

Pruritus:

- *<6 years old:* 50 mg/day orally in divided doses every 6 hourly
- *>6 years old:* 50–100 mg/day orally in divided doses every 6 hourly

ADRs:

- *Anticholinergic:* Dry mouth
- *CNS:* Drowsiness and involuntary motor activity

Clemastine

Allergic rhinitis:

- *<6 years old:* 0.05 mg/kg/day as clemastine base in divided doses every 8–12 hourly
- *6–12 years old:* 0.5–1 mg as clemastine base every 12 hours
- *>12 years old:* As in adults

Urticaria:

- *<6 years old:* 0.05 mg/kg/day as clemastine base in divided doses every 8–12 hourly
- *6–12 years old:* 0.5–1 mg clemastine base every 12 hourly
- *>12 years old:* As in adults

ADRs: CNS depression, drowsiness, sedation ranging from mild drowsiness to deep sleep (most frequent), dizziness, lassitude, disturbed coordination, muscular weakness, restlessness, insomnia, tremors, euphoria, nervousness, delirium, palpitation, epigastric distress, anorexia, nausea, vomiting, diarrhea, constipation, cholestasis, hepatitis, hepatic failure, eczema, pruritus, inflammation, papular rash, tachycardia, ECG changes (e.g., dryness of mouth, nose, and throat widened QRS) arrhythmias (e.g., extrasystole and heart block), hypotension, hypertension, dysuria, urinary retention, impotence, vertigo, visual disturbances, blurred vision, diplopia, tinnitus, acute labyrinthitis, insomnia, tremors, nervousness, irritability, facial dyskinesia, tightness of the chest, thickening of bronchial secretions, wheezing, nasal stuffiness, sweating, chills, early menses, toxic psychosis, headache, faintness, paresthesia, agranulocytosis, hemolytic anemia, leukopenia, thrombocytopenia, and pancytopenia.

Cyproheptadine

Primarily blocks 5-HT2A receptors and has additional H_1 antihistaminic, anticholinergic, and sedative properties. It has been used in allergies and is a good antipruritic, but anti 5-HT action has no role in these conditions. It increases appetite and has been also used in children and poor eaters to promote weight gain.

Hypersensitivity reaction:

- *<2 years old:* Safety and efficacy not established
- *2–6 years old:* 2 mg orally every 8–12 hours; not to exceed 12 mg/day
- *7–14 years old:* 4 mg orally every 8–12 hours; not to exceed 16 mg/day
- Alternatively, total daily dose of 0.25 mg/kg or 8 mg/m^2

ADRs: CNS depression, drowsiness, sedation, dizziness, lassitude, disturbed coordination, restlessness, insomnia, tremors, euphoria, nervousness, irritability, delirium, seizures, toxic psychosis, paresthesia, muscular weakness, palpitation, ECG changes, arrhythmias, hypotension, hypertension, dizziness, sedation, hypotension, epigastric distress, anorexia, nausea, vomiting, diarrhea, constipation, cholestasis, hepatitis, eczema, pruritus, inflammation, papular rash, erythema on exposed skin, visual disturbances, blurred vision, diplopia, tinnitus, acute labyrinthitis, dysuria, urinary retention, thickening of bronchial secretions, wheezing, nasal stuffiness, vertigo, sweating, chills, early menses, headache, impotence, dryness of mouth, nose, and throat, facial dyskinesia, tightness of chest, and faintness.

Ketotifen

- Relatively selective H_1 receptor antagonist and a mast cell stabilizer.
- *Atopic asthma (prophylactic treatment):* Children 6 months to 3 years: Initial: 0.05 mg/kg once daily or in two divided doses for 5 days; Maintenance: 0.05 mg/kg/dose twice daily (maximum dose: 1 mg twice daily)
- *Children >3 years and Adolescents:* Initial: 1 mg once daily or in two divided doses for 5 days; Maintenance: 1 mg twice daily
- *Allergic conjunctivitis in children >3 years:* 0.025% ophthalmic solution, 1 drop twice daily

ADRs: Skin rash, weight gain, abdominal pain, increased appetite, influenza, sleep disturbance, eyelid edema, epistaxis, conjunctivitis, headache, eye pain, keratitis, mydriasis, rhinitis, and photophobia.

Promethazine

Allergic conditions:

- *<2 years:* Contraindicated
- *≥2 years:* 25 mg orally at bedtime or 12.5 mg every 6 hourly

ADRs: Sedation, confusion, disorientation, blurred vision, hallucinations, dystonias, catatonic states, euphoria, excitation, extrapyramidal symptoms, tachycardia, bradycardia, leukopenia, agranulocytosis, obstructive jaundice, photosensitivity, dry mouth, angioneurotic edema, tardive, dyskinesia, urticaria, xerostomia, impotence, and urinary retention.

Second-generation (Non/Low-sedating)

The second-generation antihistaminics (SGAs) are H_1 receptor blockers marketed later have several advantages over conventional antihistaminics.

- Absence of CNS depressant property.
- *Higher H_1 selectivity:* No anticholinergic side effects.
- *Additional antiallergic mechanisms apart from histamine blockade:* Some drugs also inhibit late phase allergic reaction by modifying release/action of leukotrienes (LTs), platelet activating factor (PAF), cytokines, etc.

The newer generation antihistamines generally do not interfere with psychomotor skills, cause noticeable drowsiness, or produce subjective effects. They also do not enhance the sedative effects of benzodiazepines. While a few patients may still report feeling sleepy, the complaint is about the same as what is seen with placebo.

Cetirizine

It is a metabolite of hydroxyzine with marked affinity for peripheral H_1 receptors; penetrates brain poorly, but mild sedation and subjective somnolence is experienced by many recipients.

Allergic rhinitis:

- Infants 6 months to 1 year old—2.5 mg once a day orally
- Children 1–2 years old—2.5 mg orally initially once a day, subsequently increased to twice a day
- Children 2–5 years old—2.5 mg once or twice a day or 5 mg once a day
- Children >6 years old—5–10 mg once daily

Urticaria:

- 6 month old to 5 years old—2.5 mg IV every 24 hours
- Children 6–11 years old—5 mg or 10 mg every 24 hours IV
- Children >12 years old—10 mg IV every 24 hours

ADRs: CNS depression, fatigue, drowsiness, cardiac failure, chest pain, edema, hypertension, palpitations, syncope, acne vulgaris, alopecia, bullous rash, dermatitis, cutaneous nodules, diaphoresis, dermatitis, eczema, hypertrichosis, hyperkeratosis, photosensitivity, decreased libido, weight gain, diabetes mellitus, heavy menstrual bleeding, abdominal pain, anorexia, aphthous stomatitis, constipation, diarrhea, vomiting, cystitis, hematuria, urinary incontinence, lymphadenopathy, arthralgia, arthritis, tremor, conjunctivitis, glaucoma, and bronchospasm.

Levocetirizine

Levocetirizine is an enantiomer of cetirizine and achieves the same therapeutic benefit at roughly half the dose. It tends to cause less sedation and fewer adverse effects compared to cetirizine.

Allergic rhinitis:

- *6 months to 5 years:* 1.25 mg orally once in evening
- *6–12 years:* 2.5 mg orally once in evening
- *>12 years:* 5 mg orally once in evening

Chronic urticaria:

- *6 months to 5 years:* 1.25 mg orally once in evening
- *6–12 years:* 2.5 mg orally once in evening
- *>12 years:* 5 mg orally once in evening

ADRs: Dry mouth, fatigue, nasopharyngitis, pharyngitis, CNS depression, drowsiness, sedation, dizziness, lassitude, disturbed coordination, restlessness, insomnia, tremors, euphoria, nervousness, delirium, palpitation, seizures, epigastric distress, anorexia, nausea, vomiting, diarrhea, constipation, cholestasis, hepatitis, hepatic failure, palpitation, ECG changes, arrhythmias, hypotension, hypertension, dryness of mouth, nose, and throat, dysuria, urinary retention, impotence, vertigo, visual disturbances, blurred vision, diplopia, tinnitus, acute labyrinthitis, insomnia, tremors, nervousness, irritability, facial dyskinesia, tightness of the chest, thickening of bronchial secretions, wheezing, nasal stuffiness, sweating, chills, early menses, toxic psychosis, headache, faintness, paresthesia, agranulocytosis, hemolytic anemia, leukopenia, thrombocytopenia, and pancytopenia.

Loratadine

Loratadine is a selective, long-acting H_1 blocker that acts primarily at peripheral receptors. Because it penetrates the brain poorly, it does not cause CNS depression. Its onset of action is relatively rapid.

Allergic rhinitis:

- *2–6 years:* 5 mg orally once a day
- *>6 years:* 10 mg orally once a day

ADRs: Headache, somnolence, drowsiness, nervousness, fatigue, dry mouth, hyperkinesia, conjunctivitis, dysphonia, malaise, upper respiratory tract infection (URTI), abdominal pain, altered lacrimation, altered salivation, flushing, hypoesthesia, impotence, increased sweating, thirst, hypertension, hypotension, palpitations, supraventricular tachyarrhythmias, syncope, tachycardia, blepharospasm, dizziness, dysphonia, hypertonia, migraine, paresthesia, tremor, vertigo, altered taste, anorexia, constipation, diarrhea, dyspepsia, flatulence, gastritis, hiccup, increased appetite, loose stools, nausea, vomiting, arthralgia, myalgia, agitation, amnesia, anxiety, confusion, decreased libido, depression, impaired concentration, insomnia, irritability, breast pain, dysmenorrhea, menorrhagia, vaginitis, bronchitis, bronchospasm, coughing, dyspnea, hemoptysis, laryngitis, nasal dryness, sinusitis, sneezing, dermatitis, dry hair, dry skin, photosensitivity reaction, pruritus, purpura, urticaria, altered micturition, urinary discoloration, urinary incontinence, urinary retention, angioneurotic edema, asthenia, back pain, blurred vision, chest pain, earache, eye pain, fever, leg cramps, malaise, rigors, tinnitus, and weight gain.

Desloratadine

Desloratadine is the main active metabolite of loratadine. It is effective at about half the parent drug's dose and has been shown not to interfere with psychomotor function, with a strong record of cardiac safety.

Allergic rhinitis and urticaria:

- *6–12 months:* 1 mg orally once a day
- *1–5 years:* 1.25 mg orally once a day
- *6–12 years:* 2.5 mg orally once a day
- *12 years or older:* 5 mg orally once a day
- *6–12 years:* 2.5 mg PO once a day

ADRs: Headache, fever, irritability, diarrhea, upper respiratory infection (URI), cough, dizziness, somnolence, dizziness, fatigue, erythema, maculopapular rash, dysmenorrhea, urinary tract infection, bronchitis, and epistaxis.

Fexofenadine

Fexofenadine is derived from terfenadine, the first non-sedating second-generation antihistamine. Terfenadine was withdrawn due to dangerous side effects at higher doses or when combined with CYP3A4 inhibitors such as erythromycin, clarithromycin, ketoconazole, and itraconazole. Fexofenadine retains the benefits without these risks.

Allergic rhinitis:

- *2–12 years:* 30 mg orally twice a day
- *>12 years:* 60 mg orally twice a day or 180 mg orally once a day

Chronic idiopathic urticaria:

- *6 months to 2 years:* 15 mg orally twice a day
- *2–12 years:* 30 mg orally twice a day
- *>12 years:* 60 mg orally twice a day or 180 mg orally once a day

ADRs: Vomiting, headache, cough, diarrhea, URTI, back pain, pyrexia, dysmenorrheal, dizziness, stomach discomfort, pain in extremity, somnolence, and rhinorrhea,

Rupatadine

This recently introduced antihistaminic has additional platelet-activating factor (PAF) antagonistic property which may enhance efficacy in allergic and inflammatory pathways.

Allergic rhinitis, urticaria, and other allergic disorders:

- *≥12 years:* 10 mg once daily
- *≥2–11 years and >25 kg:* 5 mg once daily
- *≥2–11 years and 10 to ≤25 kg:* 2.5 mg once daily

ADRs: First-generation H_1 blockers often cause drowsiness, the degree of which depends on the drug's ability to cross the blood–brain barrier and its binding strength to central H_1 receptors. Individual response varies widely, so some people experience significant sedation while others are only mildly affected.

Bilastine

It binds specifically and potently to H_1 histamine receptors, with an affinity higher than cetirizine and fexofenadine. It acts as a H_1 receptor inverse agonist, reducing histamine effects, and also showing some anti-inflammatory activity.

Allergic rhinitis, urticaria, and other allergic disorders:

- *≥12 years:* 20 mg once daily
- *≥4–11 years and ≥16 kg:* 10 mg once daily

ADRs: First-generation H_1 blockers often cause drowsiness, the degree of which depends on the drug's ability to cross the blood–brain barrier and its binding strength to central H_1 receptors. Individual response varies widely, so some people experience significant sedation while others are only mildly affected.

INTRANASAL ANTIHISTAMINES

Azelastine

This newer H_1 antihistamine not only blocks histamine receptors effectively but also shows strong topical activity. In addition, it helps reduce histamine release and suppresses inflammatory responses triggered by LTs and PAF. When applied intranasally, it has been shown to decrease the expression of intracellular adhesion molecule-1 (ICAM-1) on the nasal lining. Its half-life is about 24 hours, but its effects last even longer because of its active metabolite.

Strength–0.1% 137 µg/Spray

Seasonal allergic rhinitis:

- *5 to <12 years:* One spray per nostril every 12 hours
- *≥12 years:* One to two sprays per nostril every 12 hours

Vasomotor rhinitis: ≥12 years: Two sprays per nostril every12 hours

ADRs: Bitter taste, headache, somnolence, cold symptoms/rhinitis, cough, nasal burning, sneezing, dry mouth, nausea, conjunctivitis, asthma, fatigue, rhinitis, pharyngitis, dizziness, weight gain, myalgia, amenorrhea, breast pain, constipation, contact dermatitis, eczema, flushing, glossitis, hyperkinesia, hypertension, tachycardia, vertigo, and vomiting.

Olopatadine

Olopatadine is a selective antihistamine and mast cell stabilizer used mainly to alleviate allergic eye and nasal symptoms, offering rapid relief with good tolerability.

Seasonal Allergic Rhinitis

- *6–12 years:* One spray per nostril every 12 hours
- *>12 years:* Two sprays per nostril every 12 hours

Adverse Drug Reactions

Bitter taste, epistaxis, headache, depression, fatigue, somnolence, weight gain, URTI, Pharyngolaryngeal pain, postnasal drip, cough, urinary tract infection creatine phosphokinase (CPK) elevation, dry mouth, anosmia, hyposmia, nasopharyngitis, throat irritation, and influenza.

INTRANASAL CORTICOSTEROIDS

Intranasal corticosteroids (INCSs) are formulated for potent local activity with minimal systemic effects, owing to poor absorption and significant first-pass metabolism. Common examples include beclomethasone dipropionate, budesonide, fluticasone, and ciclesonide.

Beclomethasone

Rhinitis

- *6–11 years:* One spray/nostril twice daily (168 µg/day); may increase to two sprays/nostril (336 µg/day) in patients not adequately responding or those with more severe symptoms; decrease dose to one spray/nostril twice daily once adequate control achieved
- *12 years:* As in adults; one to two sprays/nostril twice daily (total dose: 168–336 mcg/day)

Adverse Drug Reactions

Nasopharyngeal irritation, headache, nausea, light-headedness, sneezing attacks after administration, nasal congestion, nose bleeds, rhinorrhea, increased lacrimation, epistaxis, nasal mucosa ulceration, and nasal septum perforation.

Budesonide

It is a nonhalogenated glucocorticoid with high topical: systemic activity ratio. Small fraction that is absorbed is rapidly metabolized; less systemic effects are noted.

Allergic Rhinitis

- *Initial dose:* One spray/nostril per day (64 µg/day)
- *6–11 years:* Not to exceed two sprays/nostril per day (128 µg/day)
- *≥12 years:* Not to exceed four sprays/nostril per day (256 µg/day)

Adverse Drug Reactions

Epistaxis, pharyngitis, bronchospasm, cough, and nasal irritation.

Ciclesonide

This INCS uses a unique strategy to maximize local action while minimizing systemic effects. It is a prodrug, activated by esterases in the nasal and bronchial epithelium to release its active form. Although some of it is absorbed from the lungs, its oral bioavailability is <1%. In the bloodstream, it binds extensively to plasma proteins, which further reduces the amount of free active drug available to act on other tissues.

Seasonal Allergic Rhinitis

>6 years: Two sprays/nostril per day (200 μg/day)

Adverse Drug Reactions

Headache, epistaxis, nasopharyngitis, nasal discomfort, ear pain, nasal congestion, nasal ulcer, dizziness, and localized infections of nose/mouth with candida albicans.

Fluticasone

This intranasal glucocorticoid has high potency, longer duration, and negligible oral bioavailability. The dose swallowed after topical application has little propensity to produce systemic effects.

Allergic Rhinitis

- *≥4–11 years:* One spray (50 μg) in each nostril per day; may increase up to two sprays/nostril per day if not responding adequately, reduce to one spray in each nostril per day once symptoms are controlled
- *>12 years:* Two sprays in each nostril per day (i.e., 200 μg/day); reduce to one spray in each nostril per day once symptoms are controlled

Adverse Drug Reactions

Headache, URI, epistaxis, nasal congestion, pharyngitis, asthma symptoms, fever, dysphonia, cough, nasal discharge, aches and pains, flu-like syndrome, bronchitis, diarrhea, abdominal pain, and nasal ulcer.

Mometasone

A synthetic corticosteroid medication with potent anti-inflammatory, antipruritic (anti-itch), and vasoconstrictive properties. When administered nasally, mometasone furoate shows very low systemic bioavailability (<1%). This is because a large portion of the drug stays localized at the site of administration.

Allergic Rhinitis

- *2–12 years:* One spray (50 μg) in each nostril per day
- *≥12 years:* Two sprays (100 μg) in each nostril per day

Adverse Drug Reactions

Headache, pharyngitis, cough, viral infection, epistaxis, diarrhea, dyspnea, vomiting, dysmenorrhea, musculoskeletal pain, myalgia, conjunctivitis, otitis media, flu-like syndrome, anaphylaxis, angioedema, growth suppression, nasal candidiasis, taste disturbance, nasal septal perforation, nasal burning, and irritation.

Triamcinolone

Allergic Rhinitis

- *<2 years:* Safety and efficacy not established
- *2–6 years:* One spray/nostril per day (110 μg/day)
- *6–12 years:* One spray/nostril per day; may increase to two sprays/nostril per day
- *≥12 years:* Two sprays/nostril per day

Adverse Drug Reactions

Flu syndrome, pharyngitis, headache, bronchitis, dyspepsia, tooth disorder, epistaxis, excoriation, increased cough, upper abdominal pain, diarrhea, rash, asthma, and rhinorrhea.

INHALATIONAL STEROIDS

Beclomethasone

Asthma Maintenance Therapy

- *Children 4–11 years:* Initial: 40 μg twice daily; maximum dose: 80 μg twice daily.
- *Children ≥12 years and adolescents:*
    - *No previous inhaled corticosteroids:* Initial: 40–80 μg *twice daily; maximum dose:* 320 μg twice daily.
    - *Previous inhaled corticosteroid use:* Initial: 40–160 μg *twice daily; maximum dose:* 320 μg twice daily.

Adverse Drug Reactions

Headache, pharyngitis, pain, voice disorder, oral candidiasis, vomiting, diarrhea, nausea, dysmenorrhea, viral gastroenteritis, influenza, back pain, myalgia, otitis, nasopharyngitis, URTI, cough, viral URTI, oropharyngeal pain, sinusitis, allergic rhinitis, and fever.

Budesonide

Global Initiative for Asthma Guidelines

- *Children 6–11 years:*
    - *Low dose:* 100–200 μg/day

    - *Medium dose:* >200–400 μg/day
    - *High dose:* >400 μg/day.
- *Children ≥12 years and adolescents:*
    - *Low dose:* 200–400 μg/day
    - *Medium dose:* >400–800 μg/day
    - *High dose:* >800 μg/day

Adverse Drug Reactions

Otitis media, respiratory infection, rhinitis, syncope, chest pain, headache, pain, hypertonia, insomnia, voice disorder, emotional lability, fatigue, skin rash, contact dermatitis, eczema, pruritus, pustular rash, weight gain, dyspepsia, nausea, gastroenteritis, diarrhea, vomiting, abdominal pain, dysgeusia, xerostomia, anorexia, viral gastroenteritis, oral candidiasis, ecchymosis, cervical lymphadenopathy, purpura, hypersensitivity reaction, candidiasis, viral infection, herpes simplex infection, arthralgia, weakness, bone fracture, myalgia, hyperkinesias, conjunctivitis, nasopharyngitis, cough, epistaxis, and pharyngitis.

Fluticasone

Global Initiative for Asthma Guidelines Fluticasone propionate Metered-dose Inhaler

- *Children 4–5 years:*
    - *Low dose:* 100 μg/day
- *Children 6–11 years:*
    - *Low dose:* 100–200 μg/day
    - *Medium dose:* >200–500 μg/day
    - *High dose:* >500 μg/day
- *Children ≥12 years and adolescents:*
    - *Low dose:* 100–250 μg/day
    - *Medium dose:* >250–500 μg/day
    - *High dose:* >500 μg/day

Adverse Drug Reactions

Oral candidiasis, fatigue, headache, malaise, arthralgia, musculoskeletal pain, nasal congestion, rhinitis, sinusitis, throat irritation, URTI, hypertension, pruritus, skin rash, gastrointestinal distress, gastrointestinal pain, nausea and vomiting, toothache, viral gastroenteritis, viral gastrointestinal infection, malignant neoplasm of breast, abscess, influenza, viral infection, dizziness, subarachnoid hemorrhage, voice disorder, limb pain, muscle injury, muscle spasm, sprain, bronchitis, cough, epistaxis, hoarseness, nasopharyngitis, oropharyngeal candidiasis, oropharyngeal pain, pharyngitis, and respiratory tract infection.

LEUKOTRIENE RECEPTOR ANTAGONISTS

These drugs act by competitively blocking cysteinyl leukotriene-1 (CysLT1) receptors, thereby preventing LT-driven effects such as bronchoconstriction, mucus hypersecretion, increased vascular permeability, and eosinophil recruitment. In asthma patients, this leads to bronchodilation, lower sputum eosinophil counts, and suppression of airway inflammation, mucus production, and hyperreactivity. Lung function tests show variable improvement, but overall, these agents help reduce the frequency of asthma exacerbations.

Montelukast

Asthma Prophylaxis and Maintenance

- *<12 months:* Safety and efficacy not established
- *12–24 months:* 4 mg orally once daily in evening
- *2–6 years:* 4 mg orally once daily in evening
- *6–15 years:* 5 mg orally once daily in evening
- *>15 years:* 10 mg orally once daily in evening

Exercise-induced Bronchospasm Prophylaxis

- *6–15 years:* 5 mg orally 2 hours before exercise
- *>15 years:* 10 mg orally 2 hours before exercise

Allergic Rhinitis

- *6–24 months:* 4 mg orally once daily
- *2–6 years:* 4 mg orally once daily
- *6–15 years:* 5 mg orally once daily
- *>15 years:* 10 mg orally once daily

Adverse Drug Reactions

Headache, abdominal pain, eczema, influenza, laryngitis, pharyngitis, viral infection, wheezing, dental pain, dizziness, dyspepsia, elevated liver function tests, fever, gastroenteritis, nasal congestion, otitis, rash, urticaria, bronchitis, cough, sinusitis, URTI, allergic granulomatous angiitis (Churg–Strauss syndrome; rare), aggressive behavior, altered behavior, and suicidal thoughts.

Zafirlukast

Asthma

- *5–12 years:* 10 mg orally twice daily
- *>12 years:* 20 mg orally twice daily

Adverse Drug Reactions

Headache, abdominal pain, infection, nausea, diarrhea, generalized pain, vomiting, dyspepsia/gastritis, increased

ALT, infection, back pain, weakness, myalgia, eosinophilia, eosinophilic pneumonia, vasculitis, malaise, bleeding, and bruising.

MAST CELL STABILIZERS

Cromolyn Sodium

Cromolyn sodium, a chromone derivative, prevents mast cell degranulation and thereby limits the release of mediators such as histamine, LTs, PAF, and interleukins. Its mechanism may involve inhibition of a chloride channel in mast cell membranes. Long-term therapy reduces airway inflammation and hyperreactivity, and helps prevent bronchospasm triggered by allergens, irritants, cold air, or exercise. Since it is poorly absorbed orally, it is delivered by inhalation. Systemic absorption is minimal, with the absorbed fraction excreted unchanged.

Sodium cromoglycate is poorly absorbed when taken orally, so for asthma it is delivered as an aerosol via a metered-dose inhaler. Only a small portion of the inhaled dose enters systemic circulation, and that fraction is excreted unchanged in urine and bile.

Mastocytosis

- *2–12 years:* 100 mg orally four times a day
- *>12 years:* 200 mg orally four times a day

Food Allergy

- *2–12 years:* 100 mg four times daily initially
- *>12 years:* 200 mg orally four times daily

Adverse Drug Reactions

Diarrhea, headache, angioedema, premature ventricular contractions, hypoesthesia, lightheadedness, flushing, palpitation, erythema, postprandial photosensitivity, behavior changes, psychosis, esophagospasm, nausea, abdominal pain, pancytopenia, polycythemia, stomatitis, neutropenia, rash, and pruritus.

Nedocromil

Allergic Conjunctivitis

Children ≥3 years and adolescents: Ophthalmic: one to two drops in each eye twice daily throughout the period of exposure to allergen.

Adverse Drug Reactions

Unpleasant taste, headache, burning sensation of eyes, eye irritation, stinging of eyes, nasal congestion, conjunctivitis, eye redness, photophobia, asthma, and rhinitis.

Ketotifen

Ketotifen is an H_1 antihistamine that also shows cromoglycate-like activity. It reduces the activation of immune and inflammatory cells such as mast cells, macrophages, eosinophils, lymphocytes, and neutrophils, thereby decreasing the release of mediators. Unlike standard bronchodilators, ketotifen does not directly relax the airways. Its clinical use has become infrequent, but it may still be considered in patients who suffer from multiple allergic conditions.

Atopic Asthma Prophylaxis

- *Infants and children 6 months to 3 years:* Initial: 0.05 mg/kg once daily or in two divided doses for 5 days; maintenance: 0.05 mg/kg/dose twice daily (maximum dose: 1 mg twice daily)
- *Children >3 years and adolescents:* Initial: 1 mg once daily or in two divided doses for 5 days; maintenance: 1 mg twice daily

Adverse Drug Reactions

Skin rash, weight gain, abdominal pain, increased appetite, influenza, sleep disturbance, eyelid edema, epistaxis, respiratory tract infection, and increased liver enzymes.

SYSTEMIC CORTICOSTEROIDS

Glucocorticoids help in asthma mainly by suppressing inflammation. They block the production of inflammatory cytokines and limit infiltration of eosinophils and lymphocytes into the lungs. This reduces bronchial hyperreactivity, mucosal swelling, and the overall inflammatory response triggered by antigen–antibody reactions or other stimuli. Compared to bronchodilators and most other drugs, corticosteroids provide more complete and longer-lasting relief of symptoms. They improve airflow, cut down the frequency of asthma attacks, and may even slow disease progression by affecting airway remodeling. In addition, they enhance airway smooth muscle responsiveness to β_2-agonists and can restore effectiveness in patients who have become less responsive to these drugs.

That said, prolonged systemic steroid use carries significant adverse effects—sometimes more serious than asthma itself—so careful use and monitoring are essential.

Prednisolone

Asthma Exacerbations

- *Infants and children <12 years:* 1–2 mg/kg/day orally in divided doses one to two times daily; maximum daily dose: 60 mg/day for 3–10 days.
- *Children ≥12 years and adolescents:* 40–60 mg orally in divided doses one to two times daily for 3–10 days.

Adverse Drug Reactions

Bradycardia, cardiomegaly, cholesterol embolus syndrome, circulatory shock, edema, heart failure, hypertrophic cardiomyopathy (premature infants), myocardial rupture (after recent myocardial infarction), syncope, tachycardia, thromboembolism, thrombophlebitis, vasculitis, acne vulgaris, allergic dermatitis, atrophic striae, diaphoresis, dry scalp, ecchymoses, facial erythema, hyperpigmentation, hypopigmentation, inadvertent suppression of skin test reaction, skin atrophy, skin rash, thinning hair (scalp), urticaria, decreased serum potassium, fluid retention, growth retardation (children), hirsutism, hypothalamic–pituitary–adrenal (HPA)-axis suppression, hypokalemic alkalosis, impaired glucose tolerance, menstrual disease, negative nitrogen balance (due to protein catabolism), sodium retention, weight gain, hiccups, impaired intestinal carbohydrate absorption, increased appetite, nausea, pancreatic, asthenospermia, oligospermia, petechia, hepatomegaly, increased liver enzymes, nonimmune anaphylaxis, sterile abscess, abnormal sensory symptoms, amyotrophy, arachnoiditis, headache, increased intracranial pressure (with papilledema), insomnia, malaise, meningitis, myasthenia, neuritis, neuropathy, paraplegia, paresis (paraparesis), paresthesia, seizure, vertigo, aseptic necrosis of femoral head, aseptic necrosis of humeral head, Charcot arthropathy, rupture of tendon, exophthalmos, pulmonary edema, and wound healing impairment.

Methylprednisolone

Asthma Acute Exacerbation

- *Infants and children <12 years:* 1–2 mg/kg/day orally in one or two divided doses; maximum daily dose: 60 mg/day for 3–10 days
- *Children ≥12 years and adolescents:* 40–60 mg/day orally in one or two divided doses for 3–10 days

Adverse Drug Reactions

Adrenal suppression, bone growth inhibition, excitatory psychiatric disturbances, peptic ulcer, dyspepsia, gastritis, abdominal distention, and ulcerative esophagitis, cushingoid features, hyperglycemia, immunosuppression, increased infections, osteoporosis, vertebral compression fracture, glaucoma, and cataract.

Dexamethasone

Airway Edema

0.5–2 mg/kg/day PO/IV/IM divided every 6 hours, starting 24 hours before extubation and continued for four to six doses afterward.

Adverse Drug Reactions

- *Allergic reactions:* Anaphylactoid reaction, anaphylaxis, and angioedema
- *Cardiovascular:* Bradycardia, cardiac arrest, cardiac arrhythmias, cardiac enlargement, circulatory collapse, congestive heart failure, fat embolism, hypertension, hypertrophic cardiomyopathy in premature infants, myocardial rupture following recent myocardial infarction, edema, pulmonary edema, syncope, tachycardia, thromboembolism, thrombophlebitis, and vasculitis
- *Dermatologic:* Acne, allergic dermatitis, dry scaly skin, ecchymoses and petechiae, erythema, impaired wound healing, increased sweating, rash, striae, suppression of reactions to skin tests, thin fragile skin, thinning scalp hair, and urticaria
- *Endocrine:* Decreased carbohydrate and glucose tolerance, development of cushingoid state, hyperglycemia, glycosuria, hirsutism, hypertrichosis, increased requirements for insulin or oral hypoglycemic agents in diabetes, manifestations of latent diabetes mellitus, menstrual irregularities, secondary adrenocortical and pituitary unresponsiveness (particularly in times of stress, as in trauma, surgery, or illness), and suppression of growth in pediatric patients
- *Fluid and electrolyte disturbances:* Congestive heart failure in susceptible patients, fluid retention, hypokalemic alkalosis, potassium loss, sodium retention, and tumor lysis syndrome

- *Gastrointestinal:* Abdominal distention, elevation in serum liver enzyme levels (usually reversible upon discontinuation), hepatomegaly, increased appetite, nausea, pancreatitis, peptic ulcer with possible perforation and hemorrhage, perforation of the small and large intestine (particularly in patients with inflammatory bowel disease), and ulcerative esophagitis
- *Metabolic:* Negative nitrogen balance due to protein catabolism
- *Musculoskeletal:* Aseptic necrosis of femoral and humeral heads, loss of muscle mass, muscle weakness, osteoporosis, pathologic fracture of long bones, steroid myopathy, tendon rupture, and vertebral compression fractures
- *Neurological/psychiatric:* Convulsions, depression, emotional instability, euphoria, headache, increased intracranial pressure with papilledema (pseudotumor cerebri) usually following discontinuation of treatment, insomnia, mood swings, neuritis, neuropathy, paresthesia, personality changes, psychic disorders, and vertigo
- *Ophthalmic:* Exophthalmos, glaucoma, increased intraocular pressure, posterior subcapsular cataracts, and vision blurred
- *Other:* Abnormal fat deposits, decreased resistance to infection, hiccups, increased or decreased motility and number of spermatozoa, malaise, moon face, and weight gain

Hydrocortisone

Status Asthmaticus

- 1–2 mg/kg IV every 6 hours for 24 hours; not to exceed 250 mg
- *IV maintenance:* 2 mg/kg/day IV divided every 6 hours

Adverse Drug Reactions

Sodium retention, fluid retention, potassium loss, hypokalemic alkalosis, congestive heart failure in susceptible patients, increased blood pressure, muscle weakness, steroid myopathy, loss of muscle mass, osteoporosis, tendon rupture-particularly of the Achilles tendon, vertebral compression fractures, aseptic necrosis of femoral and humeral heads, pathologic fracture of long bones, peptic ulcer with possible perforation and hemorrhage, pancreatitis, abdominal distention, ulcerative esophagitis. increased liver enzymes, impaired wound healing, thin fragile skin, petechiae and ecchymoses, facial erythema, increased sweating, pseudotumor cerebri, convulsions, vertigo, headache, epidural lipomatosis, behavioral and mood changes, increased appetite and weight gain, development of cushingoid state, suppression of growth in children, secondary adrenocortical and pituitary unresponsiveness, particularly in times of stress, as in trauma, surgery or illness, menstrual irregularities, decreased carbohydrate tolerance, manifestations of latent diabetes mellitus, increased requirements for insulin or oral hypoglycemic agents in diabetics, central serous chorioretinopathy, posterior subcapsular cataracts, increased intraocular pressure, glaucoma, exophthalmos, negative nitrogen balance due to protein catabolism, and leukocytosis.

ADRENALINE

Adrenaline counteracts histamine, a key mediator in acute allergic reactions. It provides rapid relief in urticaria and angioedema and is life-saving in laryngeal edema and anaphylaxis. Its vasoconstrictor, cardiac stimulant, and bronchodilator actions all contribute to these benefits.

- Epinephrine autoinjector
- 1:1,000 solution for IM injection

Anaphylaxis

Indicated in emergency treatment of allergic reactions (type I) including anaphylaxis.

Strength–1 mg/mL solution

<30 kg: 0.01 mg/kg (0.01 mL/kg) SC/IM, not to exceed 0.3 mg (0.3 mL) per injection, repeated q5–10 min as necessary

≥30 kg: 0.3–0.5 mg (0.3–0.5 mL) SC/IM, not to exceed 0.5 mg (0.5 mL) per injection, repeated q5–10 min as necessary

Adverse Drug Reactions

Angina, anxiety, apprehensiveness, cardiac arrhythmias, dizziness, dyspnea, flushing, headache, hypertension, nausea, nervousness, pallor, palpitations, respiratory difficulties, restlessness, stress cardiomyopathy, sweating, tachycardia, tremor, vasoconstriction, vomiting, and weakness.

BIOLOGICALS

Omalizumab (Anti-immunoglobulin E)

Omalizumab is a humanized monoclonal antibody that targets immunoglobulin E (IgE). When given subcutaneously, it binds to free IgE in the circulation without triggering mast cells or other inflammatory cells. As a result, during antigen exposure, very little IgE remains attached to mast cell surface receptors, so mediator release and subsequent bronchoconstriction are minimized. In patients with severe extrinsic (allergic) asthma, omalizumab has been shown to lower the frequency of exacerbations and reduce the need for corticosteroids.

Asthma

150–375 mg SC q 2–4 weeks, depending on body weight and pretreatment serum IgE level.

Chronic Spontaneous Urticaria

- Children aged ≥12 years who remain symptomatic despite H_1 antihistamine treatment
- *≥12 years:* 150–300 mg SC every 4 weeks

IgE-mediated Food Allergy

- Use in conjunction with food allergen avoidance
- 75–600 mg SC every 2–4 weeks

Adverse Drug Reactions

Injection site reactions, viral infections, URTIs, sinusitis, headache, and pharyngitis.

Dupilumab (Anti–IL-4Rα)

Dupilumab is a monoclonal antibody that blocks interleukin-4 (IL-4) and interleukin-13 (IL-13) receptor signaling, which are important in the inflammatory pathways of several allergic and inflammatory conditions. Its mechanism involves binding to the alpha subunit of the IL-4 receptor alpha (IL-4Rα), thereby modulating signaling of both IL-4 and IL-13, reducing inflammation and immune responses that contribute to disease symptoms.

Atopic Dermatitis

- *6 months to 5 years:*
  - *5 to <15 kg:* 200 mg SC every 4 weeks
  - *15 to <30 kg:* 300 mg SC every 4 weeks
- *6–17 years:*
  - *≥60 kg:* 600 mg (i.e., two 300-mg injections) SC once, and then 300 mg SC every other week
  - *30 kg to <60 kg:* 400 mg (i.e., two 200-mg injections) SC once, and then 200 mg SC every other week
  - *15 kg to <30 kg:* 600 mg (i.e., two 300-mg injections) SC once, and then 300 mg SC every 4 weeks

Moderate-to-Severe Asthma

- *6–11 years:*
  - *15 to <30 kg:* 300 mg SC every 4 weeks
  - *≥30 kg:* 200 mg SC every 2 weeks
- *≥12 years:*
  - 400 mg SC once, then 200 mg every 2 weeks
  - 600 mg SC once, then 300 mg every 2 weeks

Adverse Drug Reactions

Injection site reactions, atopic dermatitis, injection site reactions, conjunctivitis, blepharitis, oral herpes, keratitis, pruritus, and dry eye.

Mepolizumab (Anti IL-5)

Mepolizumab is a humanized monoclonal antibody that targets interleukin-5 (IL-5), a key cytokine involved in the growth, activation, recruitment, and survival of eosinophils. By binding to IL-5, mepolizumab blocks its interaction with the alpha chain of the IL-5 receptor on eosinophils. This inhibition reduces IL-5 signaling, which in turn lowers eosinophil production and survival in the blood and tissues. Mepolizumab is primarily used as an add-on therapy for severe eosinophilic asthma.

Severe Asthma

- *6–11 years:* 40 mg SC every 4 weeks
- *≥12 years:* 100 mg SC every 4 weeks

Adverse Drug Reactions

Headache, injection site reactions, back pain, fatigue, influenza, pruritus, and eczema.

Benralizumab

Benralizumab is a humanized IgG1 monoclonal antibody that targets the alpha subunit of the interleukin-5 receptor alpha (IL-5Rα) on eosinophils. It blocks IL-5 from binding to its receptor, preventing eosinophil growth, survival, and activation. Additionally, its afucosylated structure enables strong binding to natural killer (NK) cells, triggering antibody-dependent cell-mediated cytotoxicity (ADCC) and rapid eosinophil apoptosis. This dual mechanism leads to a significant reduction of eosinophils in the blood and airways, helping control eosinophilic inflammation in severe asthma and related conditions.

Severe Asthma

6 to <12 years:

- *<35 kg:* 10 mg (one injection) SC every 4 weeks for first three doses, then every 8 weeks thereafter
- *≥35 kg:* 30 mg (one injection) SC every 4 weeks for first three doses, then every 8 weeks thereafter
- *≥12 years:* 30 mg SC every 4 weeks for the first three doses, then every 8 weeks thereafter

Adverse Drug Reactions

Headache, pharyngitis, pyrexia, and hypersensitivity reactions.

SUGGESTED READING

1. Brunton L, Knollman B, Hilal-Dandan R. Goodman & Gilman's The Pharmacological Basis of Therapeutics, 13th edition. Columbus: McGraw Hill; 2017.
2. Global Initiative for Asthma. (2024). Global Strategy for Asthma Management and Prevention. [online] Available from https://ginasthma.org/wp-content/uploads/2024/05/GINA-2024-Strategy-Report-24_05_22_WMS.pdf. [Last accessed December, 2025].
3. Joint Formulary Committee. British National Formulary (BNF87). London: Pharmaceutical Press; 2024.
4. Kliegman R. Nelson Textbook of Pediatrics, 21st edition. Amsterdam, Netherlands: Elsevier; 2019.
5. Pharmaceutical Press. Martindale: The Complete Drug Reference. [online] https://www.pharmaceuticalpress.com/products/martindale-the-complete-drug-reference/. [Last accessed December, 2025].
6. Tripathi KD. Essentials of Medical Pharmacology, 8th edition. New Delhi: Jaypee Brothers Medical Publishers (P) Ltd.; 2021.
7. World Allergy Organization (WAO). Anaphylaxis Guidelines 2023. Milwaukee, Wisconsin: World Allergy Organization; 2023.

Index

Page numbers followed by *b* refer to box, *f* refer to figure, *fc* refer to flowchart, and *t* refer to table.

B

C